Biopolymeric Controlled Release Systems

Volume II

Editor

Donald L. Wise, Ph.D.
Vice President
Dynatech R/D Company
Cambridge, Massachusetts

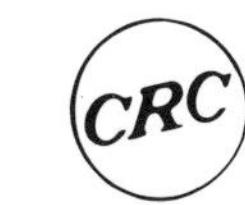

CRC Press, Inc.
Boca Raton, Florida

Library of Congress Cataloging in Publication Data
Main entry under title:

Biopolymeric controlled release systems.

Bibliography: p.
Includes indexes.
1. Drugs--Controlled release. 2. Biopolymers.
3. Pesticides--Controlled release. I. Wise, Donald
Lee, 1937- . [DNLM: 1. Delayed--Action preparations.
2. Macromolecular systems. QV 785 B6153]
RS201.C64B56 1984 615'.7 83-25276
ISBN 0-8493-5403-X (v. 1)
ISBN 0-8493-5404-8 (v. 2)

Direct all inquiries to CRC Press, Inc., 2000 Corporate Blvd., N.W., Boca Raton, Florida, 33431.

International Standard Book Number 0-8493-5403-X (Volume I)
International Standard Book Number 0-8493-5404-8 (Volume II)

Library of Congress Card Number 83-25276
Printed in the United States

PREFACE

This text has evolved from well over a decade of background in developing biopolymeric systems for the controlled release of biologically active agents. A bit of personal reminiscing and even nostalgia may be appropriate here. My work has been largely confined to developing biopolymers for implantable/injectable controlled release systems for those special situations in which patient compliance was the major driving force for this development, i.e., situations in which conventional administration of biologically active agents was simply not practical, not acceptable, or simply not carried out for the personal reasons of the patient. The funding for this early type of development work was almost totally from private foundations, agencies of the U.S. Government, and international organizations. Because of the very pointed problem of patient compliance, and the funding sources addressing these problems, the very first development programs were for controlled release systems for purposes of fertility control, treatment of narcotic addiction, and propylaxis of malaria. All this work was initiated about the same time — the early 1970s. Although treatment of alcoholism was early cited as one having potential for a controlled release application, funding (and therefore, development) was not initiated until fairly recently.

Several biopolymeric systems other than implantable/injectable systems solely for release of a biologically active agent were also initiated in the early 1970s in which the controlled release of biologically active agents was still integral to the overall objectives. For example, I initiated development work on a synthetic biopolymeric burn wound covering as a replacement for cadaver skin. Even with the initial development work, integral to the burn wound covering was the incorporation of suitable biologically active agents, for example, bactericides. Also, development work on new biopolymeric composite materials for such applications as fixation of orthopedic surgical implants and repair of avulsive combat-type maxillofacial injuries always implied the ultimate incorporation of selected biologically active agents into the biopolymeric matrix even if initial development work was focused on the synthesis and evaluation of the biopolymeric material.

A further application of biopolymeric systems for controlled release of biologically active agents was that of selected broadcast applications such as herbicides, larvacides, molluscicides, etc. For broadcast applications the cost of the biopolymeric material is of significance; for human implants the biopolymer cost is almost not a consideration at all.

The selection of the biopolymer has been of special interest to me. Early development work focused on the synthesis of copolymers of lactic and glycolic acids because these were known at the time to be biodegradable, i.e., to hydrolyze and be metabolized. Therefore, these products of glycolysis were simply used early in the development of controlled release systems because it was a practical starting point for investigating the concept of controlled release. Later, other monomers of the human metabolism were investigated as ones to be synthesized into polymers for use as biodegradable implants. For example, work was initiated on using monomers of the Krebs cycle and on using selected amino acids to synthesize biopolymers of such a nature that they would breakdown to the parent monomer. The reasoning in using all these monomers, i.e., using products of glycolysis such as lactic and glycolic acid, using Krebs cycle monomers, using amino acids, was that upon synthesis, these biopolymers would maintain what was termed biocompatibility, i.e., tissue reaction would be minimum. Clearly for broadcast applications the question of tissue compability is not a problem, but environmental acceptance is a question to be addressed.

A further consideration in the design of biopolymeric systems for the controlled release of biologically active agent is that of mechanism of release. The development work has been primarily focused on matrix type systems, ones in which the biopolymer and the biologically active agent are intimately mixed in a physical matrix much as gravel or sand is mixed in cement. Further, both diffusion of the active agent and hydrolysis of the polymer occur simultaneously to achieve the controlled release. As a result a mathematical description of the mechanism has been difficult and essentially empirical relationships have evolved for predicting release.

With this background a brief overview of the material and arrangement in the text is in order. The material is primarily arranged under topical headings of the area in which biopolymeric controlled release systems have been under development. Thus, there are chapters including work on (1) antimalarials, (2) narcotic antagonists, (3) fertility control, (4) alcoholism, and (5) broadcast applications. Several chapters address the question of mechanisms for controlled release. A final section of chapters on alternative applications is enclosed.

It is anticipated that this text will be most useful as a guide to those industrial and academic research directors and program managers who are exploring the potential of biopolymeric controlled release for application to their own problems. For this reason as much detail has been preserved as has been practical in preparing a reference text. This has been done in order that people actually involved in system development and in problem solving may be able to follow well the topical material presented. I hope you find the material presented to be helpful to you!

Donald L. Wise, Ph.D.
1984

THE EDITOR

Donald L. Wise, Ph.D., is Vice President, Dynatech R/D Company, Cambridge, Mass. Dr. Wise received his B.S., M.S., and Ph.D. degrees in chemical engineering at the University of Pittsburgh. Dr. Wise is a specialist in biotechnology including advanced biomaterials development. While an Associate Professor of Engineering at Widener University in Chester, Pa., Dr. Wise carried out research as Principal Investigator for the National Institute of Health and was an NIH Special Research Fellow in Biochemical Engineering, Department of Nutrition and Food Science, Massachusetts Institute of Technology, Cambridge, Mass. Part of his work there concerned diffusion studies in microbial systems. Dr. Wise received a Corporate Appointment to Harvard University as a Research Fellow in the Division of Engineering and Applied Physics. At Dynatech, he has developed a unique program area in biotechnology. This work has been in both biomaterials and bioconversion, including specialized work on enzyme stabilization.

Dr. Wise initiated a project for development of a unique implantable sustained release contraceptive with the Population Council of The Rockefeller University and has continued this program with the World Health Organization and the U.S. Agency for International Development; human testing is now scheduled. He was Principal Investigator on a program to develop a sustained release implant for the chemotherapeutic treatment of malaria for the Walter Reed Army Institute of Research and has continued this work with WHO. He was also Principal Investigator on the program for development of an implantable sustained release drug antagonist for treatment of drug addiction patients with the National Institute for Drug Abuse; human testing is being carried out. Dr. Wise is working on biopolymers for selectively binding antigens/antibodies for improved sensitivity of diagnostic systems and is working with the U.S. Army Institute of Dental Research on a biopolymeric repair material for avulsive combat-type maxillofacial injuries. He has a project with the U.S. Army Medical R&D Command to synthesize an "enzyme fragment" or peptide for selectively binding chemical agents. In a related biomaterials area, he initiated a program with the Office of Naval Research (Naval Medical Research Institute, Bethesda, Md.) for development of a biocompatible synthetic polymer for the treatment of burn patients.

CONTRIBUTORS

David Bergbreiter
Dynatech R/D Company
Cambridge, Massachusetts

Stephen C. Crooker
Group Laboratory Supervisor
Department of Chemical Engineering
Dynatech R/D Company
Cambridge, Massachusetts

Edmund W. J. de Maar
Senior Programme Officer
Special Programme for Research and Training in Tropical Diseases
World Health Organization
Geneva, Switzerland

John B. Gregory
Dynatech R/D Company
Cambridge, Massachusetts

Joseph D. Gresser, Ph.D.
Dynatech R/D Company
Cambridge, Massachusetts

John F. Howes, Ph.D.
Key Pharmaceuticals, Inc.
Miami, Florida

Judith P. Kitchell, Ph.D.
Manager, Biosystems Programs
Biosystems Division
Dynatech R/D Company
Cambridge, Massachusetts

Oliver Midler
Dynatech R/D Company
Cambridge, Massachusetts

James L. Olsen, Ph.D.
Division of Pharmaceutics
School of Pharmacy
University of North Carolina
Chapel Hill, North Carolina

Michael Phillips, M.D.
Associate Professor of Medicine
Chief, Joint Division of General Medicine and Clinical Pharmacology
The Chicago Medical School
North Chicago, Illinois

Richard H. Reuning, Ph.D.
Professor and Chairman
Division of Pharmacy Practice
College of Pharmacy
The Ohio State University
Columbus, Ohio

Hani M. Sadek, Ph.D.
Banner Gelatin Products Co.
Chatsworth, California

Shafik E. Sadek, Ph.D.
Dynatech R/D Company
Cambridge, Massachusetts

John E. Sanderson, Ph.D.
Dynatech R/D Company
Cambridge, Massachusetts

A. Carl Sharon
Dynatech R/D Company
Cambridge, Massachusetts

Ralph L. Wentworth
Dynatech R/D Company
Cambridge, Massachusetts

Donald L. Wise, Ph.D.
Vice President
Dynatech R/D Company
Cambridge, Massachusetts

Donald F. Worth
Warner-Lambert
Pharmaceutical Research Division
Ann Arbor, Michigan

TABLE OF CONTENTS

Volume II

ALTERNATIVE APPLICATIONS

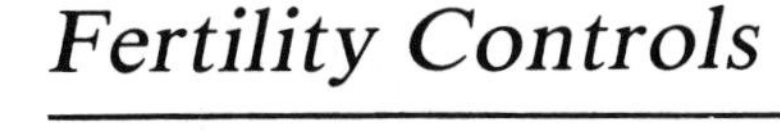

Fertility Controls

Chapter 1

BIODEGRADABLE CYLINDRICAL IMPLANTS FOR FERTILITY CONTROL

A. Carl Sharon, Donald L. Wise, and John F. Howes

TABLE OF CONTENTS

I. INTRODUCTION

The technical background for the work described in this chapter is based on an experimental search at Dynatech R/D Company (Cambridge, Mass.) over a period of years for a suitable biodegradable cylindrical implant for fertility control. Levonorgestrel (courtesy of Wyeth) has been used as the fertility controlling agent. The progressive results of this work are of interest and are summarized chronologically as follows. In addition, reagent results of original research are presented.

II. BACKGROUND

The work at Dynatech on sustained release was initiated by the Population Council of Rockefeller University. In this study,[1] in which thin films of levonorgestrel in polymer of L(−)-lactic acid were used, it was postulated that the findings might relate to cylindrically shaped implants. Due to the lower rate of polymer hydrolysis with respect to steroid release discovered by that study, an investigation was then carried out using polymers with greater susceptibility to degradation, i.e., an effective lifetime of 6 months to 1 year. This continuing work was sponsored by the National Institute for Child Health and Human Development (NICHD).

Under this NICHD contract, biodegradable, cylindrical, subdermal implants for fertility control were evaluated in beagle dogs.[2] Dog testing was carried out at the Massachusetts Institute of Technology (MIT) under the direction of Dr. Paul M. Newberne. Polymers of L(+)-lactic, dl-lactic, and glycolic acids were synthesized with weight ratios of 75dl/25G, 75L(−)/25G, 90dl/10G, 100dl, 50dl/50L(−), and 100L(−), and at selected molecular weights from 46,000 to 260,000. The hormonal steroid, levonorgestrel, was incorporated into these polymers as a physical matrix at several weight ratios of polymer to steroid and extruded into cylinders of 1.5 mm diameter. These cylinders were inserted subcutaneously by trochar in the area of the right femoral groove of each dog. After experiencing some initial mild edema, the dogs tolerated the cylinders well. Radioactive assays of urine, as well as some feces, were used to evaluate the steroid release and, to a lesser extent, polymer hydrolysis.

The release of steroid was found to follow directly the polymer susceptibility to degradation. The approximate ranking of polymers in order of most rapid biodegradation was 75dl/25G, 75L(−)/25G, 90dl/10G, 100dl, 50dl/50L(−), and 100L(−). The 100dl and 50dl/50L(−) type materials appeared to have potential for a delivery system with a lifetime of 6 months to 1 year; consequently, the other materials were excluded from further investigation because they degraded too rapidly.

In general, lower molecular weight polymers and higher steroid loadings of the implant appeared to result in faster steroid release. Overcoating of cylinders with pure polymer reduced initial peaks of steroid released, however, a later higher release was noted when the polymer coatings hydrolyzed; the effect of overcoating depended on polymer composition. Only a minor later peak was observed when the overcoat was the most hydrolysis resistant [50L(−)/50dl copolymer]. Ratios of excreted vs. implanted ^{3}H (polymer) and ^{14}C (steroid) suggested that some lactide oligomer was possibly associated with levonorgestrel fragments. All of the dogs were examined post-mortem, and none showed any tissue reaction at the implant site. Necropsy and histopathological studies showed no abnormalities attributable to the implants.

While all results were ranked with respect to polymer composition, attention also was called to both polymer molecular weight and levonorgestrel loading in the implant. Although the 100L(−) polymer system tested was excluded as not being within the range of desired results, it was noted that this system had a polymer of high molecular weight and a low steroid loading relative to the other systems. Likewise, compared with the other systems tested, the more promising 50dl/50L(−) system was also prepared from high molecular weight polymer and had a low loading of steroid. On the other hand, the 100dl system, which appeared to have an overall equivalence with the 50dl/50L(−) system, employed a polymer with one of the lowest molecular weights used and contained one of the highest steroid loadings tested.

Upon necropsy, very little polymer or drug was found to remain at the implant site. Based on the favorable biological results of all systems, it was concluded that select biodegradable cylindrical subdermal implants have potential for fertility control.

Late in this program a copolymer of 90L(−)/10G was prepared and tested in rats and rabbits. At the conclusion of the NICHD contract, implants following the experimental design listed below were recommended for testing:

Composition			**Percent by weight d-norgestrel**		
dl	**L(+)**	**G**	**20**	**33**	**50**
100	—	—	√	√	√
—	90	10	√	√	√
50	50	—	√	√	√

Of the implants prepared and delivered at the end of the contract, testing in rats had been carried out on these implants:

	Composition			**Percent by weight d-norgestrel**	
Order of testing	**dl**	**L(−)**	**G**	**33**	**50**
1	—	90	10	—	√
2	50	50	—	—	√
3 and 4	—	90	10	√	√

As a result of these recommendations, biodegradable subdermal implants consisting of a physical matrix of levonorgestrel and copolymers of lactic and glycolic acids were evaluated in rats. Two copolymers were prepared: one from 90 parts L(−)-lactide/10 parts glycolide by weight [90L(−)/10G] of 220,000 mol wt and one from 50 parts dl-lactide/50 parts L(−)-lactide by weight [50dl/50L(−)] of 180,000 mol wt. These copolymers were solvent blended with ^{14}C-labeled levonorgestrel, cast into thin films, extruded into 1/32-in. diameter cylinders, and implanted subcutaneously in the scapular region of rats. The drug loading in the 50dl/50L(−) rods was 50% by weight, while implants using the 90L(−)/10G copolymer were prepared at 33 and 50% by weight levonorgestrel.

Results of the release rate from the implants were determined by measuring the ^{14}C from levonorgestrel in the urine and feces of the rats.[3] A plot of cumulative release rate is given in Figure 1. It was found that all animals experienced a sharp burst in release of ^{14}C from levonorgestrel within approximately 12 days postimplantation, and that this burst was approximately 10 times the longer-term release rate. Longer-term release was measured for at least 90 days and up to 328 days. Except for the initial burst, release of ^{14}C from d-norgestrel was found to be approximately zero order for the periods measured. For some of the implant systems tested, over 50% of the total implanted ^{14}C was released during this period measured.

Absolute values of the longer-term release ranged from approximately 10 to 40 μg/day. The 90L(−)/10G system with 33% d-norgestrel provided the lowest release rate of 10 μg/day,

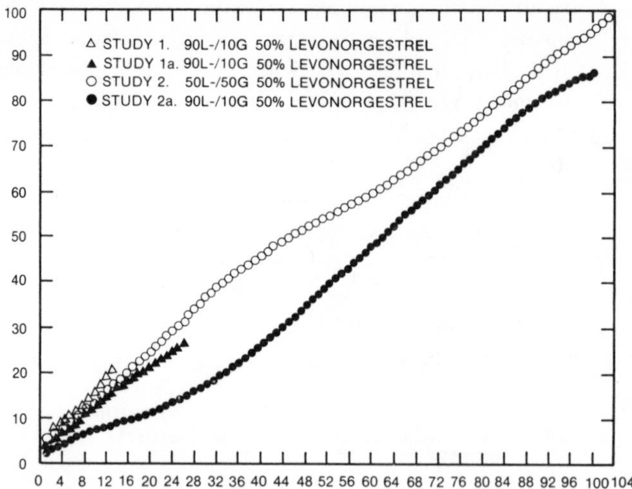

FIGURE 1. Cumulative release of ^{14}C from levonorgestrel in the urine and feces (total) of rats for the four implant systems tested.

while the 90L(−)/10G system with 50% levonorgestrel provided the highest release rate of 40 μg/day. The system of 50dl/50L(−) with 50% levonorgestrel released 25 μg/day. Fecal to urinary ratio of ^{14}C from d-norgestrel correlated, in general, with measured release rates. Specifically, the fecal to urinary release was 22:1 for the 90L(−)/10G rods at 50% drug releasing 40 μg/day and was 8:1 for the 90L(−)/10G rods at 33% drug releasing 10 μg/day. It is significant to note that no tissue irritation or adverse effect on the animals was observed.

From the sequence of developmental programs outlined above, it appeared clear that an implantable biodegradable cylinder was ready for advanced animal testing. The system selected was the 1/32-in. diameter cylinder using 90L(−)/10G copolymer of 200,000 mol wt and 50% by weight levonorgestrel. From Figure 1 it is seen that all implants selected for testing under this program design appeared to merit further development. However, one may reject the 50dl/50L(−) polymer because of possible concern over using a d form of lactic acid. The implant of 33% levonorgestrel using the 90L(−)/10G implant may be rejected as having too low a drug loading. On the basis of these considerations, the 90L(−)/10G implant of 50% levonorgestrel was selected for advanced testing. This work was carried out under the sponsoring of the Program for Applied Research for Fertility Regulation (PARFR).

A long-term delivery system for the fertility control steroid, levonorgestrel, was fabricated and tested in baboons and rats. The system consisted of the ^{14}C-labeled steroid, levonorgestrel, physically dispersed at 50 wt % loading in a tritium-labeled polymer excipient. The polymer, a polyester of 257,000 weight average molecular weight, was synthesized from 10 wt % glycolide and 90 wt % tritium-labeled lactide. Polymerization was initiated with triethyl aluminum.

The drug/polymer composite was extruded as a 1/32-in. (0.08 cm) diameter rod and cut into convenient 1-cm lengths for subcutaneous implantation. Four baboons were each implanted at four sites parallel to the median line with 217 mg of composite rods to deliver 111 mg of steroid. Eight rats were implanted in the scapular region with 39 mg of composite delivering 20 mg of the drug.

Feces and urine from both groups of animals were periodically monitored for radiolabeled materials derived from both steroid and polymer. Analysis was performed by liquid scintillation counting of samples combusted to $^{14}CO_2$ and ^3H_2O. Cumulative excretion of steroid-derived materials by both baboons and rats was linear with time.

For baboons the daily total rate of excretion (in urine plus feces), averaged over each week, varied between 28.9 and 60.2 μg/day during weeks 5 to 35. Fecal excretion in this period varied between 11.6 and 29.2 μg/day; thus fecal and urinary excretion rates were almost equal. Maximum excretion rates occurred during week 4. Rods were surgically excised on day 237 postimplantation. At this time 10.6 mg (9.5% of the initial dose) had been recovered. Tritium excretion was erratic; on removal of the rods a mean of 22 mg of polymer had been recovered.

Rods remained in rats for a maximum of 197 days. In this interval, rats had excreted 2.05 mg (14.7% of the initial dose). Most of this, 2.59 mg, was recovered in feces. No tritium was observed in rats' excreta until days 184 to 197 when only two rats passed some in feces.

Concomitant with excretion analyses, blood samples were taken from baboons for radioimmunoassay. Analyses indicated mean serum norgestrel levels varying between 2 and 8 μg/mℓ while implants were in place. Following removal, serum levels declined to zero within several days.

While implants were in place, normal ovarian cycling as judged by sex skin turgescence was completely inhibited. Breakthrough bleeding did, however, occur in all four cases for 17, 22, 31, and 67 days. Normal cycling was resumed within 5 to 10 days after removal of the rods.

Rods excised from both groups of animals were examined by scanning electron microscopy (SEM) and by gel permeation chromatography (GPC). SEM did not reveal any gross structural differences at high magnification (1000 to 5000 ×), but did show marked cracking and fissures at lower magnification (~100 ×).

GPC showed a large drop in polymer molecular weight. The original values ($\overline{M}_w$ = 257,200; $\overline{M}_n$ = 85,000) had declined to a mean of $\overline{M}_w$ = 10,400 ± 4000 (S.E.), $\overline{M}_n$ = 4300 ± 2500 for baboons. Rods removed from rats had a $\overline{M}_w$ = 6800 ± 4200; $\overline{M}_n$ = 2500 ± 1340. A t test applied to the difference between the means of $\overline{M}_w$ indicated a probability of 25% that the difference was due to random variation.

Polyester hydrolysis in solution was studied in order to determine the effect of the lactide to glycolide ratio, molecular weight, and initiator on hydrolysis rate. Results indicate that these factors do not affect rates.

Based on these results, work was continued under PARFR sponsorship. This work is summarized as follows and is presented in more detail in this chapter.

Five formulations of sustained-release systems for levonorgestrel were manufactured at Dynatech and were tested in rats at SISA Inc. (Cambridge, Mass.). The objective of examining several formulations was to determine which parameters (drug loading, polymer composition, polymer molecular weight) exerted the most influence on levonorgestrel release rate. All systems were in the form of 0.8-mm (1/32-in.) diameter cylindrical rods. The five systems were composed of two different drug loadings, 50 and 70% by weight, and three different polymers: 165,000 $\overline{M}_w$ 90/10 poly-[L(−)-lactic-co-glycolic acid] (PLGA), 40,000 $\overline{M}_w$ 90/10 PLGA, and 45,000 $\overline{M}_w$ 75/25 PLGA. The two 90/10 PLGAs were each loaded to 50 and 70% levonorgestrel, and the 75/25 PLGA loaded to 50%. Thus, the effects of the three parameters listed above could be evaluated.

Release rates as determined by combustion and scintillation counting of urine and feces collected periodically from rats implanted with the five dosage forms are summarized below.

Drug content by weight (%)	Polymer composition	Polymer ($\bar{M}_w$)	Release rate (μg/day)	Combined rates
50	90/10	165,000	4.9	5.4
50	90/10	40,000	5.9	5.4
50	75/25	45,000	11.2	11.2
70	90/10	165,000	8.2	8.0
70	90/10	40,000	7.8	8.0

Because of scatter in the experimental data, differences in the release rate of levonorgestrel of ±10% of the mean were considered insignificant. Polymer molecular weight was seen to make little difference in levonorgestrel release rate for the two 50% samples (4.9 μg/day for the 165,000 $\overline{M}_w$ polymer, 5.9 μg/day for the 40,000 $\overline{M}_w$ polymer), and less for the two 70% loaded samples (8.2 μg/day for the 165,000 $\overline{M}_w$ polymer, 7.8 μg/day for the 40,000 $\overline{M}_w$ polymer). Large differences in release rate were seen between dosage forms of different drug loadings and different polymer compositions. The sample composed of 50% drug and 75/25 PLGA was seen to release drug at a rate 2.1 times as fast as the sample with the same drug loading, but using a polymer composed of 90 parts lactide and 10 parts glycolide. The samples loaded to 70% drug released levonorgestrel at a rate of 1.5 times that of those loaded to 50% with drug.

These results indicate that a wide range of release rates may be obtained from levonorgestrel/PLGA rods, and that the release rate of a given dosage form can be controlled by varying polymer composition and drug loading of the sustained release device.

A. Summary of Present Research Program

Five formulations of sustained release systems for levonorgestrel were manufactured at Dynatech and tested for excretion rates in rats at SISA Inc. The objective of examining several formulations was to determine which parameters (drug loading, polymer composition, polymer molecular weight) exerted the most influence on levonorgestrel release rate. All systems were in the form of 0.8-mm (1/32-in.) diameter cylindrical rods. An appropriate mass of a single length of rod (containing approximately 7 mg of drug) was implanted in each animal. Four rats were implanted with each dosage form; thus a total of twenty animals were involved in the testing.

The levonorgestrel incorporated into these sustained release devices was labeled with ^{14}C to make excretion rate analysis possible by collection and combustion of the animals' urine and feces. The polymer excipient in these formulations was not labeled with any radioactive isotope.

The compositions of the five levonorgestrel sustained release formulations are presented in Table 1.

Specific activities of the matrices were determined by dissolution of samples in dioxane followed by liquid scintillation counting of aliquots of the solutions. Specific activities of the two drug dilutions were also determined in the same manner. The latter drug (specific activity 1.84 mCi/g) was incorporated into matrix sample 07440. The other drug (specific activity 1.00 mCi/g) was incorporated into the other formulations.

Drug content of the matrices as determined by gravimetric measure and reported in percent by weight, as well as the drug content as determined by specific activity, are shown in Table 2. Agreement between these two values was very good. Calculations of excretion rates were based on the gravimetric measures of 50 and 70% and the measured specific activities.

Table 1
COMPOSITIONS OF THE FIVE LEVONORGESTREL DOSAGE FORMS

Sample	Drug content by weight (%)	Specific activity (mCi/g)	Drug content from specific activity (%)	Polymer composition	Polymer ($\overline{M}_w$)
07440	50	0.93	50	90/10	165,000
07444	70	0.61	61	90/10	165,000
07446	50	0.51	51	75/25	45,000
07447	50	0.52	52	90/10	40,000
07448	70	0.68	68	90/10	40,000

Table 2
GEL PERMEATION CHROMATOGRAPHIC DATA FOR POLYMER A

Retention time (min)	Elution volume (mℓ)	Chromatogram height (cm)	Molecular weight	Weight of fraction (%)
16.0	28.16	0.50	1,237,033	1.35
16.5	29.04	1.80	634,318	4.86
17.0	29.92	4.00	325,262	10.80
17.5	30.80	6.05	180,408	16.33
18.0	31.68	7.15	127,101	19.30
18.5	32.56	6.75	89,545	18.22
19.0	33.44	5.20	63,086	14.04
19.5	34.32	2.80	44,445	7.56
20.0	35.20	1.50	31,312	4.05
20.5	36.08	0.90	22,060	2.43
21.0	36.96	0.40	15,541	1.08
Totals		37.05		100.02

III. METHODOLOGY: POLYMER PREPARATION AND CHARACTERIZATION (THREE POLYMERS — A, B, AND C)

A. High Molecular Weight Polymer

A 20-g batch of 90L/10G poly-[L(+)-lactic-co-glycolic acid] (PLGA), catalyzed with triethyl aluminum (TEAL), with a weight average molecular weight ($\overline{M}_w$) of 167,000, was prepared and characterized. The GPC data for this polymer are tabulated in Table 2. Weight average molecular weight of this polymer is seen to be 167,000; $\overline{M}_n$ is 84,000; and the dispersity is 1.99.

B. Moderate Molecular Weight Polymer

A 20-g batch of 90L/10G PLGA, catalyzed with p-toluenesulfonic acid (PTSA) with a weight average molecular weight of 33,900 was prepared and characterized. PTSA-catalyzed polymers are prepared by charging L(−)-lactide and glycolide in a 9:1 ratio by weight, along with 1% by weight PTSA catalyst, into a reaction vessel, and placing the vessel in a 120 ± 1°C oven for 5 days while continuously evacuating the vessel to 0.1 Torr. Moderate molecular weight polymer is recovered and purified in the same manner as high molecular weight polymer. The GPC data for this polymer are tabulated in Table 3. The $\overline{M}_w$ for this polymer is 33,900; the $\overline{M}_n$ is 16,600; and the dispersity is 2.04.

Table 3
GEL PERMEATION CHROMATOGRAPHIC DATA FOR POLYMER B

Retention time (min)	Elution volume (mℓ)	Chromatogram height (cm)	Molecular weight	Weight of fraction (%)
17.75	31.51	0.60	136,201	1.40
18.25	32.39	2.00	95,760	4.68
18.75	33.28	4.40	67,200	10.29
19.25	34.17	6.60	47,203	15.43
19.75	35.06	7.44	33,156	17.40
20.25	35.94	6.61	23,289	15.46
20.75	36.83	5.34	16,359	12.49
21.25	37.72	3.91	11.490	9.14
21.75	38.61	2.53	8,071	5.92
22.25	39.49	1.50	5,669	3.51
22.75	40.38	0.98	3,982	2.29
23.25	41.27	0.60	2,797	1.40
23.75	42.16	0.25	1,981	0.58
Totals		42.76		99.99

Table 4
GEL PERMEATION CHROMATOGRAPHIC DATA FOR POLYMER C

Retention time (min)	Elution volume (mℓ)	Chromatogram height (cm)	Molecular weight	Weight of fraction (%)
18.20	30.94	0.20	170,600	1.03
18.70	31.79	0.90	121,700	4.63
19.20	32.64	2.40	86,700	12.34
19.70	33.49	3.20	61,800	16.45
20.20	34.34	3.40	44,100	17.48
20.70	35.19	3.00	31,400	15.42
21.20	36.04	2.20	22,400	11.31
21.70	36.89	1.60	16,000	8.23
22.20	37.74	1.10	11,400	5.66
22.70	38.59	0.65	8,100	3.34
23.20	39.44	0.40	5,800	2.06
23.70	40.29	0.30	4,150	1.54
24.20	41.14	0.10	2,950	0.51
Totals		19.45		100.00

Note: $\overline{M}_w$ = 45,800; $\overline{M}_n$ = 24,000; and D = 1.91.

C. 75L/25G Polymer

A 20-g batch of 75L/25G PLGA with a $\overline{M}_w$ = 45,000 and catalyzed with PTSA was prepared and characterized. The 75L/25G PLGA was synthesized by charging a reaction vessel with L(−)-lactide and glycolide in a 9:1 ratio by weight, and 0.9% by weight PTSA catalyst, evacuating the vessel to 0.1 Torr, sealing it, and placing the sealed vessel into a 120 ± 2°C oven for 5 days. This polymer was recovered and purified in the same manner as the 90L/10G polymer preparation. The GPC data for this polymer are tabulated in Table 4. The $\overline{M}_w$ for the polymer is 45,800; the $\overline{M}_n$ is 24,000; and the dispersity is 1.91.

D. ^{14}C-Labeled Levonorgestrel Synthesis

^{14}C-labeled levonorgestrel was custom synthesized for Dynatech by Amersham Corporation, Chicago. Specific activity of the synthesized material was 109 mCi/mmol. Obtained from Amersham was 5 mCi of the ^{14}C-labeled levonorgestrel in 9:1 toluene to ethanol solution. This levonorgestrel was diluted to approximately 2 mCi/g with unlabeled levonorgestrel (courtesy of Wyeth, Radnor, Pa.). This quantity of diluted levonorgestrel was sufficient to prepare system 1 of the levonorgestrel/PLGA sustained delivery preparations. An additional 10 mCi of ^{14}C-labeled levonorgestrel was ordered from Amersham. This additional material was diluted to 1 mCi/g and incorporated into the other implantable, biodegradable sustained-release device formulations.

1. Drug Dilution

The specific activity of the 5 mCi of ^{14}C-labeled levonorgestrel obtained from Amersham was 35 μCi/mg. The ^{14}C-labeled levonorgestrel was shipped dissolved in a 9:1 toluene:ethanol solution. The 5 mCi of ^{14}C-labeled levonorgestrel was combined with 2.4845 g of unlabeled levonorgestrel in 135 mℓ of GPC-grade tetrahydrofuran (THF). After complete dissolution was achieved, the solvent was rotary evaporated to recover the 2.5 g of solid levonorgestrel. The solid, diluted, ^{14}C-labeled levonorgestrel was then vacuum desiccated at 60°C overnight. A total of 2.53 g of levonorgestrel was recovered. Quintuple samples of the ^{14}C-labeled levonorgestrel were assayed for specific activity by a Beckman® LS100 scintillation counter. Specific aciticity of the sample was determined at 1.87 mCi/g.

2. Preparation of 90L/10G PLGA//^{14}C-Levonorgestrel Matrix

Two sets of 90L/10G PLGA//levonorgestrel matrix were prepared, one with ^{14}C-labeled levonorgestrel, the other with unlabeled levonorgestrel. Both matrices contained 50% w/w steroid and 50% w/w PLGA. The unlabeled matrix was prepared to test extrusion conditions prior to extrusion of the valuable ^{14}C-labeled levonorgestrel/PLGA casting. In both cases, 2.00 g of PLGA (B04493) and 2.00 g of levonorgestrel were charged to 4-oz jars with 65 mℓ of Fisher ACS grade toluene. Previous implantable levonorgestrel/PLGA matrices formulated during this program were blended with benzene. Toluene was substituted because of its lower toxicity, yet similar solvent characteristics. Glass beads and porcelain balls were placed in the jars to grind the levonorgestrel to particles in the 1- to 10-μm size range. The jars were sealed and rolled on a ball mill for 2 days.

The levonorgestrel suspensions were then cast on glass plates to allow solvent evaporation, then scraped from the plates and vacuum desiccated at 60°C to remove traces of toluene solvent. The castings were analyzed for residual solvent content and extruded into 1/32-in. diameter cylindrical dosage forms.

3. Preparation of Dosage Forms

Three batches of polymer were prepared for incorporation into the different formulations of levonorgestrel sustained delivery devices. Polymer sample numbers and characteristics are summarized in Table 5 below.

Polymer/levonorgestrel matrices were prepared by dissolving the polymer in toluene or benzene, adding the appropriate amount of drug to the solution, then ball milling the mixture for 48 to 60 hr to grind the drug particles to ≤5 μm. Levonorgestrel is insoluble in benzene and toluene. After ball milling, the suspensions were cast in thin films on glass plates to evaporate off the solvent. The polymer/drug films were then removed from the glass plates and vacuum desiccated at ~60°C for at least 48 hr to remove residual solvent. Table 6 summarizes the matrix compositions and blending and casting conditions.

Table 5
SUMMARY OF POLYMER CHARACTERISTICS

Sample polymer	Polymer composition	Polymer molecular weight	Catalyst
A	90% w/w lactide 10% w/w glycolide	165,000	TEAL
B	90% w/w lactide 10% w/w glycolide	33,000	PTSA
C	75% w/w lactide 25% w/w glycolide	45,000	PTSA

Table 6
SUMMARY OF PLGA/LEVONORGESTREL MATRIX COMPOSITIONS AND BLENDING AND CASTING CONDITIONS

Sample	Polymer and composition	Drug content by weight	Solvent	Ball mill duration (hr)	Drying time and temperature
07440	04493 90L/10G	50% ^{14}C-levonorgestrel	Fisher ACS grade toluene	48	16 days at 60°C
07444	04493 90L/10G	70% ^{14}C-levonorgestrel	Fisher ACS grade toluene	48	~16 days at 60°C
07446	07425 75L/25G	50% ^{14}C-levonorgestrel	Benzene	48	48 hr at 60°C
07447	07405 90L/10G	50% ^{14}C-levonorgestrel	Benzene	~60	~60 hr at 60°C
07448	07405 90L/10G	70% ^{14}C-levonorgestrel	Benzene	~60	~60 hr at 60°C

E. Excretion of ^{14}C-Labeled Materials by Rats

1. Implantation

The five formulations of levonorgestrel sustained delivery systems were tested in rats for excretion rate. Samples of each formulation were implanted in four rats. A total of 20 rats was employed in this test.

Each rat received approximately 7 mg of levonorgestrel. Cut from the 70% by weight formulations were 17-mm lengths of the 0.8-mm diameter rods (about 10 mg) and 23-mm lengths (about 14 mg) were cut from the 50% by weight formulations for insertion into rats. Precise weights of the rods are given in Table 7.

Each rat was anesthetized with Penthrane®, incised in the scapular region, and implanted subcutaneously with a single rod. The wound was then closed with two wound clips, and the animal was allowed to recover. Each animal was numbered and implanted with a rod corresponding to the number. This correspondence is noted in Table 7.

Urine and feces of each animal were collected daily for 4 days, pooled from the 5th to the 7th days of the experiment, and pooled and collected weekly thereafter. After collection, each sample was homogenized and an aliquot taken for combustion and liquid scintillation counting. The release of ^{14}C-levonorgestrel from the implanted rods can therefore be measured by monitoring the excretion of ^{14}C-labeled levonorgestrel and metabolites.

2. Research Findings and Their Significance

a. Results

Excretion of ^{14}C-labeled material from rats is shown graphically in Figures 2 through 4. Figure 2 shows the cumulative recovery of ^{14}C from rats implanted with 07440 rods composed of 50% by weight levonorgestrel and 50% 165,000 $\overline{M}_w$ 90/10 PLGA. This formulation is

Table 7
WEIGHT OF IMPLANTED RODS

Sample	Weight (mg)	Drug content by weight (%)	Polymer composition	Polymer molecular weight	Implanted in rat no.
07440-1	14.1	50	90% lactide	165,000	1
07440-2	14.1		10% glycolide		2
07440-3	14.0				3
07440-4	14.1				4
07440-5	14.0				
07444-1	10.2	70	90% lactide	165,000	5
07444-2	10.1		10% glycolide		6
07444-3	10.1				7
07444-4	10.2				8
07444-5	10.2				
07446-1	14.1	50	75% lactide	45,000	9
07446-2	13.9		25% glycolide		10
07446-3	14.1				11
07446-4	13.8				12
07446-5	14.1				
07447-1	14.0	50	90% lactide	40,000	13
07447-2	13.8		10% glycolide		14
07447-3	13.7				15
07447-4	13.5				16
07447-5	14.0				
07448-1	10.0	70	90% lactide	40,000	17
07448-2	10.2		10% glycolide		18
07448-3	10.0				19
07448-4	10.3				20
07448-5	10.2				

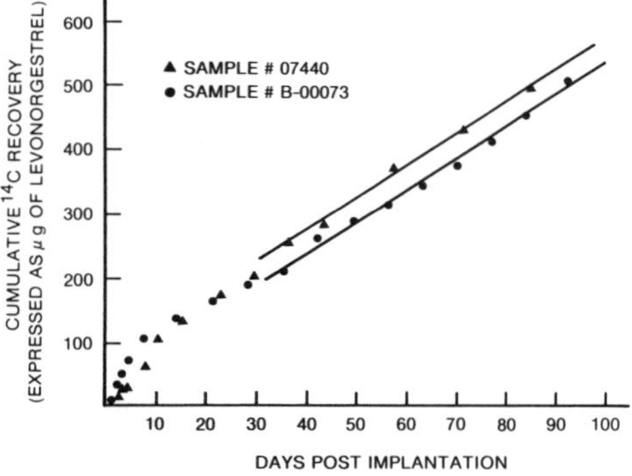

FIGURE 2. Comparison of current and previous levonorgestrel excretion by rats.

similar in composition to a previous Dynatech formulations identified as B00073. In vivo levonorgestrel release data from rats implanted with the B00073 rods are also shown in Figure 2. Since rats were implanted with 20 mg of levonorgestrel for the previous test (B00073 rods), and 7 mg of levonorgestrel for the current test, the previous data was multiplied by 7/20 to normalize it with the present data. Although this may not be a rigorously correct method of normalizing the data, it serves as a useful approximation to allow comparison of the two tests.

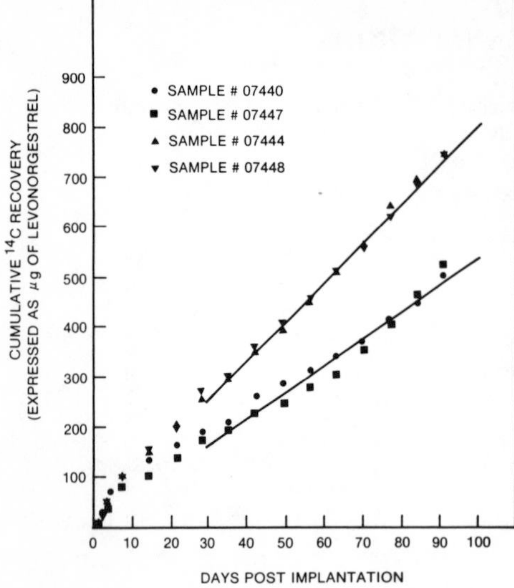

FIGURE 3. Variation of cumulative excretion of ^{14}C-labeled materials from rats with drug loading and polymer $\overline{M}_w$.

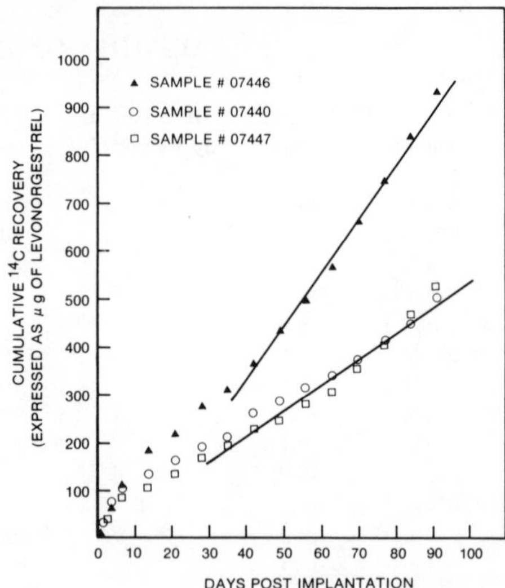

FIGURE 4. Variation of cumulative excretion of ^{14}C-labeled materials from rats with polymer composition.

Cumulative ^{14}C recovery is seen to be nearly identical in rats implanted with the two preparations. This similarity of release from the two preparations is important as it demonstrates reproducibility of release from dosage forms manufactured more than 2 years apart.

The excretion rates reported here are taken from the slope of a linear regression performed on rat ^{14}C-excretion data from days 29 to 91 postimplantation. Monolithic sustained release devices such as this levonorgestrel/PLGA system often display a "burst" or rapid release of drug immediately postimplantation. Release of drug then slowed to a more or less constant rate. Days 29 to 91 were chosen as a convenient time period for data analysis since all the formulations had completed their "bursts", and ^{14}C release had become nearly constant with time.

Figure 2 shows that the release data obtained in the current set of tests are comparable to those obtained in previous in vivo studies.

Figure 3 is a graph of the variation of cumulative excretion of ^{14}C-labeled material from rats with drug loading and polymer molecular weight. Excretion rates from dosage forms composed of two drug loadings of 50 and 70% by weight and two polymer molecular weights, ~40,000 and ~165,000, are compared in this figure. It is immediately apparent that polymer molecular weight has almost no effect on drug release rate. Samples 07444 (165,000 $\overline{M}_w$) and 07448 (40,000 $\overline{M}_w$) both contain 70% w/w drug and show identical release rates. Similarly, the two samples containing 50% w/w drug, 07440 (with 165,000 $\overline{M}_w$ polymer) and 07447 (with 40,000 $\overline{M}_w$ polymer), show nearly identical release rates. The polymer composition in all cases was 90% by weight lactide and 10% glycolide.

While Figure 3 reveals that polymer molecular weight has almost no effect on drug excretion rate, it shows that drug content of the rod has a significant effect. Excretion rates were determined by linear regression through data points for each drug loading; data points for both polymer molecular weights were included in each drug loading. The analysis reveals that rods loaded to 70% with drug released at a rate (8.0 μg/day) approximately 1.5 times that of the rods loaded to 50% with levonorgestrel (5.4 μg/day).

Figure 4 is a graph of the variation of cumulative excretion of ^{14}C-labeled materials from rats with polymer composition. Rods loaded to 50% by weight with levonorgestrel were

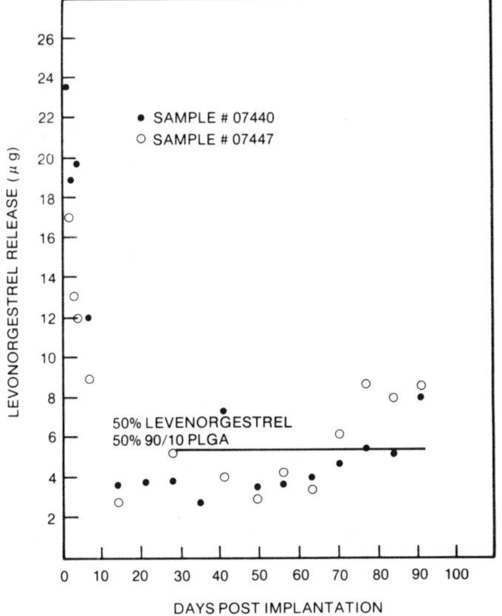

FIGURE 5. Average daily excretion of ^{14}C-labeled materials excreted by rats, expressed as micrograms of levonorgestrel.

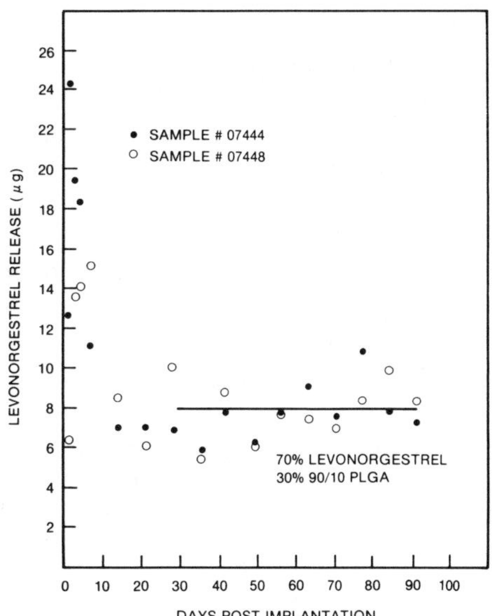

FIGURE 6. Average daily excretion of ^{14}C-labeled materials by rats, expressed as micrograms of levonorgestrel.

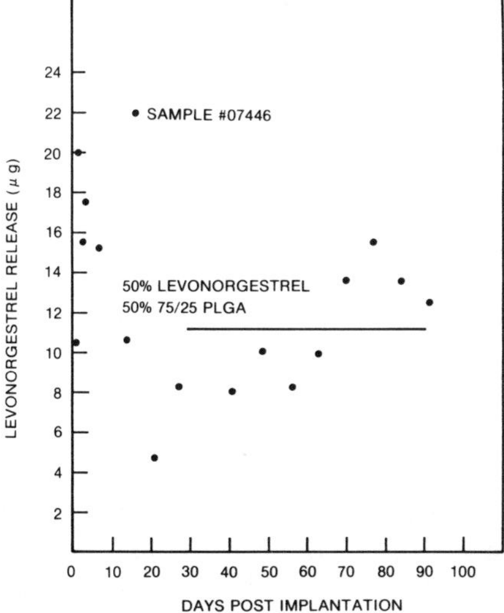

FIGURE 7. Average daily excretion of ^{14}C-labeled materials by rats, expressed as micrograms of levonorgestrel.

made with 90/10 PLGA (of 40,000 and 165,000 $\overline{M}_w$) and with 75/25 PLGA display an excretion rate of about 11.2 μg/day, while those comprised of 90/10 PLGA release at about 5.4 μg/day. Polymer composition has a very significant effect on drug release rate from rods, with the 75/25 rods releasing about 2.1 times as fast as the 90/10 rods.

Figures 5 to 7 present the average daily release of levonorgestrel from all of the samples.

b. Discussion

The "first-generation" levonorgestrel sustained release system (B-00073), composed of 50% by weight drug and 50% 257,000 $\overline{M}_w$ 90/10 PLGA, sustained the delivery of drug for 2 years in rats. This system was deemed too long lasting for practical application. The current work at Dynatech is aimed at revealing the parameters which affect release rate in this particular drug/polymer composite in order to design a dosage form which will deliver steroid for 6 months to 1 year.

Table 8 summarizes the results. It presents a comparison of release characteristics from the several levonorgestrel sustained delivery systems formulated and tested recently and the "first-generation" system. The first three columns of Table 8 describe the different systems; the final three give the drug release rate and duration from the samples.

The excretion rate figures are determined from the slope of a linear regression of days 29 to 91 of cumulative excretion data from rats implanted with the samples. This time period is selected because data was obtained 91 days postimplantation. The projected lifetime of the system is the amount of time which would be required to release all the drug implanted in an animal, assuming the excretion rate remained constant throughout the system lifetime:

$$\text{Projected lifetime} = \frac{\text{implanted dose}}{\text{excretion rate (days 29—91)}}$$

The "anticipated lifetime" is defined here as the expected lifetime of the system in rats, based on the B00073 rods which were tested to exhaustion and released levonorgestrel for 2 years. The anticipated lifetime is calculated by taking the ratio of the excretion rate from a current sample to the excretion rate of B00073, and multiplying it by 2 years:

$$\text{Anticipated lifetime} = \frac{\begin{array}{c}\text{excretion rate of sample}\\ \text{(days 29—91)}\end{array}}{\begin{array}{c}\text{excretion rate of B00073}\\ \text{(days 30—85)}\end{array}} \times 2 \text{ years}$$

The B00073 rods are the only ones that have been tested to exhaustion in rats.

System lifetime in baboons for the Dynatech "first-generation" system (B00073) appeared to be somewhat longer than in rats. Based on excretion data for ^{14}C-labeled levonorgestrel, and with a rate calculated from about the same time period, a lifetime of 6.2 years was projected. It is likely that matrix degradation with time would increase the release rate and reduce the system lifetime, but these tests were run for only 6 months.

The significance of the current work is that two parameters, drug loading and polymer composition, have been shown to affect levonorgestrel release rate from these drug/polymer systems significantly. If these effects are additive, and as they are independent they appear to be so, an even larger range of release duration and rates from levonorgestrel/PLGA dosage forms is possible.

Since the increase in release rate due to the increase of drug loading from 50 to 70% is a factor of 1.5, and the increase in release rate due to changing the polymer composition to 75L/25G from 90L/10G is 2.1, a dosage form composed of 70% levonorgestrel in 75L/25G PLGA will result in an increase in release rate of $1.5 \times 2.1 = 3.1$, a factor of 3.1 over that of the first-generation system. This, in turn, will result in an excretion rate (days 29 to 91) of 3.1×5.4 μg/day $=$ 17 μg/day per 7-mg implant and a projected system lifetime of 3.6/3.1 years or 14 months. Based on an actual lifetime in rats for the first-generation system, a 3.1-fold increase in release rate would yield an implant with a lifetime of about 7 months.

Based on the current work, it appears that an implant with a lifetime of from 6 to 12 months would be obtained from a dosage form composed of 70% levonorgestrel and 30%

Table 8
SUMMARY OF LEVONORGESTREL RELEASE FROM SEVERAL SUSTAINED RELEASE FORMULATIONS

		Polymer		In vivo in rats		
Sample	**Levonorgestrel content**	**Composition**	$\overline{M}_w$	**Excretion rate (days 29 to 91)**	**Projected lifetime**	**Anticipated lifetime**[a]
B00073	50% w/w	90L/10G	257,000	4.9 μg/day	1,429 days (3.9 years)	2.0 years
07440	50% w/w	90L/10G	165,000	5.4 μg/day	1,296 days (3.6 years)	1.8 years
07447	50% w/w	90L/10G	40,000	5.4 μg/day	1,296 days (3.6 years)	1.8 years
07444	70% w/w	90L/10G	165,000	8.0 μg/day	875 days (2.4 years)	1.2 years
07448	70% w/w	90L/10G	40,000	8.0 μg/day	875 days (2.4 years)	1.2 years
07446	50% w/w	75L/25G	45,000	11.2 μg/day	625 days (1.7 years)	0.9 years
Proposed system combination of variables in 07448 and 07446	70% w/w	75L/25G	40,000	~17 μg/day	411 days (1.1 years)	0.6 years, 7.0 months

[a] Anticipated lifetime is based on a previous in vivo test in rats. This test was run to exhaustion with B00073 rods. The anticipated lifetime is determined by taking the ratio of excretion rates of the current samples to that of sample B00073 and multiplying this ratio by the actual lifetime of the B00073 rods.

75/25 PLGA by weight. This system would meet design objectives for 6- to 12-month sustained delivery fertility control implant.

A reservation about the use of 75L/25G PLGA for levonorgestrel/PLGA dosage forms springs from past experience with this polymer. Under the program with the Population Council, several sustained release systems were examined in rats. The system composed of 75/25 PLGA showed a dramatic increase in levonorgestrel release rate after several weeks, after which the rate decreased. This system displayed release characteristics very different from the constant release rate desired. The current set of experiments shows an increasing release rate with time for the 75/25 PLGA composite. Further animal testing should be conducted for 6 months to a year in order to identify possible problems with an increasing levonorgestrel release rate from PLGA sustained release systems.

The results of the current program indicate the potential for PLGA/levonorgestrel rods to provide a range of drug release rates and durations. Rate and duration of release have been modified by changing the polymer composition and drug loading of the sustained release dosage forms. These results also indicate the broader utility of PLGA/drug matrices as a means of sustaining, moderating, and controlling the in vivo delivery of drug to a patient.

ACKNOWLEDGMENT

This work was carried out under Contract 91N from the Program for Applied Research on Fertility Regulation (PARFR). The continued support of Gerald I. Zatuchni, M.D., is acknowledged with appreciation.

REFERENCES

1. **Jackanicz, T. M., Nash, H. A., Wise, D. L., and Gregory, J. B.,** Polyactic acid as a biodegradable carrier for contraceptive steroids, *Contraception,* 8(2), 227, 1973.
2. **Wise, D. L., Gregory, J. B., Newburne, P. M., Bartholow, L. C., and Stanburg, J. B.,** Results on biodegradable cylindrical subdermal implants for fertility control, in *Polymeric Delivery Systems,* Kostelnik, R. J., Ed., Gordon & Breach, New York, 1978, 121.
3. **Wise, D. L., Rosenkrantz, H., Gregory, J. B., and Esber, H. J.,** *J. Pharm. Pharmacol.,* 32, 399, 1980.

Chapter 2

PRELIMINARY PRODUCTION COST ESTIMATES FOR AN INJECTABLE SUSTAINED RELEASE FERTILITY CONTROL SYSTEM

John B. Sanderson

TABLE OF CONTENTS

I. INTRODUCTION

This chapter describes the preliminary process engineering, facilities design, and cost estimates associated with the production of sufficient quantity of material to produce 4 million doses per year of an injectable controlled release fertility control system. Such a quantity of material could be produced and packaged in a light industrial building with a usable area of approximately 2000 ft^2. A work force of 10 individuals working 2000 hr/year would be required. The manufacture would be carried out using a mixture of small-scale pilot plant equipment and large-scale laboratory equipment. The packaging would be performed on an automatic packaging line under sterile conditions. The capital required to build such a plant is estimated at less than $600,000, not including land. The annual operating costs for producing 4 million units is estimated at less than $1 million, giving a unit cost of less than $0.25 per dose.

II. PRELIMINARY PROCESS AND FACILITY DESIGN

Preliminary process and facility design has been completed for the production of 4 million doses per year of an injectable controlled release fertility control system. Norethisterone is used as an example drug. The process is divisible into five steps: (1) lactide-glycolide preparation; (2) polymerization; (3) polymer-norethisterone blending; (4) particle formation; and (5) packaging.

Figure 1* is a process flow sheet showing these five steps and the various materials and possible unit operations involved in them. The lactide and glycolide (cyclic dimers of lactic and glycolic acids, respectively) are made in a vapor phase cyclization process in the vacuum distillation of lactic or glycolic acid. It is necessary to convert the lactic and glycolic acids into their cyclic dimeric form in order to achieve the desired molecular weight of the resulting polymer. Only low molecular weight polymers have been produced by the direct condensation polymerization of lactic and glycolic acids.

The next step is to purify the resulting lactide or glycolide. The possible methods for obtaining sufficiently pure lactide or glycolide are recrystallization or sublimation. Recrystallization has been shown to be the more effective method. At this point the product is checked for purity and is repurified if necessary.

The pure lactide and glycolide are combined with triethyl aluminum (TEAL) initiator and a melt polymerization is carried out. The crude polymer is dissolved in an appropriate solvent, filtered to remove insoluble matter, and coagulated in a nonsolvent under high shear. Once dried the polymer is checked for purity and molecular weight.

The polymer is then dissolved in a solvent which will not dissolve the norethisterone, and the drug is milled into the polymer solution. It has been found that a more uniform blend of drug and polymer can be obtained in this way than if the drug is also dissolved.

Conversion of this norethisterone suspension into final particles is currently being accomplished by casting the suspension into a film, extruding the film into a rod, and cryogenically grinding the rod into particles. However, a number of alternative routes may be used which produce particles of the proper size without further classification. One of these is the use of an air impact pulverizer or micronizer on the shredded film. The other is pelletization of the cast film, wherein the polymer is extruded into fibers and the fibers are cut to give cylinders of the appropriate size. A technique for producing particles without going through the film casting route is to spray dry the suspension. Generally spray drying has produced particles smaller than those desired, but by proper specification of suspension rheology,

* Figures and tables appear at the end of the text.

nozzle geometry, and air velocity it is conceivable to produce particles in the proper size range. In any case spray drying is an alternate way to film casting to prepare polymer for pelletization.

Classification is currently accomplished by sifting, with the coarse particles being reground and the fine particles redissolved. If classification is required in the final process it could be accomplished by air elutriation, wherein the particles are fractionated based on their surface-to-mass ratio.

At this point it is necessary to ensure that the particles are of the desired size, and that the proper drug loading has been achieved. If the product is acceptable, it is packaged. Basically, two methods of packaging seem feasible. One is to package a weighed dose of particles in a vacuum-formed container, accompanied by a vial containing the suspending solution. This approach has the advantage that the particles could be sterilized with ethylene oxide in the sealed container, but a fair amount of effort will be required on the part of the user to combine the two materials and prepare the suspension. The alternate method is to provide the particles and the suspending solution in a two-chambered mixer vial, such as those used for injectable preparations including B-complex vitamins and certain water-sensitive derivatives of hydrocortisone and methylprednisolone. This method of packaging provides relative ease of suspension preparation, but the possibility of sterilization in the sealed container is unlikely. Alternatively, the product could be handled from some point in the process where sterility could be demonstrated under conditions designed to prevent recontamination. For example, if pelletization is used to produce the particles, they would be sterile as they are made because of the high temperature and long residence time required. Since packaging would be done under clean room conditions, recontamination could be prevented.

Figure 2 is a conceptual layout showing the kind of equipment required to produce this product according to the process which most nearly approximates the method of preparing research quantities in the laboratory and in the amounts required for 4 million doses per year. The equipment shown is a mixture of small-scale pilot plant equipment with large-scale laboratory equipment. The packaging, on the other hand, must be done on a substantial scale. The process is visualized as an intermittent conveyor with automatic filling and capping equipment designed to operate at a rate of 32 packages per minute. The conveyor would be hand loaded and unloaded. The packages would be hand labeled and hand cartoned. It is easily the most labor intensive part of the operation. No provision is made for the preparation of the suspension fluid as it is assumed that it will be prepared elsewhere. However, preparation of the suspension fluid is relatively simple, and provision for preparing it on site could be made.

Figure 3 is a floor plan of a plant which would be capable of producing this product. It covers about 2000 ft^2 and consists of a production area, sterile packaging room, quality control room, and supporting facilities. Figure 4 shows the same layout in isometric projection.

The plant is designed to produce 4 million doses per year, operating on a 1-shift, 5-day-week basis. Production could be increased up to fourfold by operating on a 24-hr, 7-day-week basis. Any further increase in production would require additional and/or more sophisticated packaging equipment.

III. PRELIMINARY COST ESTIMATES

Table 1 contains a list of the process equipment illustrated in Figure 2, along with the costs for this equipment, and with estimates for the costs of installation of each piece of equipment if required. The capital requirement for this process is estimated to be $360,624. Some of the alternate unit operations included in Figure 1 would require equipment which is somewhat more expensive than the pieces they replace, but a substitution would not be made unless a tangible benefit could be demonstrated, such as an improvement in quality or yield or a reduction in the amount of materials or labor required. In any case a capital requirement in excess of $400,000 for process equipment is not anticipated.

Table 2 lists the capital requirements for the physical plant. The building, in addition to what is shown in Figures 3 and 4, would also include a partial lower level or outbuilding to house a boiler, a compressor, and a 70 kVA transformer. It is anticipated that the air handling equipment would be mounted on the roof. A freezer is included for use in recrystallization of lactide and glycolide.

The capital requirement for physical plant, not including land but with provision for some exterior improvements to the site such as driveways and parking lots, is estimated to be $121,500.

Table 3 lists some other capital requirements such as office furniture, material handling equipment, and initial inventory and start-up costs. An allowance of $38,500 is made for these items.

Table 4 gives the total capital requirement of $520,324, excluding land.

Table 5 presents a breakdown of the anticipated annual operating costs associated with producing 4 million units per year. The annual cost for raw materials is estimated to be $169,000, the bulk of which is for the norethisterone. The next item listed is packaging materials costing $472,000/year, approximately 75% of which is for mixer vials. Alternate methods of packaging, as described earlier, would reduce the packaging costs considerably.

The utility expense, lab and office supplies, solvent disposal, local taxes and insurance (5% of investment), depreciation (10-year straight line), and labor add an additional $288,500 to the annual operating expense.

Table 6 summarizes the total annual operating expense at $929,500. Such a cost to produce 4 million doses per year gives a unit cost of $0.232 per dose. This calculation is shown in Table 7.

Table 8 lists the work force required to operate this plant. The estimate of $200,000/year for the cost of labor presented in Table 5 is based on this work force.

It should be noted that a number of items in both the capital requirements and the annual operating costs are sensitive to the location of the plant. Some of the more important factors are labor, including the labor portion of the building costs and installation of equipment, import duties on capital equipment, and local taxes. In spite of these variations, however, it is not anticipated that the total capital requirement, excluding land, would exceed $600,000, nor that the annual operating costs would exceed $1 million, or $0.25 per unit.

ACKNOWLEDGMENT

This chapter was prepared from Dynatech Report No. 1396 (Dynatech R/D Company, Cambridge, Mass.) to the World Health Organization, Task Force: WHO Expanded Programme of Research, Development and Research Training in Human Reproduction, relevant to production costs of an injectable fertility control system.

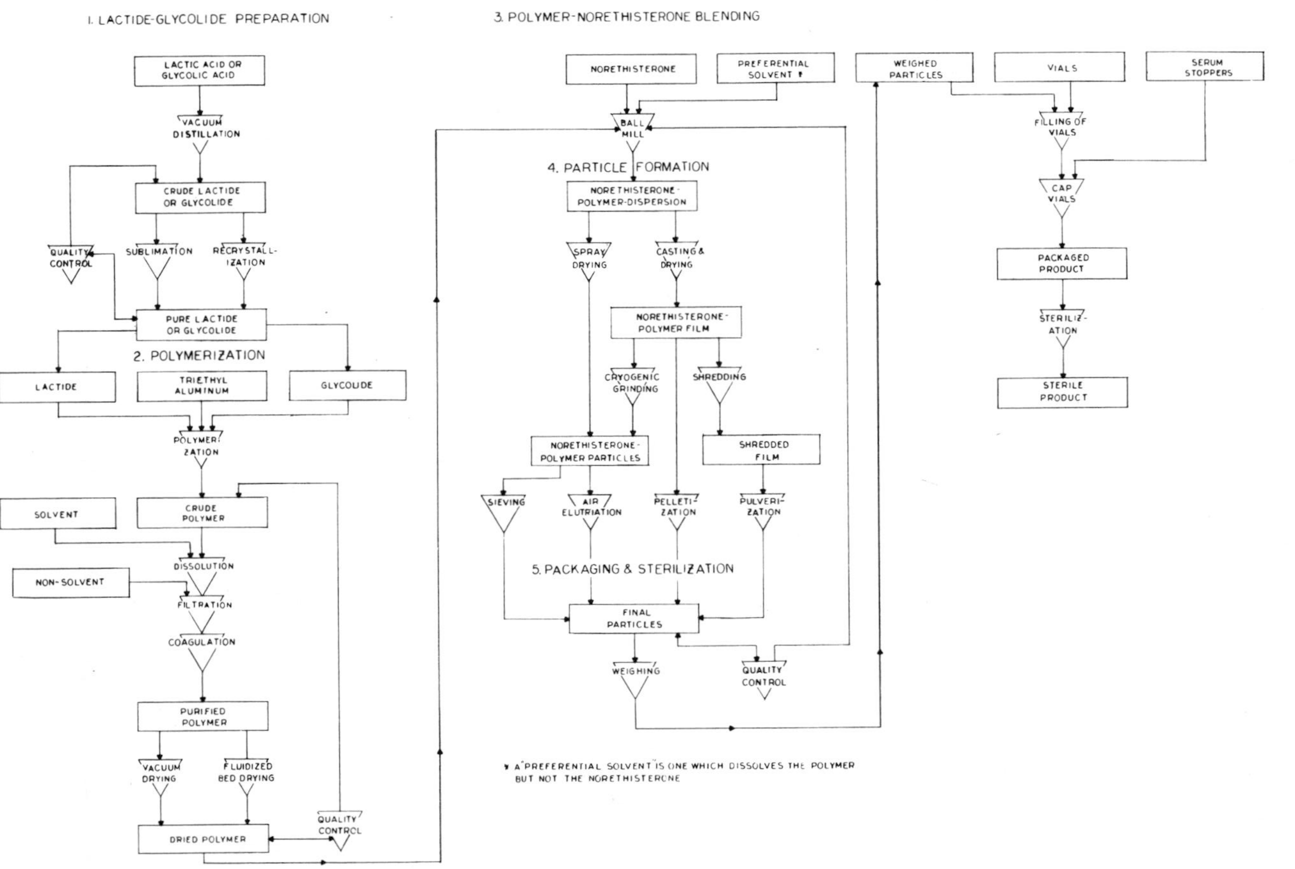

FIGURE 1. Flow sheet for production of injectable sustained release norethisterone.

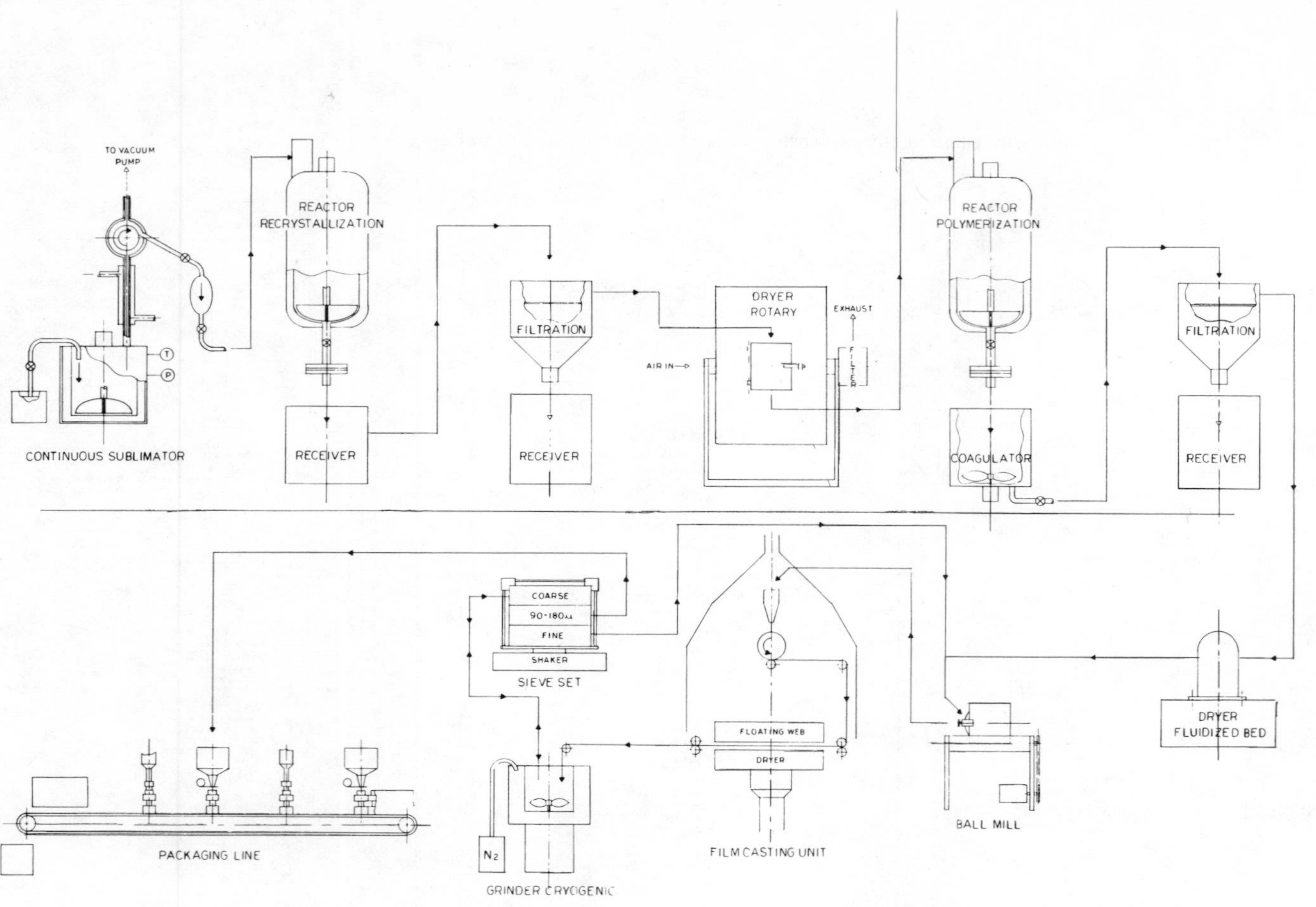

FIGURE 2. Production of injectable sustained release norethisterone conceptual layout.

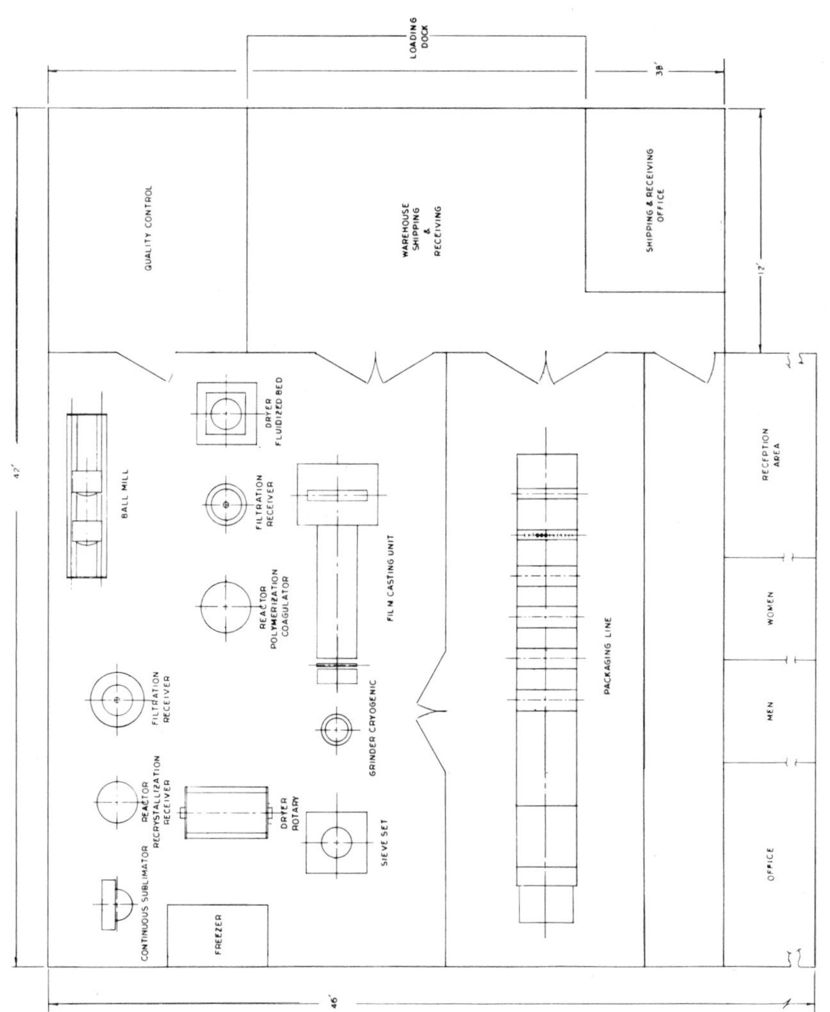

FIGURE 3. Production of injectable sustained release norethisterone conceptual layout.

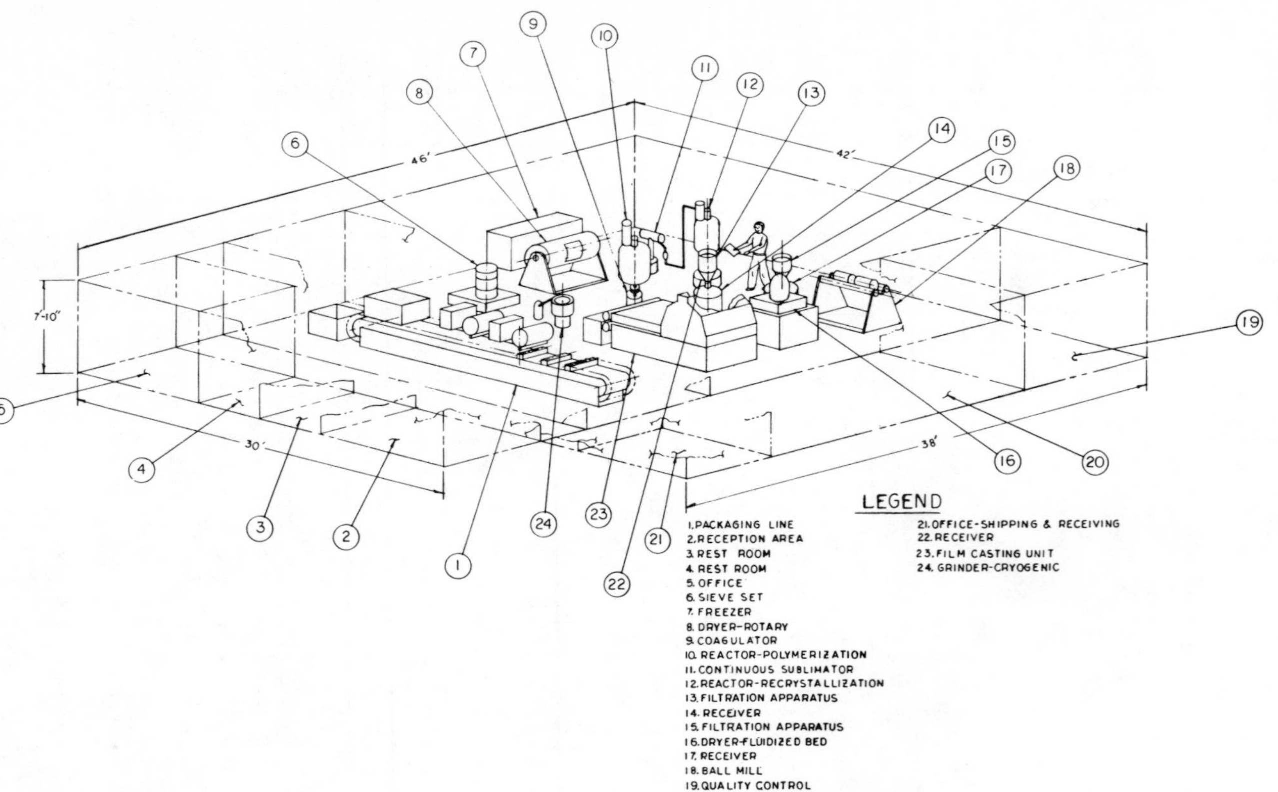

FIGURE 4. Production of injectable sustained release norethisterone conceptual design.

Table 1
CAPITAL REQUIREMENTS: PROCESS EQUIPMENT

Item	$ Price	$ Installation	$ Total cost
Lactide-glycolide preparation			
Continuous sublimator with vacuum pump, electric heat exchanger, and traps	50,000	3,000	53,000
Reactor, 20 gal, jacketed, with turbine agitator and explosion proof drive, reflux condenser baffles, flush valve, ball valve, and in-line flange filter	16,500	3,000	19,500
3 receiving tanks, HDPE, 15-gal capacity	120	—	120
Filtration apparati consisting of 2 325-mm bench top büchner funnels plus 4 10-gal carboys	230	250	470
Rotary dryer, 5 lb/hr capacity	6,694	400	7,094
Totals	73,544	6,650	80,184
Polymerization			
Reactor, 20 gal, jacketed, with anchor-helix agitator and explosion-proof drive, ammeter, flush valve, ball valve, and flange filter	19,500	3,000	22,500
Coagulator, consisting of a 3 hp explosion-proof high-shear mixer with 5 in. impeller and 15-gal 316 stainless-steel container	2,450	500	2,950
Filtration apparati consisting of 2 325-mm bench top büchner funnels plus 4 10-gal carboys	230	250	480
Dryer — fluidized bed — 75-lb capacity	8,500	800	9,300
Totals	30,680	4,550	35,230
Polymer-drug blending			
Ball mill, 1 hp with 6 6-gal 316 SS-baffled jars with 1-in. 316 SS balls	1,800	100	1,900
Totals	1,800	100	1,900
Particle formation			
Casting unit consisting of heated casting drum, floating web dryer, and draw rolls, enclosed in exhaust hood	35,000	5,000	40,000
Cryogenic grinding apparatus, pin mill, 5 hp, variable speed, 316 stainless steel	7,400	400	7,800
Sieve set with 18-in. sieves	1,200	100	1,300
Totals	43,600	5,500	49,100
Packaging equipment			
Intermittent conveyorized packaging line with automatic filling and capping equipment to process 32 packages per minute	150,000	150,000	165,000
Totals	150,000	150,000	165,000
Other process equipment			
Balances, pumps, benches	2,400	—	2,400
Quality control equipment	14,000	2,000	16,000
Totals	16,400	2,000	18,400
Total process equipment	$326,024	$168,800	$349,814

Table 2
CAPITAL REQUIREMENTS: PHYSICAL PLANT

Item	Estimated cost ($)
Building	
Structure 2000 ft^2 at $25/$ft^2$, partial lower level for boiler, compressor, transformers, etc.	50,000
Electrical service, 70 kVA	8,000
Heating-air conditioning system, 15 ton	15,000
Freezer, explosion proof, 0°F, 50 ft^3	4,000
Air filtration and sterilization system for packaging area	20,000
Boiler, 500,000 BTU/hr	10,000
Compressor, 100 cfm at 100 psi	4,500
Exterior improvements to site	10,000
Total physical plant	$121,500

Table 3
CAPITAL REQUIREMENTS: OTHER

Item	Estimated cost ($)
Office furniture and equipment	10,000
Material handling equipment	6,000
Miscellaneous	2,500
Initial inventory and start-up costs	20,000
Total other	$38,500

Table 4
TOTAL CAPITAL REQUIREMENT (EXCLUDING LAND)

Item	Requirement ($)
Process equipment	360,324
Physical plant	121,500
Other	38,500
Total capital requirement (excluding land)	$520,324

Table 5
ANNUAL OPERATING COSTS

Item	Cost ($)
Raw materials	
Lactic acid/glycolic acid, 2500 lb at $5.00/lb	12,500
Triethyl aluminum, 5 lb at $50/lb	250
Solvents, 5000 gal at $2.00/gal	10,000
Norethisterone 1000 lb at $145/lb	145,000
Liquid nitrogen 3 lb/lb product 9000 lb at $0.139/lb	1,250
Total raw materials	$169,000
Packaging materials	
Mixer vials 4 million/year at $0.09/vial	360,000
Stoppers for 4 million vials at $0.02/vial	80,000
Labels, inserts, etc., 4 million × $0.003	12,000
Cartons and cases, 4 million × $0.005	20,000
Total packaging	$472,000
Utilities	
Electricity, 50,000 kWh/year at $0.05/kWh	2,500
Oil (or equivalent), 2 × 10^8 BTU/year ÷ 875,000 BTU/$	1,100
Water, 1,600,000 gal/year at $0.25/1000 gal	400
Total utilities	$4,000
Other	
Lab and office supplies	6,000
Solvent disposal, $0.10/gal × 5000 gal	500
Local taxes and insurance, 5%	26,000
Depreciation, 10-year straight line	52,000
Direct labor (see Table 8)	200,000
Total other	$284,500

Table 6
TOTAL ANNUAL OPERATING COSTS

Item	Cost ($)
Raw materials	169,000
Packaging materials	472,000
Utilities	4,000
Other	284,500
Total annual operating costs	$929,500

Table 7
PER-UNIT-COST ESTIMATE

Total estimated annual costs (I)	$929,500
Total output (II)	4 million units
Per unit cost (I/II)	$0.232/unit

Table 8
LABOR REQUIREMENT

Position	No. required
Manager	1
Quality control chemist	1
Maintenance man	1
Shipping/receiving man	1
Plant operator	2
Secretary/receptionist	1
Packager	3
Total labor	10

Chapter 3

EXAMPLE OF GOOD MANUFACTURING PRACTICES (GMP) PROTOCOLS

Judith P. Kitchell

TABLE OF CONTENTS

I. FLOW CHART: OVERVIEW OF PROJECT

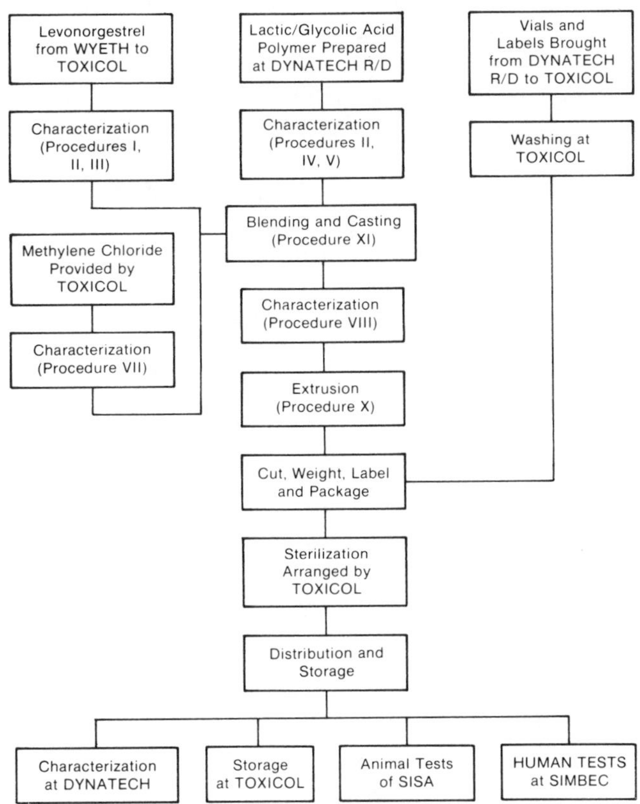

II. BATCH PRODUCTION RECORD

A. Definition of Terms

Batch — The final product rods made from a single blending process (procedure XI). A single batch may include several castings from one blend of levonorgestrel and polymer, and several rod extrusions from the castings.

Batch number — The number assigned to a batch. This number is the laboratory notebook page number that contains the first reference to the levonorgestrel/polymer blending process. This number is also assigned to all ingredients used in making the final product (i.e., levonorgestrel, polymer, methylene chloride, and packaging materials).

Package number — The number assigned to each sealed vial of final product. These are consecutive, beginning with "1".

Lot number — The manufacturer-assigned lot or batch number used to identify an ingredient.

Lab identification number — The laboratory notebook page number which contains the first reference to an ingredient.

Ingredient — One of the four starting materials used to make the final product, namely, levonorgestrel, polymer, methylene chloride, or packaging material.

B. Abbreviations

Abbreviations used are GPC, gel permeation chromatography; PLGA, polylactic/glycolic acid; PTSA, para-toluene sulfonic acid; THF, tetrahydrofuran; RI, refractive index; IR, infrared; and VVS, variable voltage source.

1. Ingredient Analysis Check Sheet for Levonorgestrel

Batch Control No.:________Lab. I.D. No.:____________________

Procedure	Performed by	Date
1. Enter the manufacturer, manufacturer's reported melting point, date received from manufacturer, levonorgestrel lot no., lab i.d. no., and batch control no. into the levonorgestrel ingredient analysis report form (see Section I.C).	__________	_____
2. Determine the melting point of a sample of levonorgestrel from this lot as detailed in procedure 1, and record it on the levonorgestrel ingredient analysis report form (see Section I.C).	__________	_____
3. Determine the extinction coefficient of this lot as detailed in procedure III, and record on the levonorgestrel ingredient analysis report form (see Section I.C).	__________	_____
4. Prepare an IR spectrum of this levonorgestrel lot as detailed in procedure II, using levonorgestrel in place of polymer. (Compare the spectrum obtained with that shown in Figure 4.) If no extraneous peaks are seen, the lot may be accepted.	__________	_____
5. Initial and date the master formula record upon completion of the tests and acceptance of this batch.	__________	_____

2. Ingredient Analysis Report Form for Levonorgestrel

Batch Control No.:________Levonogestrel Lot No.:____________________

Manufacturer:______________________________________

Manufacturer's Reported Melting Point:________________________

Date Received from Manufacturer:______Lab I.D. No.:________________

Date	Test	Results	Limits	Performed by	Checked by
	Identity by:				
	IR spectrum (procedure II)				
	Melting Point (procedure I)				
	Extinction coefficient at 242 nm (procedure III)				

Comments:

Batch Accepted:____Rejected:____for use.
By:__________(Project Manager) Date:__________
Reason for Rejection:__________
____

Approved by:__________Date:______
Principal Investigator or Department Manager

3. Ingredient Analysis Check Sheet for Polymer
Batch Control No.:______Lab I.D. No.:__________

Procedure	Performed by	Date
1. Enter the batch control no., polymer lot no., lab i.d. no., and date manufactured onto the polymer ingredient analysis report form (see Section I.E).	______	____
2. Determine the weight average molecular weight (Mw) of the polymer by gel permeation chromatography as detailed in procedure IV. Record the Mw in the polymer ingredient analysis report form (see Section I.E).	______	____
3. Determine the optical rotation and L-lactide concentration of the polymer as detailed in procedure V. acceptable limits are 75 ± 3% L-lactide.	______	____
4. Prepare an IR spectrum of the polymer and compare it to a standard spectrum by procedure II. The polymer is acceptable if no extraneous peaks appear in the spectrum.	______	____
5. Polymer lot is acceptable if all analytical test results are within the specified limit. Initial and date the master formula record upon completion of these tests and acceptance of this batch.	______	____

4. Ingredient Analysis Report Form for 75/25 PLGA Polymer
Batch Control No.:______Polymer Lot No.:__________
Manufacturer:__________
Date Manufactured:______Lab I.D. No.:__________

Date	Test	Results	Limits	Performed by	Checked by
	Molecular weight (by GPC, procedure IV)				
	Identity by spectrum (procedure II)				
	Optical rotation (procedure V)				
	L-lactide concentration				

Comments:

Batch Accepted:____Rejected:____for use.
By:____________(Project Manager) Date:____________
Reason for Rejection:____________

Approved by:____________Date:____
Principal Investigator or Department Manager

5. Ingredient Analysis Check Sheet for Methylene Chloride
Batch Control No.:________Lab. I.D. No.:____________

Procedure	Performed by	Date
1. Enter the manufacturer, manufacturer's lot or batch no., lab. i.d. no., and date received into the methylene chloride ingredient analysis report form (see Section I.G).	________	____
2. Measure the refractive index of this methylene chloride lot by procedure VII. Record the value obtained on the methylene chloride ingredient analysis report form (see Section I.G). This batch of methylene chloride is acceptable if the observed refractive index is equal to 1.424 ± 0.002.	________	____
3. Initial and date the master formula record upon completion of analyses and acceptance of this batch.	________	____

6. Ingredient Analysis Report Form for Methylene Chloride
Batch Control No.:________Methylene Chloride Lot No.:____________
Manufacturer:____________
Date Received from Manufacturer:________Lab. I.D. No.:____________

Date	Test	Results	Limits	Performed by	Checked by
	Identity: Refractive index at 20°C (by procedure VII)				

Comments:

Batch Accepted:____Rejected:____for use.

By:____________Date:____________
Project Manager
Reason for Rejection:____________

Approved by:____________Date:____
Principal Investigator or Department Manager

7. Manufacturing Check Sheet for Blending and Casting

Batch Control No.: ____________

Levonorgestrel Lab. I.D. No.: ____________ Weight ____________

Polymer Lab. I.D. No.: ____________ Weight ____________

CH_2Cl_2 Lab. I.D. No.: ____________ Volume ____________

Date Mixed ____________ Date Cast ____________

Date Drying Completed ____________ Date Assayed ____________

% w/w Methylene Chloride after Evacuation ____________

% w/w Levonorgestrel from Assay ____________ Date ____________

Procedure	Performed by	Date
1. After ingredient assays have been performed, and the ingredients released for use, enter the batch control no. and lab. i.d. nos. for each ingredient in the appropriate spaces above.	____________	____
2. Select an appropriate batch size and levonorgestrel loading percent, then weigh the necessary amounts of levonorgestrel and polymer to the nearest 0.1 mg. Record these weights above and on the master formula record.	____________	____
3. Dissolve weighed levonorgestrel and polymer in methylene chloride (procedure XI).	____________	____
4. Clean enough flat glass plates to spread the entire solution volume by thoroughly washing with Alconox® Laboratory cleanser, and rinsing with distilled water, until the water flows smoothly across the entire surface. Dry the plates in a 150°C oven.	____________	____
5. Pressure filter the solution through a 5 μ Teflon® Millipore® filter and cast the solution onto the plates (procedure XI). Record data above.	____________	____
6. Peel the dry film from glass plates and vacuum dessicate for 3 days (as in procedure XI). Record drying completion data above.	____________	____
7. Clean glass plates thoroughly in methylene chloride after removal of the film.	____________	____
8. Assay each batch for percent methylene chloride after evacuation (procedure VIII). Vacuum dessicate the film at 65°C for an additional 24 hr if more than 0.2% w/w methylene chloride is present. Repeat assay after reevacuating and record percent methylene chloride above.	____________	____
9. Accept the batch for use if methylene chloride content is less than 2000 ppm and levonorgestrel % w/w is ±10% of the desired proportion.	____________	____
10. Store film in a dessicator.	____________	____

Copy Approved by: ______________________________ Date: ________
Project Manager

Copy Approved by: ______________________________ Date: ________
Principal Investigator
or Department Manager

8. Manufacturing Check Sheet for Extruding Rods (Complete One Form for Each Extrusion)
Casting Batch No.: ________ Weight % Levonorgestrel ________________
Polymer Mw: ________ Molding No. ________ Date: ________________

Procedure	Performed by	Date
1. Clean mold in the ultrasonic cleaner with methylene chloride.	________	____
2. Prepare extrusion mold as described in procedure X.	________	____
3. Weigh a glass jar with lid.	________	____
4. Apply ~4 g of casting to mold, extrude rods as described in procedure X.	________	____
5. As rod is extruded, catch in glass jar, breaking off ~30-cm pieces as they emerge from mold.	________	____
6. Reweigh jar of rods with lid.	________	____
7. Weight of mold hold-up:	________	____
8. Temporarily store rods in the jar clearly labeled with date, batch no., no. of rods, and a description of rods. Include a dessicator stick in the jar.	________	____

Copy Approved by: ______________________________ Date: ________
Project Manager

Copy Approved by: ______________________________ Date: ________
Principal Investigator
or Department Manager

9. Manufacturing Check Sheet for Container Cleaning
Batch Control No.: ______________________________
Control No.: ________ Lab. I.D. No.: ________ Manufacturer's Lot No.: ________
Manufacturer: ______________________________
Description: 5-mℓ Glass Vials with Rubber Stopper Seals and Crimp-On/Tear-Off Aluminum Tops

Procedure	Performed by	Date
1. Enter manufacturer, manufacturer's lot no., batch control no., and lab i.d. no. above.	________	____
2. Select the appropriate number of vials for the batch size (10% more than necessary).	________	____
3. Load the vials, two at a time, onto a cuvette washer, wash for 14 sec with a solution of Alconox® laboratory glassware cleaner, then rinse with distilled water.	________	____

4. Place the glass vials into a 150°C oven for 4 hr to dry. ________ ____
5. Manually agitate the vial caps (rubber stoppers) in Alconox® laboratory glassware cleaning solution, then rinse with distilled water. ________ ____
6. Place the vial caps in a 100°C oven for 4 hr to dry. ________ ____
7. Remove vials and caps using asbestos gloves, allow them to cool, then close them to prevent dust accumulation within the vials. ________ ____

I certify that the vials and caps used for batch____were washed, rinsed, and dried as above.

Signed:____Date:________
Project Manager

Number of Vials Prepared:____
Witness to the Above:____Date:________

10. Manufacturing Check Sheet for Cutting Rods
Molding Batch No.:____Date:________

Procedure	Performed by	Date
1. Clean a lab bench area of all chemicals and equipment, and cover it with clean, lint-free paper.	________	____
2. Weigh two glass jars with lids: label one "rejects", label one "accepted, cut pieces", "batch no. ____".	________	____
3. Open one jar of extruded rods and remove one piece of rod.	________	____
4. Visually inspect for roughness or holes. If the rod is not acceptable, place it in the "reject" jar.	________	____
5. If the rod is accepted, use a clean razor blade to trim one end of the rod, then cut it into 3.5-cm (±0.5 cm) pieces.	________	____
6. Place all pieces of this size into the "accepted" jar. Place all others into the "rejected" jar.	________	____
7. When all rods are cut, weigh the jars and record weight of cut pieces (____g) and rejected rods (____g).	________	____

Copy Approved by:____Date:________
Project Manager

Copy Approved by:____Date:________
Principal Investigator
or Department Manager

11. Manufacturing Check Sheet for Packaging and Labeling

Batch Control No.:_______ Batch No. on Labels:______________________________

Date:__________________

Procedure	Performed by	Date
1. Clean a lab bench area of all chemicals and equipment, and cover it with clean, lint-free paper.	__________	____
2. Enter bach control no. and batch no. printed on labels, and date, above.	__________	____
3. Arrange cleaned vials, jars of cut rods, and printed labels on the cleaned lab bench.	__________	____
4. Remove four cut rod pieces and weigh. Record weight on label.	__________	____
5. Open one vial. Place four weighed rods in the vial, and insert its rubber stopper to seal.	__________	____
6. Peel the self-adhering label from the sheet and place it on the vial containing four rods.	__________	____
7. Wrap a piece of transparent cellophane tape around the label to secure it.	__________	____
8. Set the closed, labeled vial in a separate box.	__________	____
9. Repeat steps 4 through 8 until vials are exhausted or all rods have been packaged.	__________	____
10. Secure the rubber stopper on each vial with a crimp-on aluminum cap.	__________	____
11. Enter the total number of rods and filled vials into the appropriate spaces of this form.	__________	____

Label Accounting

Copy of Final Label

No. Prepared:____________________

No. Used: ____________________

No. Retained:____________________

Disposition of Excess:______________

____

Signed:____ Date:_______

I certify that the final label applied to this product agrees in every respect with the master formula and specific product data.

Signed:________________________

Project Manager

Date:________________________

Copy Approved by:______________________________ Date:__________
Project Manager

Copy Approved by:______________________________ Date:__________
Principal Investigator
or Department Manager

12. Final Product Assay Report
Batch Control No.:______________________________

Date	**Test**	**Results**	**Limits**	**Performed by**	**Checked by**
	Measure absorbance at 242 nm				
	Levonorgestrel content from assay (by procedure IX)				
	Polymer molecular weight (by GPC procedure IV)				
	Sterility (see procedure XII) (certification attached)				
	Residual solvent (by procedure VIII)				

Conclusion:

Batch Approved:______ Rejected:______ By:______ Date:____________________

Label Accounting

Copy of Final Label

No. Prepared:______ No. Used:____________
No. Retained:________________________
Disposition of Excess:__________________
____

Signed:__________________________________ Date:______________

I certify that the final label applied to this product agrees in every respect with the master formula and specific product data.

Copy Approved by: ______________________________ Date:__________
Project Manager

Copy Approved by: ______________________________ Date: __________
Principal Investigator
or Department Manager

13. Reservation of Active Ingredient and Final Product

Product: ____________________

Ingredient: Levonorgestrel

Manufacturer: ____________________

Date Received from Manufacturer: ______ Lab. I.D. No.: ____________________

Batch Control No.: ________ Levonorgestrel Lot. No.: ____________________

Date of Product Batch Manufacture: ____________________

Date of Final Distribution of Product, Batch No.: ______ : ____________________

Amount of Levonorgestrel Reserved: ____________________

I certify that ______ g of batch no. ____________________
of levonorgestral has been reserved, labeled, and stored at ____________________

Signed: ____________________ Date: ________

Witnessed by: ____________________ Date: ________
Project Manager

I certify that ______ containers of batch no. ____________________
of final product have been reserved, labeled, and stored at ____________________

Signed: ____________________ Date: ________

Witnessed by: ____________________ Date: ________
Project Manager

14. Product Distribution Record

Product: ____________________

Active Ingredient: Levonorgestrel

Date of Manufacture: ________ Batch No.: ____________________

Distributed to: ____________________

Address: ____________________
____
____

Quantity Sent: ____________________

Date Sent: ____________________

Physical Description of Product and Container: ____________________
____
____

I certify that the above stated information is correct.

Signed: ____________________ Date: ________

Witnessed by: ____________________ Date: ________
Project Manager

Copy Approved by: ____________________ Date: ________
Project Manager

Copy Approved by: ____________________ Date: ________
Principal Investigator
or Department Manager

III. MANUFACTURING AND QUALITY CONTROL PROCEDURES

A. Melting Point Determination

1. Apparatus

Thomas Hoover melting point apparatus with periscopic thermometer — Arthur H. Thomas, Cat. No. 6427-H10 or equivalent.

2. Preliminary Determination

Place melting point tube filled with enough powdered sample to occupy 1/8 to 1/4 in. at the bottom (after tapping to pack the sample) in the melting point apparatus. To determine approximate melting point, set heat dial so temperature rises at a rate of about 20°C/min. Observe melting point range. Note heat dial setting in your notebook.

3. Actual Determination

Turn heat dial to "off" and allow the apparatus to cool to at least 10°C below the observed melting point. Set heat dial so temperature rise is 5°C/min or less, then turn heat dial to "on" and repeat observations described above. When you approach the melting point, decrease rate of rise to 2°C/min and start recording the temperature and what happens. Note particularly the temperatures at which the first slump, first appearance of liquid, and final complete melting occur. Tabulate the results in your notebook as you do the work as follows:

Variac setting	Temperature	Observations

When measuring lactide and glycolide melting points, set heat dial to 6.0 and allow temperature to rise 10°C below the expected melting point, and then use the following heat dial settings:

	Setting
L-lactide	2.8
dl Lactide	3.5
Glycolide	2.4

B. Identification of L-Lactide/Glycolide Copolymers and Levonorgestrel by IR Spectroscopy

Prepare an IR spectrum of polymer by spreading a solution of the polymer in a volatile solvent on the prism of the instrument used, and allowing the solvent to evaporate.

Compare the spectrum to those presented in Figures 1 to 3 by superimposing it on a light box and note whether or not it matches any of the three. Figures 1 to 3 are spectra for L-lactide homopolymer, 90/100 L-lactide/glycolide copolymer, and 75/25 L-lactide/glycolide copolymer, respectively. Note that the ratio of the lactide peak heights at 6.85 and the glycolide peak height at 7 can be used to estimate the ratio of L-lactide to glycolide.

The IR spectrum of levonorgestrel is reproduced as Figure 4.

C. Determination of Levonorgestrel Extinction Coefficient in Ethanol

1. Levonorgestrel has a molar extinction coefficient of 16,900 at 242 nm in ethanol. Using Beer's law (shown below), a 2.96×10^{-5} M solution should have an absorbance of 0.5 in a 1-cm cell. The molecular weight of levonorgestrel is 312.44. Prepare a 2.96×10^{-5} M solution of levonorgestrel in absolute ethanol (0.0092 mg/l mℓ) as follows: (1) dissolve 92 mg levonorgestrel in 10 mℓ of ethanol, and (2) dilute 0.025 mℓ of this solution to 25 mℓ in a 25-mℓ volumetric flask.

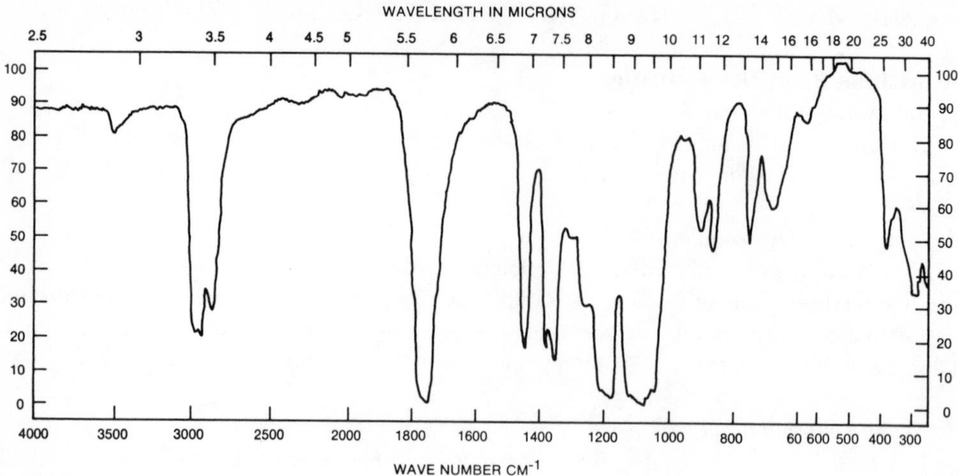

FIGURE 1. IR spectrum of L-lactide homopolymer.

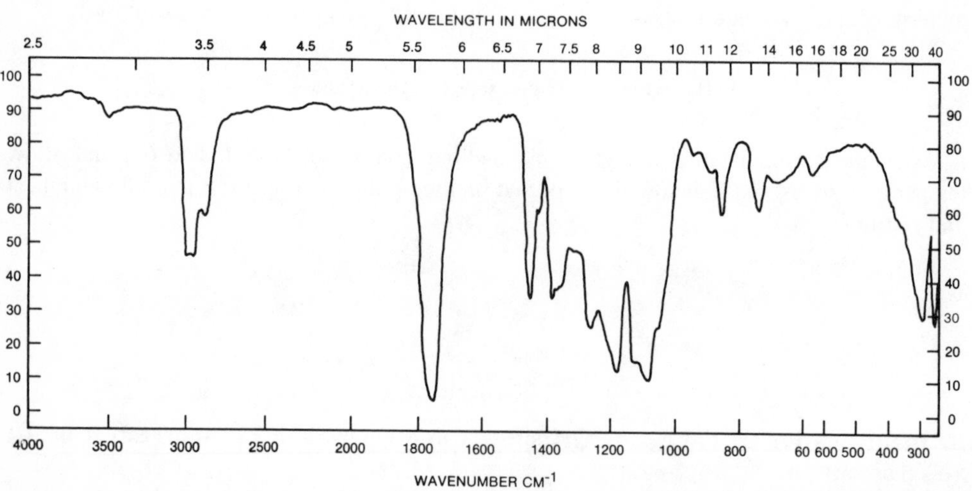

FIGURE 2. IR spectrum of 90/100 L-lactide/glycolide copolymer.

2. Measure the absorbance of this solution at a wavelength of 242 nm using a Perkin-Elmer double-beam spectrophotometer (Coleman 124D) or equivalent. Calculate the mass extinction coefficient ϵ from Beer's law, $A = \epsilon LC$, where A = absorbance; L = path length = 1 cm; C = concentration in mol/ℓ; and $\epsilon = A/LC$ = extinction coefficient.
3. The literature value for ϵ is 16,900 in ethanol. Repeat the determination if the experimental value of ϵ is not within 10% of this value.

D. Determination of Molecular Weight by Gel Permeation Chromatography

1. Equipment

1. Sonicor Ultrasonic Cleaner Model G-580 or equivalent

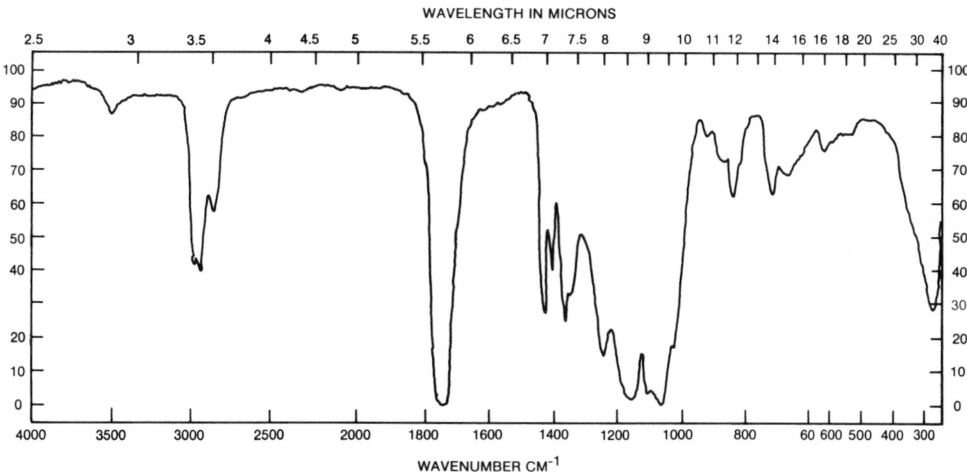

FIGURE 3. IR spectrum of 75/25 L-lactic/glycolide copolymer.

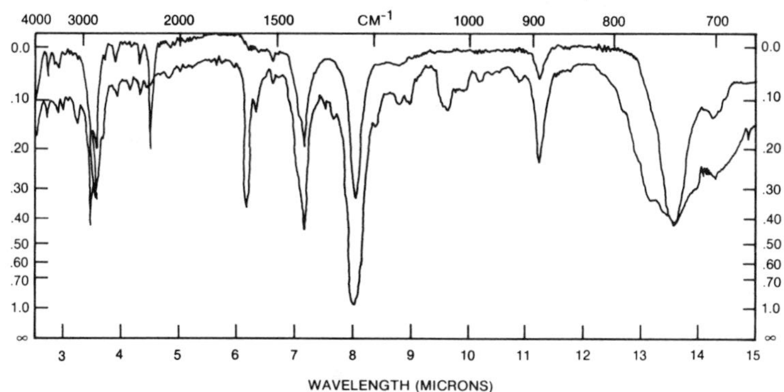

FIGURE 4. IR spectrum of levonorgestrel.

2. Teflon® Millipore® Filters FHLP02500
3. 10-mℓ B & D glass syringe with Luer Lock, Fisher Scientific 14-823-10C or equivalent
4. Millipore® filter holder, Luer inlet XX3002500
5. Hypodermic needles
6. 1-mℓ gas-tight syringe
7. 11-mℓ glass specimen bottles with aluminum foil-lined caps
8. Magnetic stirrer
9. Spectrograde THF (Burdick & Jackson, Muskegon, Mich.) or equivalent
10. Methylene chloride
11. 50-mℓ buret
12. Houston Instrument Omniscribe® Recorder or equivalent
13. Waters® GPC consisting of: Milton Roy® Mini Pump or equivalent; Model 6UK Injector; Model 440 Absorbance Detector UV detector); columns with μm Styragel® packing (as necessary to cover range of interest, such as Water® 10^5, 10^4, 10^3, 500, and 100Å in series); and differential refractometer [refractive index (RI) detector].
14. GPC calibration kit containing eight polystyrene standards: 2.7×10^6; 4.7×10^5; 2×10^5; 1.1×10^5; 3.5×10^4; 1.75×10^4; 3.6×10^3; 2.35×10^3.

2. Calibration of Chromatograph Using Polystyrene Standards

Both direct and indirect methods of calibrating GPC columns have been used to obtain molecular weight averages. With polymers for which narrow molecular weight distribution standards are commercially available (e.g., polystyrene), a direct calibration on the basis of molecular weight can be made. If standards are not commercially available, they must either be prepared or indirect methods (based on, e.g., other known polymers and respective Q factors) used.

Direct method — Prepare fresh calibration standards in the same manner as samples, but use 0.1% concentrations of the polystyrene standards obtained from Waters Associates, Milford, Mass. As many standards as possible should be run in the range of interest. If the sample is totally unknown, it may be necessary to chromatograph it first to determine the estimated range. Be sure each injection point is clearly marked. With the Model U6K Universal Injector this is done automatically. Measure the retention volume or time of each standard from the start of injection to the maximum of the chromatographic peak. Plot this value (on the linear x axis) on semilog paper vs. the corresponding value (on the logarithmic y axis) of the peak molecular weight, peak M (listed on the standard), for each standard. Draw a smooth curve through the points plotted to obtain the calibration curve. (The apparatus should be recalibrated at least yearly, and after any changes of tubing, fittings, filters, columns, etc. in the sample path.)

3. Sample Preparation

Weigh to the nearest 0.1 mg approximately 0.035 g of dry polymer into a new 11-mℓ specimen bottle and dissolve in 10 mℓ of spectrograde THF obtained via the pump draw-off valve. Use foil-lined caps on vials! *Note:* polymer samples must be completely dry. If in any doubt, evacuate sample in a dessicator overnight at 75 mmHg before weighing. If polymer does not dissolve completely right away, heat to boiling. After cooling, add additional THF to maintain the original volume. Record sample weights in the GPC notebook, giving the sample a GPC notebook number and referencing the source of the sample by notebook number and any other information necessary to completely identify the sample.

Clean filter holders and 10-mℓ syringe by placing them in a clean Sonicor for 10 min in fresh methylene chloride. Filter specimen solution through 0.45-μm Millipore® filter into a new 11-mℓ specimen bottle. Mark with sample number.

4. Instrument Start-Up and Operation

The time for start-up and equilibration required to achieve a stable baseline takes 2 to 3 hr, therefore, start flushing the apparatus early in the morning.

The RI detector should be turned on 1 day in advance, and left on between runs, as it requires up to 8 hr to stabilize. Flush, in sequence, the injector sample and bypass loops, for at least 10 min each; flush the RI detector reference cell for at least 15 min; finally, flush the column assembly (through the RI detector sample cell) until a flat baseline is obtained. Repeat flushing sequence to recheck solvent homogeneity.

A few hours before injecting a sample, turn on recorder power and drive, place pens in down position on chart, set chart speed at *10 cm/min* to check for a stable baseline. If baseline is not stable after 60 min, check and retighten valves, and perform other standard troubleshooting techniques.

5. Determining Molecular Weight

Using the 1-mℓ Hamilton syringe, withdraw about 0.7 mℓ of sample, hold with needle upright, and tap barrel with finger so any air present will collect near the opening and expel air and enough sample so volume in syringe is 0.50 mℓ. Flip upper level on injector to ''load'', and flip bottom lever down. Remove pin in injector port, insert syringe needle into injector port, and inject sample. Replace the pin, reset lower lever, and close stopcock on 50-mℓ buret (Figure 1). Set recorder speed to 10 cm/10 min. As soon as the THF reaches the 50-mℓ mark on the buret, flip upper level on injector to "inject". Record date, GPC number, sample number, recorder speed, RI detector attenuation, pump pressure ranges, and any other necessary information on chart. After primary peak has eluted, pressure the "chart marker" button and simultaneously note the THF volume in the buret. Repeat after 1 or 2 more mℓ. Measure the distance on the chart in centimeters from the start of the run to the marks placed on the chart. The flow rate in milliliters per centimeter is the average of the two values of retention volume divided by the distance in centimeters.

When all injections have been made, turn off the stirrer, pump, and Omniscribe® Recorder. *Note:* the Differential refractometer and UV detector are left on at all times, as more than 8 hr warm-up time is required for these instruments.

6. *Computation of Number Average and Weight Average of an Unknown Polymer Sample*

On the chromatogram, mark the retention volumes for the start V_i and finish (V_t) of the polymer of the polymer chromatogram. Draw a linear baseline from before V_i to after V_t. (If the baseline is drawn from V_i to V_t, small rises might be overlooked.)

a. Computation by Hand

Once the baseline has been determined, measure peak heights in centimeters to the nearest 0.5 cm at ±0.5-cm intervals from the peak maxima along the GPC curve until peak height from baseline becomes less than 0.25 cm. Tabulate these data under the headings shown below.

1	2	3	4	5	6
No. of cm from V_i to mark	**Retention volume (mℓ)**	**Height of curve at mark (H)**	**Molecular length at mark A**	**Col 3/col 4**	**Col 3 × col 4**

Note: Col 3 = H = NA; col 5 = NA/A = N; col 6 = NA × A = NA^2.

Determine molecular lengths by reference to calibration curve and Q factors (see below), then list molecular lengths in column four and determine molecular length averages by the following equations:

$$A_N = \Sigma \text{ column } 3/\Sigma \text{ column } 5 = \frac{\Sigma NA}{N}$$

$$A_w = \Sigma \text{ column } 6/\Sigma \text{ column } 3 = \frac{\Sigma NA^2}{NA}$$

The retention volume is related directly to A, the molecular length in angstroms, and the amplitude of the curve is directly related to the length of the molecules present and hence, N, the number of molecules present times their molecular length or NA.

(*Note:* a computer program has been written for the HP-97 calculator. If this is used, only the first and third columns need be recorded in the notebook. The flow rate must also be recorded.)

The calculator will compute and print out the values for columns 2 and 4, and will automatically calculate and store:

Σ heights	Col 3	$= \Sigma NA$
Σ heights/molecular length	Col 5	$= \Sigma N$
Σ heights × molecular length	Col 6	$= \Sigma NA_2$

The calculator will then determine and print out $\overline{M}_n$, $\overline{M}_w$, and $D = \overline{M}_w, \overline{M}_n$, in that order. If the factor Q for a given polymer is known, the actual molecular lengths can be calculated:

$$\overline{A}_n = \overline{M}_n/Q$$

$$\overline{A}_w = \overline{A}_w/Q$$

The following Q values can be used:

	Q in g/Å
Polystyrene	41.4
Polylactic acid	45

A program has been written to calculate $\overline{M}_n$ and $\overline{M}_w$ for polystyrene only. This is usually used for polylactic acid polymers and copolymers since the error is only about 10%. [$\overline{M}_x$ (for polylactic acid) $=$ $\overline{M}_s$ (as calculated for polystyrene) $\times$ $\frac{Q_{\text{Polylactic acid}}}{Q_{\text{Polystyrene}}}$].

(Assuming use of polystyrene program card.)

b. Procedure for Using Calculator

1. Turn on calculator and set switches at "run" and "norm".
2. Load program from magnetic card.
3. For each chromatogram, do the following: punch D to load registers with constants; store flow rate in register 8 (units mℓ/cm); load distance to first point in centimeters and punch "enter", load value for corresponding peak height in centimeters and punch "A"; wait for calculator to finish calculation and enter the rest of the data pairs; when all pairs have been entered punch "C" to calculate and print out $\overline{M}_n$, $\overline{M}_w$, and D.

E. Determination of Percent Lactide in L-Lactide/Glycolide Copolymers by Polarimetry

1. Equipment

Model 51 Visual Polarimeter (Rudolph Instruments Engineering Co.) or equivalent.

*2. Procedure**

1. Turn lamp on.
2. Loosen thumb screw no. 1 and rotate lamp until lamp aperature is in alignment with the optic axis of the polarimeter. Tighten thumb screw no. 1 so that the lamp cannot turn.
3. Remove any sample cells that may be in the trough of the polarimeter.
4. Look into the telescope eyepiece and bring the fine dividing line of the circular half-shade image field into sharp focus by slowly sliding the eyepiece in and out, using a turning motion.
5. Loosen thumb screws no. 2 and slide lamp and lamp mounting plate laterally so that the lamp axis and optic axis intersect to obtain maximum uniform image field brightness. Tighten the two thumb screws no. 2 so that lamp cannot move laterally.

* Refer to Figure 5 to identify capitalized items.

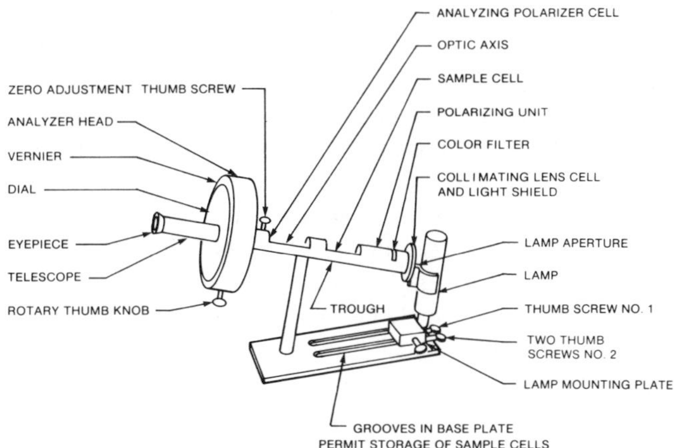

FIGURE 5. Rudolph Model 51 Visual Polarimeter.

6. Turn rotary thumb knob thereby simultaneously turning Vernier and analyzing polarizer, until the half-shade image field is "matched" or has equal brightness in both halves. Since a 180° rotation of the analyzing polarizer yields three actual matchpoints, two of high brightness and one of low brightness, care must be taken to select the match point of low brightness since this is the more sensitive one and the one which will yield settings of 0.05° reproducibility.
7. Read the analyzer dial and note the angular degree setting to the nearest 0.05°, using the conventional Vernier method.
8. Repeat steps 6 and 7 at least three times and average these readings. If the average is 0.00°, no zero adjustment is necessary. If the average is not 0.00°, one may use the average value obtained as the nominal blank value of the instrument and make the appropriate correction by either adding or subtracting this nominal "blank value" to or from the optical rotation values measured, or one may take a physical zero adjustment of the analyzing polarizer.
9. Zero adjustment is made by rotating the analyzing polarizer cell in its mounting, thereby changing the azimuth position of the analyzing polarizer with respect to the Vernier. Ordinarily only a very slight adjustment is necessary since all these polarimeters are factory adjusted to give a 0.00° reading with the empty or "blank" instrument. To loosen the polarizing analyzer cell for this purpose, loosen zero adjustment thumb screw and rotate it counterclockwise until the analyzing polarizer cell may be freely turned by light finger tip pressure on its knurled edge. Now turn the rotary thumb knob until the Vernier indicates exactly 0.00° on the dial. Next look into the telescope eyepiece and turn the analyzing polarizer cell until the low brightness match point is obtained, and tighten the zero adjust thumb screw by turning it clockwise, thereby locking the analyzing polarizer cell so that it cannot turn in its mounting.
10. Repeat steps 6 through 9 as often as necessary to obtain a satisfactory "blank" reading.

3. Operation

1. Turn light on and perform steps 6 to 8 of the calibration procedure to make sure that the correct "blank value" is obtained (i.e., 0.00° or the nominal "blank value" if the zero was not adjusted when the instrument was calibrated). If in doubt, repeat entire calibration procedure.
2. Fill a sample cell with methylene chloride, insert in the trough, and slide it down against the polarizing unit. Be sure that there is no bubble large enough to block the

light path inside the sample cell. It may now be necessary to refocus the telescope eyepiece in order to hold the half-shade image field in sharp focus. Also, it may be necessary to wait until the liquid in the sample cell becomes "homogeneous" or of uniform refractive index. This may require 5 to 10 min, depending on the viscosity, in case of thermal gradients or nonuniform solute concentrations.

3. Repeat steps 6 to 8 of the calibration procedure. There may be a slight difference in readings obtained with the empty instrument and with the optically inactive solvent-filled sample cell. However, readings must remain constant as the sample cell is rotated in the trough, either end for end or about the optic axis. If there is appreciable change due to such rotation, the sample cell windows probably contain stress birefringence which may be caused by tightening the sample cell screw caps too tightly or which may be inherent in the glass of the windows. If the former is the case, simply loosening the screw caps will correct this condition. If the latter is the case, the sample cell windows must be discarded and must be replaced by "optically homogeneous" ones.
4. Repeat steps 2 and 3 with a 2.0% w/v solution of the copolymer in methylene chloride in the sample cell. The difference in readings obtained with the "blank" and with the "sample" is the "optical rotation" or "optical rotary power" of the sample in angular degrees.

4. Calculation

$$[\propto]_{D}^{25} = \frac{RV}{NL}$$

where R = observed rotation in degrees; N = grams of substance in V milliliters of solvent; and L = length of sample cell in decimeters.

Using a 2-dm cell, the specific rotation of a 2% w/v solution of L-lactide homopolymer is − 160° in benzene. Therefore:

$$\text{Mole \% L-lactide} = \frac{[\propto]\text{ sample} \times 100}{[\propto]\text{ L-lactide pol}} = \frac{[\propto]\text{S} \times 100}{-160}$$

F. Final Product Storage

All vials of product shall be placed in sealed bags and stored at 0 to − 20°C until needed. Location of the vials shall be recorded on the "Reservation of Active Ingredient and Final Product" form. When any vials are distributed, a product distribution record shall be completed.

G. Measuring Refractive Index of Liquids

1. Equipment

Refractometer (Fisher Scientific Cat. No. 13-947) or equivalent.

2. Calibration Procedure

Note: calibrate the refractometer prior to initial use, after the prism is replaced, or if the eyepiece is moved for any reason by using the following procedure.

1. Pivot nameplate of instrument to one side and remove prism from felt-lined storage recess.
2. Carefully clean the prism and the glass plate of eyepiece with a Kimwipe®. If necessary, wet Kimwipe® with distilled water, or any readily volatile solvent.
3. Place prism on eyepiece under the spring clamp so that the beveled edge of prism forms a V-shaped well with the lower edge of the bevel bisecting the small hole behind the permanently mounted glass plate.

4. Place some distilled water in the prism well. Distilled water has a refractive index of 1.333 at 22 ± 2°C.
5. Loosen setscrew that holds eyepiece in position, and move eyepiece in or out until correct reading is obtained. Then tighten setscrew without moving eyepiece.
6. If planning to make determinations, proceed to step 2 under Operation section; otherwise clean prism and glass plate of eyepiece, then return prism to storage recess.

3. Operation

1. If making a determination following initial installation or shutdown, perform steps 1 through 5 of calibration procedure (above).
2. Make sure temperature of instrument is 22 ± 2°C. Carefully clean prism and glass plate with a Kimwipe®. If necessary, wet Kimwipe® with distilled water or any readily volatile solvent.
3. Place prism on eyepiece under spring clamp so that the beveled edge of the prism forms a V-shaped well with a lower edge of the bevel bisecting the small hole behind the permanently mounted glass plate.
4. Place a small amount of sample liquid into the V-shaped well, such that liquid is drawn into the apex to form a liquid prism.
5. Depress light switch at back of instrument and take index reading. *Note:* for substances having low dispersion, the virtual image seen is a white image as narrow as the slit itself. For substances having appreciable dispersive powers, the image obtained is not a line image, but rather a multicolored band. The scale of the instrument has been so constructed that the reading of the yellow portion of the spectral band formed indicates the refractive index of the medium. this yellow portion is generally sharply defined as the narrow region between the brillant red and green portions of the image.
6. Repeat steps 2 through 5 for remaining samples.
7. Clean prism and glass plate of eyepiece as directed by step 2, then replace prism in felt-lined recess underneath nameplate.

4. Refractive Index of Various Solvents at 22 ± 2°C

Acetone	1.350
Anhydrous methanol	1.329
Anhydrous isopropanol	1.378
Dioxane	1.423
Methylene chloride	1.424
THF	1.408
Nitromethane	1.380

H. Determination of Residual Solvent in Polymers and Polymer/Drug Matrices

1. Equipment

1. 250-mℓ Short Neck Flat Bottom Flask 24/40 (SGA F-9124 or equivalent)
2. Adapter Straight Nose Connector 24/40 (SGA A3030 or equivalent)
3. 250-mℓ gas sampling tubes
4. Rubber septums
5. Gow Mac Model 750 gas chromatograph (GC) with flame ionization detector or equivalent
6. 10 × 1/8 in. diameter 5% SE-30 or 80/100 Chron W. Column for Gow Mac Model 750 GC (Applied Science Labs, State College, Pa.) or equivalent
7. 10-μℓ syringe
8. 1- and 10-mℓ gas-tight syringes

2. Volume Calibration of 250-mℓ Flasks and Adapters

Assemble the flask and adapter and measure the volume to the nearest milliliter by filling the water and pouring the contents into a graduated cylinder.

3. Procedure — Residual Solvent

Weigh 0.1 g of sample to the nearest 0.1 mg, place in a clean, dry 250-mℓ flask of known volume (determined as above), and purge for 1 min with a stream of nitrogen. Attach the volume-calibrated adapter. With stopcock open, evacuate the flask to about 10 Torr and close the stopcock. Decompose the polymer and drive any residual solvent into the vapor phase by heating the flask at 150°C for 1 hr in an oven. Allow the flask to cool, and backfill with nitrogen. Close the stopcock and place a rubber septum over the adapter outlet.

Prepare 10,000- and 100-ppm standards as follows.

4. Preparation of 10,000- and 100-ppm Standards

Clean two 250-mℓ gas sampling tubes. Rinse thoroughly with distilled H_2O and finally with acetone. Place in 60°C oven to dry for several hours. Remove from oven, allow to cool, and flush each sampling tube for several minutes with a moderate N_2 flow. Evacuate each tube and backfill with N_2. The tubes are now ready for use in standards preparation.

a. 10,000-ppm Standard

A measured amount of solvent corresponding to 10,000 ppm is injected with a 10-μℓ syringe into one of the 250-mℓ gas sampling tubes through the rubber septum. The amount of solvent needed is calculated through the use of the following equations:

1. Amount of vapor required for 10,000 ppm $\approx 10^4/10^6 \times 250$ mℓ $= 2.5$ mℓ $= 2.5 \times 10^3$ μℓ of vapor.
2. # mℓ of vapor contained in 1 mol at 20°C $= 22{,}400$ mℓ/mol $\times 293/273 = 24{,}041 \times 10^3$ mℓ/mol at 20°C.
3. # μℓ of CH_2Cl_2 needed for 10,000 ppm $= 84$ g/mol mol wt $\times$ 1 mℓ/1.33 g solvent density $\times 2.5 \times 10^3$ μℓ/24.041 $\times 10^3$ mℓ/mol $= 6.4$ μℓ of CH_2Cl_2 required for 10,000 ppm.

b. 100-ppm Standard

From the 10,000-ppm standard 2.5 μℓ of vapor is quantitatively transferred with a gas-tight syringe through the rubber septum to the second 250-mℓ gas sampling tube filled with N_2. The 100-fold dilution of 10,000-ppm standard forms a 100-ppm standard.

Inject a 0.5-mℓ sample taken from the flask containing the polymer into the GC by opening the adapter stopcock and inserting the needle of the 1-mℓ syringe through the septum and stopcock into the flask. The syringe plunger should be pulled out to 1 mℓ and depressed to 0 several times before taking the sample. Withdraw an excess for a count of 10, depress to 0.5 mℓ and then inject into the GC. Repeat injections until three similar peak heights have been obtained. Repeat the injection sequence, obtaining three peaks of similar height for the 100- and 10,000-ppm standards.

Approximate GC operating parameters for analysis of THF, dioxane, benzene, and methylene chloride:

Gas flow

H_2	65
Air	45
N_2	2

Temperature (°C)

Port	164
Column	104

Calculations are as follows:

$$\%\ \text{solvent in polymer} = \frac{\dfrac{\text{peak height of sample*}}{\text{peak height of sample*}} \times \dfrac{\text{weight of solvent in standard}}{250\ \text{m}\ell} \times \text{vol (m}\ell\text{) of flask and adapter}}{\text{sample weight}} \times 100$$

* Corrected for attenuation

A sample calculation follows:

$$\%\ CH_2Cl_2\ \text{in polymer} = \frac{\dfrac{15.9\ \text{cm}}{8.5\ \text{cm}} \times \dfrac{8.5\ \text{mg}}{250\ \text{m}\ell} \times 270\ \text{m}\ell}{765.3\ \text{mg}} \times 100 = 2.24\%$$

I. Assay for Levonorgestrel Weight Percent in Polymer Matrix

1. Grind about 200 mg of levonorgestrel polymer matrix preparation with a mortar and pestle until particles are <200 μm in size. Reflux the powder in 10 mℓ of absolute ethanol for 8 hr. Cool the solution and vacuum filter it through Whatman® #42 filter paper to remove matrix particles. Dilute 0.01 mℓ of filtered solution to 10 mℓ in a volumetric flask.
2. Repeat with 130 mg of levonorgestrel (final concentration will be 4.2×10^{-5} m).
3. Measure and record the absorbances (A) of these solutions at 242 nm in a cuvette with 1-cm path length using a Perkin-Elmer double-beam spectrophotometer (Coleman 124D) or equivalent.
4. Find ϵ, the refluxed levonorgestrel sample, using Beer's law: $\epsilon = A/cL$ = extinction coefficient (Beer's law); A = absorbance; L = path length = 1 cm; C = concentration of drug [=] moles/liter.
5. Using ϵ from part 4 and Beer's law, find the concentration (C) of levonorgestrel in the levonorgestrel/polymer extract.
6. Find the weight percent of levonorgestrel in the polymer matrix using the concentration found in above.
   a. The concentration found in 5 above is the number of moles in a liter. The number of moles in the 10-mℓ sample is C × 0.01 ℓ. This solution is a 1000-fold dilution from the initial refluxed solution so the number of moles in the 200-mg levonorgestrel/polymer sample is C × 0.01 ℓ × 1000.
   b. The molecular weight of levonorgestrel is 312.44. Find the weight of levonorgestrel in the 200-mg levonorgestrel/polymer sample by multiplying the number of moles formation part (A) by the molecular weight, i.e., # mol × 312.44 g/mol = weight of levonorgestrel in cooling matrix.
   c. Find the weight percent by dividing the answer from part (b) (weight of levonorgestrel in the 200-mg matrix sample in milligrams) by 200 mg, i.e., mg levonorgestrel per 200 mg = weight percent of levonorgestrel.

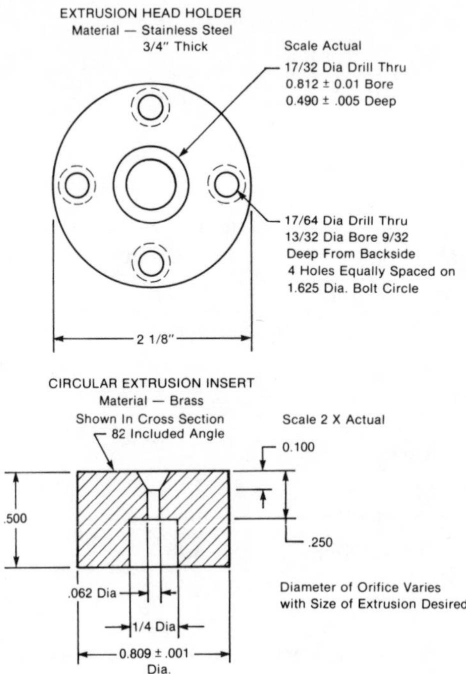

FIGURE 6. Extrusion head holder.

J. Extrusion of Rods

1. Apparatus

1. Hydraulic Press (3 × 8 in. platens, 4 in. ram with 20 in. daylight between platens with 0- to 200-psi auxiliary gauge and 10-in.^{3} capacity hydraulic accumulator Parket Hannifin model A2A0010A1K connected to compressed nitrogen cylinder equipped with gas pressure regulator or equivalent
2. Variable voltage source (VVS)
3. Thermocouples with digital temperature readout
4. Extruder support — channel iron $1^1/_2$ × 10-in. long, squared ends
5. Extruder — see Figures 6 to 9
6. Band heater — Chromalox Model HBZ 12224 circular band heater
7. O-rings — Parker sizes 2-012 and 2-016 or equivalent, silicone rubber
8. Silicone Rubber Harness 70 Shore A
9. Ultrasonic cleaner filled with methylene chloride

2. Procedure

1. Assemble extruder with extrusion insert of desired size, with mold extension (Figure 9) if needed, with size 2-016 O-ring in place and thermocouple inserted in thermocouple well in extrusion cylinder. Load 1 + g of casting into extruder and insert piston fitted with size 2-012 O-ring into extruder end toward polymer. Slip heater around extruder and adjust so band is flush with face of the extrusion head holder.
2. Connect thermocouple to digital readout.
3. Connect a full cylinder of nitrogen to pressurize the accumulator on the press as shown in Figure 10.
4. Make sure that the 2-in. diameter cylinder in the accumulator in the press is at the top. This is done by closing the press by hand pumping with the valves on the press

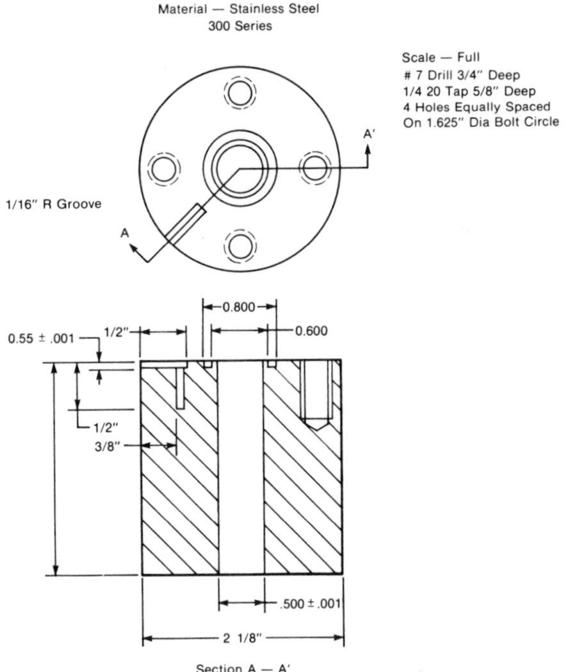

FIGURE 7. Material — stainless steel, 300 series.

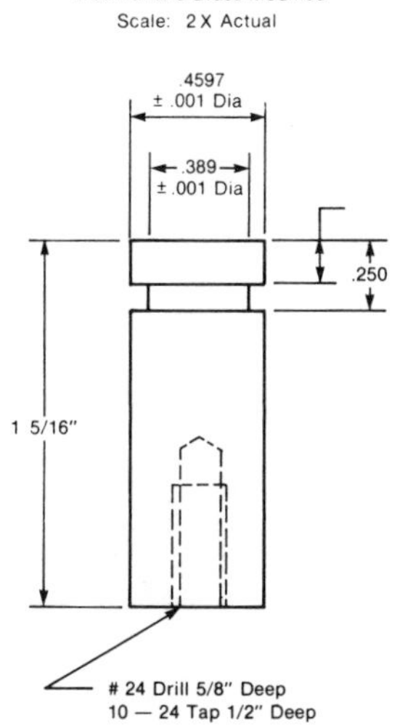

FIGURE 8. Piston.

leading to the auxiliary gauge and to the accumulator in the open position with the accumulator needle valve in the open (down) position with the line valve open and with the main bleed valve next to this valve open. Pump until the press holds 100 psi pressure on the auxiliary pressure gauge. Drop the lower press platen by opening the main valve in the pump hydraulic system, and mount the extruder in the press with the channel iron beneath it and the extrusion head holder pointed downwards (see

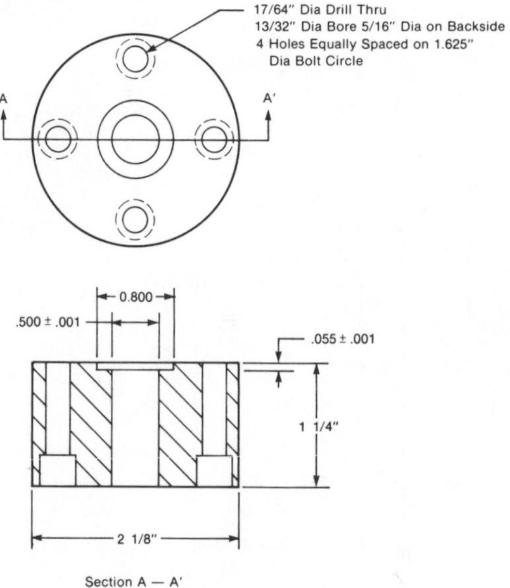

FIGURE 9. Mold cylinder extension.

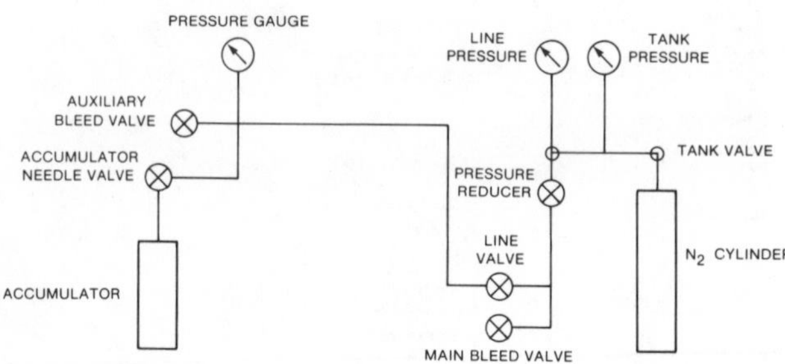

FIGURE 10. Schematic drawing of extrusion system.

Figure 11). Close the press by hand, pumping until the auxiliary pressure gauge on the press reads 20 psi. This will set the piston and hold the mold in position.

5. Set appropriate voltage for extrusion temperature on variable voltage source (VVS).
6. Move the switch on the VVS to the ''on'' position and when the extrusion temperature is reached as read by the thermocouple in the thermocouple well in the extrusion cylinder, reduce voltage by 5 to 10 V, close the main bleed valve, open the tank valve on the nitrogen tank with the pressure regulator preset at extrusion pressure (see note 2), and allow material to extrude. (Line valve should still be ''open''.) Recover polymer rod as it extrudes; pulling with tweezers to keep the rod as straight as possible. (See Figure 11.) If the rod extrudes too fast, open the auxiliary bleed valve slightly and remember to adjust pressure reducer to lower pressure for next run. When extrusion is completed, *close tank valve*. If necessary to drop press platens, *open main valve* in press hydraulic system.

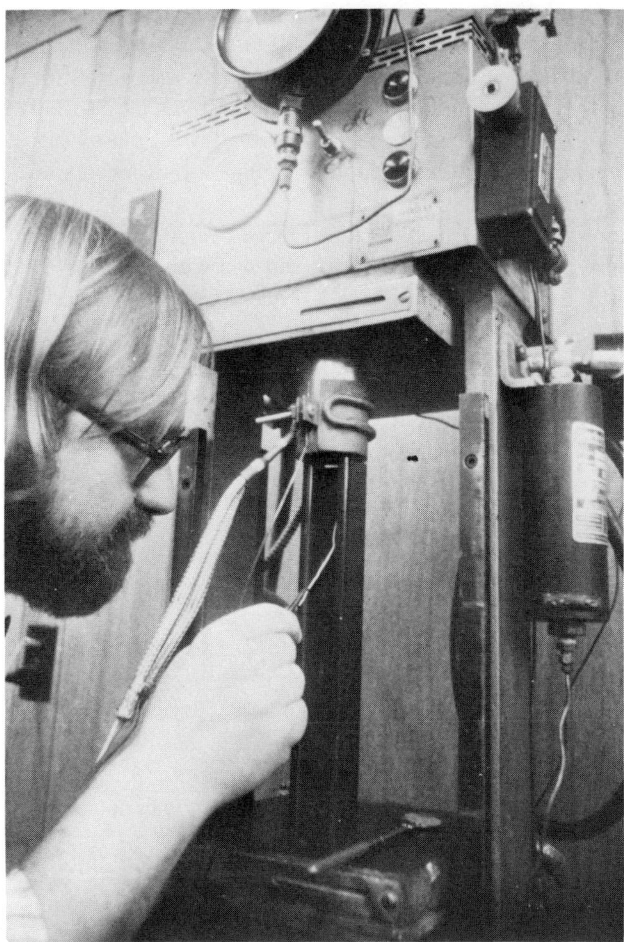

FIGURE 11. Typical set-up for extruding rods of levonorgestrel-loaded polymers.

3. Notes

1. If extrusion temperature is not known, select an estimated temperature. If the rod does not extrude at this temperature at a pressure of up to 200 psig on the auxiliary gauge, raise the voltage on VVS enough to raise temperature until extrusion occurs. Record the temperatures and VVS settings for future reference. If the extruded rod appears to be too soft and flexible, lower the VVS setting. Clean out the extruder and make another run starting with a cold extruder using the new setting.
2. To adjust pressure, *close* line valve and *main bleed valve*. Open tank valve and adjust *pressure reducer* to give desired line pressure. For example, if the desired extrusion pressure is 150 psig on the auxiliary gauge, the pressure regulator should be set to give a line pressure of about 600 psig. *Open* and *close main bleed valve* and check *line* pressure. Gauge should still read desired pressure. If not, adjust *pressure reducer* accordingly. If the *line pressure* climbs after opening and closing main bleed valve, the pressure reducer leaks and should be replaced.

To remove ristor from mold, remove heater and extrusion head holder. Support the inverted assembly on channel iron and press the plunger out using an appropriate push rod. Clean out residual polymer. Finally clean in methylene chloride using Sonicor.

K. Blending and Casting Levonorgestrel Base with Polymer

Dissolve poly [L(+)-lactic-co-glycolic acid](PLGA) in methylene chloride in a jar with a tight cover and polyethylene film liner to the appropriate viscosity. Roll the container until all the polymer has gone into solution. Pressure filter through a 0.5-μm Teflon® Millipore® filter into a second clean jar containing ~1/3 vol of ~1/4-in. glass beads and ~1 dozen 1/2-in. diameter porcelain rolls. Add the appropriate amount of levonorgestrel, and ball mill polymer and drug overnight.

Cast this solution directly onto a clean, level piece of flat plate glass, spread the solution to a thickness of not over 0.625 mm (25 mil), and wet with a Boston-Bradley® Adjustable Blade. Peel the drug films from the plate glass, and vacuum dessicate.

L. Radiation Sterilization

The rods are sterilized after they are sealed in labeled vials. The sealed vials are placed in cartons labeled with the product label and shipped to:

Radiated Products, LTD.
Moray Road
Eligrin Industrial Estate
Swindon, Wiltshire SN2-6DU
ENGLAND

A random sampling of the sterilized vials is shipped to North American Sciences Associates, Toledo, Ohio for bioburden testing. A copy of their report is to be attached to the final product assay report.

M. Final Product Assay Report

This report will certify the levonorgestrel content, polymer molecular weight, residual solvent content, and sterility of the final product.

Testing will be performed as soon as practicable after sterilization. The levonorgestrel content and polymer molecular weight will be remeasured after 6 months.

III. MASTER FORMULA RECORD

A. Description of Product

The final product is a sealed, radiation-treated vial containing 4 rods with a total length of 14.0 ± 0.5 cm. The rod composition is 50% levonorgestrel and 50% polymer (w/w). The polymer is 75:25 lactic/glycolic acids, copolymerized.

B. Weight of Active Ingredient per Dosage Unit

The amount of active ingredient (levonorgestrel) in each vial is 100 ± 5 mg.

C. Component Register

Ingredient	Reference no.	Amount	Accepted by	Date
Levonorgestrel				
75:25 PLGA				
Methylene chloride				
Packaging material				

IV. SUMMARY

One practical aspect in any medical research and development project that has ultimate application to use by humans is that of preparing the material according to good manufacturing practices (GMP). Often the details of this work are overlooked by the research worker. In the area of sustained release, a number of other factors involving the polymer, release rate, mechanism of release, etc. are discussed; only late in a project is attention given to GMP documentation. This chapter is presented as a guide to those who will be preparing GMP documentation.

ACKNOWLEDGMENTS

This material was prepared as part of a project with the Program for Applied Research on Fertility Regulation (PARFR), Chicago, Ill. Our appreciation for support is extended to Gerald I. Zatuchni, M.D., Medical Director.

Alcoholism

Chapter 4

TREATMENT OF ALCOHOLISM WITH SUSTAINED RELEASE DISULFIRAM IMPLANTS

Michael Phillips

Anyone involved in the treatment of alcoholic patients soon encounters a fundamental schism that splits therapists into two camps: it hinges on whether one believes alcoholism to be a disease (like diabetes or pneumonia) or a bad habit (like cheating at cards or spitting on the floor).

Those who embrace the disease concept tend to regard alcoholism as a legitimate subject of biomedical research, with the implicit assumption that, like diabetes or pneumonia, it is a condition with a definite etiology and pathogenesis. Hence it follows that as the disease is better understood, it should be possible to design a rational plan of drug treatment.

There are many who do not accept this so-called "medical model" of alcoholism. In their view, alcoholism is not so much a disease but a bad habit, best treated by education, persuasion, and moral uplift. Extreme adherents to this view see no role for drug therapy in alcoholism, regarding it as irrelevant at best and pernicious at worst.

It is not my intention, in this short paper, to resolve a controversy which has raged for more than a century. I suspect, like many other issues which have generated vehemently polarized and conflicting opinions, the truth lies somewhere between the two extremes.

Whatever the truth may be, it could well be another hundred years or more before we know it. In the meantime, physicians are confronted with the immediate daily reality of having to cope with the pressing problem of treating patients suffering miserably from their alcoholism.

One immediate and attractive approach is the use of drugs for the treatment of alcoholism. Ideally, a drug should treat the underlying cause of a disease rather than its symptoms. For instance, patients with pneumonia often suffer with a painful cough which, even a hundred years ago, could be treated effectively with narcotic cough suppressants. However, it was not until the invention of penicillin that the underlying cause of the cough — the bacteria multiplying in the lungs — could be effectively treated. We are in a roughly analogous position with alcoholism: we do not really know the underlying causes of the disease, but we have a very powerful drug to block the major symptom, the drinking of alcohol.

Disulfiram has been used in industry for many years in the vulcanization of rubber. However, its medical role was not suspected until 1948, when it was discovered by a curious accident. Two Danish researchers — Hald and Jacobsen — were looking for a new treatment for intestinal parasitic infections. They knew, from laboratory studies, that the helminthic parasites required divalent cations in order to grow. This led them to an ingenious hypothesis: what if they treated the infected patient with a drug that could "mop up" divalent cations in the intestinal lumen? Would this perhaps starve the helminths of a vital nutrient and kill them?

After reviewing the known in vitro properties of several chemical compounds, Hald and Jacobsen selected disulfiram as a substance which appeared to fit their requirements because of its demonstrated capacity to avidly chelate divalent cations such as zinc and copper.

Drug research, in those days, was not inhibited by the governmental and institutional regulations that we enjoy today. The only limitation upon researchers, before entering into a clinical trial of a drug, was their ethical commitment to make sure that the drug was not toxic to humans.

Hald and Jacobsen approached this problem head on by testing the drug upon themselves. Each took a large dose orally, and after observing no apparent ill effects they went out for dinner. In Copenhagen, meals are frequently accompanied by Aqua Vite, a national beverage celebrated for its flavor and high alcohol content. The two researchers drank a toast to the promising progress of their endeavors, and shortly afterwards they entered medical history as each was gripped by what we now recognize as a disulfiram-ethanol reaction — facial flushing, a rapid heart beat and respiration, followed by a sensation of nausea, progressing to vomiting.

They immediately recognized the potential clinical application of their discovery, and performed a study under controlled laboratory conditions.[1] They recruited a group of normal volunteers and dosed them with 1.0 to 1.5 g of disulfiram. The next day, they challenged them with a dose of 10 to 20 g of ethanol. All of their subjects experienced a similar disulfiram-ethanol reaction (DER). At the same time, they noted a pungent smell of acetaldehyde on the breath.

This suggested that accumulation of acetaldehyde in the blood might be responsible for the DER. Their colleague Asmussen[2] tested this hypothesis by infusing a solution of acetaldehyde into normal volunteers by intravenous injection. Since it is highly unlikely that any human experimentation committee in the U.S. would approve such a study today, we are fortunate that Asmussen recorded his findings so well. In fact, he virtually duplicated all the symptoms and clinical signs that Hald and Jacobsen observed during the DER, confirming that acetaldehyde was the responsible agent.

During the past 30 years, these findings have been confirmed many times over in different laboratories.[3,4] The most widely accepted explanation is that disulfiram blocks the normal metabolic breakdown of alcohol in the liver:

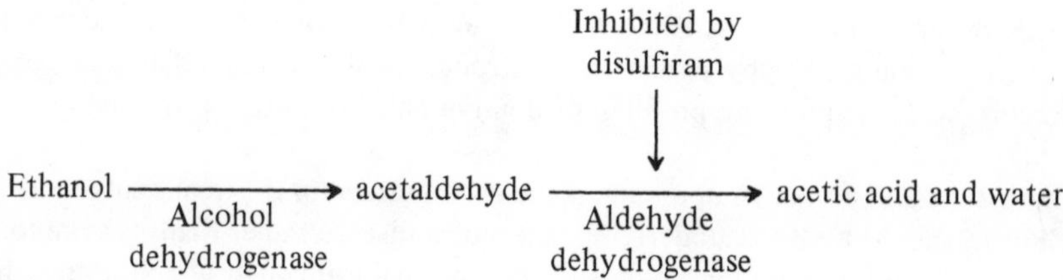

This scheme suggests that disulfiram inhibits the oxidation of acetaldehyde in the liver, resulting in an accumulation of acetaldehyde in the body. Aldehyde dehydrogenase is a heterogeneous enzyme occurring in the hepatic mitochondria, microsomes, and cytosol. Numerous studies have demonstrated that disulfiram inhibits this enzyme in vitro.[4] The process is one of noncompetitive inhibition, irreversibly inactivating the enzyme by a disulfide interchange reaction with essential thiol groups.[5]

The announcement of these findings generated considerable enthusiasm and optimism. Some went so far as to hail disulfiram as "the cure for alcoholism". Sadly, this was not the case. Physicians soon discovered that though disulfiram was an extremely potent agent, it suffered from one major limitation: the willingness of the patient to keep on taking the drug. It became apparent that many patients decided, on their own volition, to discontinue their daily disulfiram tablet, and resume drinking as soon as the effects wore off. The situation was further complicated by the difficulty of determining whether or not the patient was taking disulfiram, since there was no clinically useful assay for measuring drug levels in the blood.

In the early 1950s, this problem led a French physician, Marie, to advocate a new approach to the problem — surgical implantation of disulfiram under the skin. At operation, under general anesthetic, he implanted 1 g of sterile disulfiram under the skin of the abdomen of chronic alcoholics. He reasoned that the drug would be slowly absorbed from the depot site, thus effectively treating the patient for several months.[6]

It has taken the passage of nearly 30 years to learn that this approach does not work. The problem is that the disulfiram is mobilized extremely poorly (if at all) from the implant site. The implant is often "rejected" as a foreign body — it may become surrounded by fibrous tissue and "walled off" from the circulation. In some cases, extrusion through the skin has been observed. It seems highly unlikely that sufficient quantities of disulfiram were ever mobilized from the implant to generate a pharmacologic effect.[6]

If the disulfiram implant merely sits under the skin as an inert lump, why has implantation been so popular for so many years? I suspect there are a number of factors at work. First, the implanted drug has an extremely powerful placebo effect. Patients can roll the tablets between finger and thumb, feeling them through the skin, to constantly remind themselves that "something" is there in their body to stop them drinking. This has a tremendous psychological impact; some patients have requested repeated implants to bolster their resolve to abstain. Another aspect of the placebo effect is that many patients with disulfiram implants have claimed to feel severely uncomfortable after drinking alcohol. However, controlled drinking studies in a laboratory setting have failed to reproduce the classic disulfiram-ethanol reaction in implant patients. Nonetheless, faith and expectation have led many patients (and their physicians) to believe that the implants really work, despite the lack of any objective supporting evidence.

Second, studies with disulfiram implants have been plagued with methodological difficulties: the drop-out rate of alcoholics (often more than 50%), the near impossibility of measuring serum levels of disulfiram or its metabolites, and finally, poor experimental design (most studies have lacked a placebo treatment control group). In one study performed with placebo-treated controls, the evidence for a real clinical effect of the disulfiram implants was not convincing.[7]

In the face of all this negative information, has not the time finally arrived to completely abandon the practice of disulfiram implantation?

I suggest the answer to this is both yes and no.

It is certainly time to abandon the practice of subcutaneous implantation of plain tablets of sterile disulfiram. Though this practice lives on among a few sturdy enthusiasts (mainly in Western Europe and Scandinavia), there is really little convincing evidence that it is anything more than an "active placebo".

But what if we could improve the implant so that it really worked pharmacologically? We might finally realize Marie's dream — that with one single procedure, a patient might be truly protected from alcohol for a period of weeks or months. However, this requires that the drug be delivered into the circulation at a predictable rate for a prolonged period.

I believe that the technology is now available to achieve this objective. However, I must enter a caveat that much of what follows is speculation and fantasy, not yet supported by experimental data.

Disulfiram taken by mouth is a pharmacologically effective drug; nobody disputes this. However, in order for an implant to be pharmacologically effective, a drug delivery system is required which will regulate the rate of release of drug into the circulation.

Such a delivery system is now available in the form of a biodegradable polymer of polylactic-glycolic acid (PLGA). PLGA provides a matrix from which a bound drug may be released into the circulation, as the polymer breaks down in the body. Used initially as a biodegradable material for absorbable surgical sutures, there is now good evidence from animal studies that PLGA implants can deliver drugs into the circulation at a steady rate for a period of several weeks or months.

Funded by a grant from the National Institute on Alcohol Abuse and Alcoholism, and working in conjunction with Dynatech R/D Company, Cambridge, Mass., the author is currently investigating the possibility of developing a PLGA/disulfiram combination, with the specific objective of using it in the treatment of alcoholic humans.

Where all this will lead is still too early to say. Treatment of alcoholism is still an empirical, frustrating activity, often ending in failure. Since nothing much seems to work clinically, it is tempting to hope that sustained release pharmacotherapy offers some potential assistance for alcoholics. One might consider the daily life of an alcoholic as being a series of decisions: shall I or shall I not take a drink right now? He or she faces this question several times a day. The advent of oral disulfiram reduced this to one decision a day (resolved by taking or not taking the pill). An effective implant might extend this time period to one decision every 3 or more months. Thus an alcoholic might build a ''chemical wall'' around himself, effectively making alcohol consumption impossible for long periods.

Even if such a treatment could be developed, it raises a series of fascinating questions. How will patients respond to such treatment? Will it truly have any impact on their life and work and happiness? Would it have any effect on their desire for alcohol? Might not life without alcohol become intolerably depressing for some? Or could this drug provide a new beginning, a way to lead an alcohol-free life for the first time in years?

Researchers tend to be enthusiastic about new technology, and it is sometimes easy to overlook the human implications of one's work. Sustained release pharmacotherapy is a dazzling new technology with awesome potential for modifying and controlling human behavior. The major question now facing researchers in this infant field: Can it be made to work on humans?

I suggest that this is not enough; we should never forget to add: And if it works, is this treatment in the patient's best interests?

REFERENCES

1. **Hald, J. and Jacobsen, E.,** A drug sensitizing the organism to ethyl alcohol, *Lancet,* 2, 1001, 1948.
2. **Asmussen, E., Hald, J., and Larsen, V.,** The pharmacological action of acetaldehyde in the human organism, *Acta Pharmacol. Toxicol.,* 4, 311, 1948.
3. **Lundwall, L., et al.,** Disulfiram treatment of alcohol: a review, *J. Nerv. Ment. Dis.,* 158, 381, 1971.
4. **Kitson, T. M.,** The disulfiram-ethanol reaction, *J. Stud. Alcohol,* 30, 96, 1977.
5. **Deitrich, R. A.,** Diphosphopyridine nucleotide-linked aldehyde dehydrogenase. III. Sulfhydryl characteristics of the enzyme, *Arch. Biochem. Biophys.,* 119, 253, 1957.
6. **Kitson, T. M.,** On the probability of implanted disulfiram's causing a reaction to ethanol, *J. Stud. Alcohol,* 39, 183, 1978.
7. **Kline, S. A. and Kingstone, E.,** Disulfiram implants: the right treatment but the wrong drug?, *CMA J.,* 116, 1382, 1977.

Chapter 5

PRELIMINARY TESTING OF AN IMPLANTABLE SYSTEM FOR SUSTAINED DELIVERY OF DISULFIRAM FOR THE TREATMENT OF ALCOHOLISM

Joseph D. Gresser

TABLE OF CONTENTS

I. INTRODUCTION

A. Sample Preparation

Two composites were prepared containing 20 and 50% by weight of ^{14}C-disulfiram in a polymer matrix. The polymer was synthesized from L-lactic and glycolic acids in a weight ratio of 9:1. Its weight average molecular weight was ~34,400. Dose form preparation required compaction and extrusion of these matrix systems under pressure at temperatures above the glass transition temperatures.

The matrix containing 20% by weight of the drug was successfully extruded as 1/8-in. diameter cylindrical rods. This composite extruded at 75 to 80°C and appeared to be slightly plasticized by the drug. Some difficulties were encountered with this extrusion. Temperatures had to be kept as low as possible to prevent melting of the disulfiram. However, below approximately 75°C the composite was insufficiently plastic for extrusion. This problem was exacerbated with the matrix containing 50% by weight of the drug. The matrix could not be extruded at temperatures sufficiently low to prevent melting of the drug. No in vivo experiments were conducted with the higher-loaded matrix.

B. In Vivo Results

Rods of the composite containing 20% by weight of ^{14}C-disulfiram were implanted in the scapular region of five Wistar CD-1 rats. Each rat received 500 mg of rod, sufficient to contain 100 mg of drug. Five additional rats served as controls, each receiving 100 mg of powdered pure labeled drug. The rate of excretion in both urine and feces was monitored by liquid scintillation counting to day 88 postimplantation.

By day 88, controls (group 2) had released a mean total of 80.5 mg in urine and feces. Of this a mean of 71.3 mg has been recovered by day 18. Almost all appeared in urine; at the end of the period of observation urinary excretion accounted for 75.8 mg of the 80.5 mg (94.2%).

In contrast, by day 88 rats implanted with the sustained release rods (group 1), had excreted the equivalent of only 17.4 mg of which 16.3 mg (93.7%) appeared in the urine.

Rods were excised from group 1 rats. These were analyzed for residual drug in order to complete a material balance. Total recovery including excreted materials was 73.0 mg, in good agreement with the controls. No attempt was made to account for ^{14}C expired as $^{14}CO_2$.

Tissue excised from the implant site was prepared for histological analysis. No abnormalities were found. No encapsulation of the rods was observed.

II. SAMPLE PREPARATION

A. Polymer Synthesis and Characterization

The polyester prepared by Dynatech R/D Company (Cambridge, Mass.) for this program was synthesized in bulk from L-lactide and glycolide using p-toluenesulfonic acid monohydrate as a catalyst.

The catalyst and monomers were introduced into a glass reaction flask equipped with a constriction to facilitate sealing under vacuum. The mixture was degassed for 45 min to less than 0.05 mmHg. The reaction flask was sealed and then rotated to mix ingredients and placed in a constant temperature oven at 118°C. After 2 hr, the flask was removed temporarily. The now liquid reactants were thoroughly mixed by shaking and the flask replaced.

The reactants were allowed to react for 10 days at 118 ± 2°C.

After removal and cooling, tetrahydrofuran (THF) was introduced to the flask to dissolve the polymer. The solution was filtered through glass wool to remove particulates.

The polymer was recovered by precipitation in a large excess of distilled water. The THF solution was poured slowly with constant stirring into water. The polymer precipitated as

Table 1
POLYMER SYNTHESIS

Polymer synthesis			
Material	Sample no.	MP (°C)	Weight (g)
Glycolide	013109	81.0—82.0	10.00
L-Lactide	011627-2A	96.0—97.5	90.00
PTSA			1.000

Reaction conditions	
Pressure	0.05 mmHg
Temperature	118 ± 2°C
Time	10 days

Precipitation	
Polymer solvent	THF (550 mℓ)
Precipitant	~10.4 ℓ distilled H_2O

Results: polymer No. 013973-A, -B		
$\overline{M}_w$	33,550; 35,306	mean = 34428 ± 877 (A.D.)
$\overline{M}_n$	13,177; 14,007	mean = 13592 ± 415 (A.D.)
d	2.55; 2.52	mean = 2.54 ± 0.02 (A.D.)
Yield	~90%	

fibrous strands which collected as cocoon-shaped deposits on the glass stirring rods. After addition of approximately 100 mℓ of the THF solution into approximately 1/2 gal of water, the water began to develop a slight milkiness due to suspended colloidal particles of polymer. At this point the precipitation was continued in fresh water. This process was continued until all polymer had been recovered.

The cocoons being extremely porous, were allowed to drain to remove entrained solvent, and air dried prior to exhaustive vacuum drying.

Prior to sample preparation, the polymer molecular weight distribution was determined by gel permeation chromatography (GPC). These measurements were made on a Waters Associates (Milford, Mass.) System equipped with three μ-Styragel® columns, 30 cm × 5 mm, covering 10^5, 10^4, and 10^3 Å ranges. Both carrier and sample solvents were THF, with a sample concentration of ~5 mg/mℓ. The instrument is equipped with a differential refractive index detector.

The weight average molecular weight ($\overline{M}_w$) was 34,428 ± 878 (mean and average deviation of two determinations). This value is well within the range selected for the polymer used in a Dynatech program conducted for the World Health Organization. (The goal of this WHO program was to prepare a sustained delivery system for an antimalarial drug.) The polymer selected was also a 90L/10G (90% dilactide, 10% glycolide) with a $\overline{M}_w$ of 40,000 ± 8000 (i.e., ±20%).

Data relevant to polymer synthesis are included in Table 1.

B. Disulfiram Dilution

Unlabeled disulfiram (USP) was obtained from Ayerst Laboratories, New York. Five millicuries (5.0 mCi) of labeled disulfiram, tetra-[1-^{14}C]-ethylthiuram disulfide, was obtained from Amersham Corporation, Chicago. The structure is as pictured.

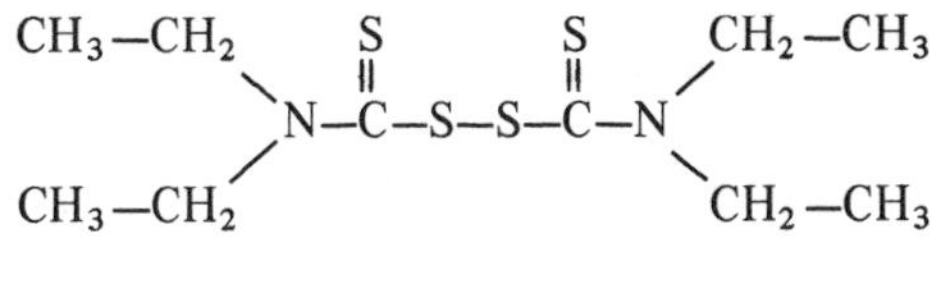

$$(CH_3{-}CH_2)_2N{-}\overset{\overset{S}{\|}}{C}{-}S{-}S{-}\overset{\overset{S}{\|}}{C}{-}N(CH_2{-}CH_3)_2$$

tetra-[1-^{14}C]-ethylthiuram disulfide (disulfiram)

Table 2
DISULFIRAM DILUTION

^{14}C-disulfiram:[a]	5.0 mCi
Disulfiram:[b]	14.9991 g
Dissolved in 650 mℓ ethanol[c]	
Recovered disulfiram (sample no. 013958-2)	
Weight = 14.9860 g	
Specific activity = 336 μCi/g	

[a] Amersham Corp. CFQ 2868, Dynatech aquisition no. 13-166.
[b] Ayerst Laboratories, lot no. 81-6357-8; D700ZTZ.
[c] Reagent grade, Fisher.

The radiolabeled drug (specific activity >1 mCi/mmol) was dissolved in 650 mℓ of reagent-grade ethanol (Fisher). To this was added 14.9991 g of unlabeled disulfiram. The disulfiram dissolved completely after 2 hr of stirring at room temperature.

The disulfiram was recovered by evaporating 250- to 300-mℓ aliquot samples of the solution to dryness. After combining the recovered portion and vacuum drying the diluted disulfiram at 60°C for 10 days, the weight of recovered drug was 14.9860 g.

Specific activity of the diluted drug was measured on a Beckman® LS-100C liquid scintillation counter. Two samples, each measured in triplicate, gave a mean specific activity of 336 μCi/g. [The calculated specific activity (5.0 mCi/15.0 g) (1000 μCi/mCi) = 333 μCi/g.]

Data on disulfiram dilution are given in Table 2.

C. Composite Fabrication and Characterization

The method chosen for preparation of composites required preparation of cosolutions of polymer and ^{14}C-disulfiram in methylene chloride. First the polymer was dissolved and this solution pressure filtered through a Millipore® Type LS (5-μM Teflon®) filter. Then to this was added the requisite quantity of drug, adjusted for loss of polymer via filtering. Solutions were cast on clean glass surfaces as thin films. Film thickness was adjusted to 0.025 in. with a Boston-Bradley® film spreader to facilitate drying. Films were allowed to air dry prior to exhaustive vacuum drying at 45°C.

Prior to making these castings with ^{14}C-disulfiram several experiments were conducted with cold drug/polymer solutions. The purpose was to determine conditions for casting which would result in a homogeneous composite. Homogeneity requires that drug precipitation in the drying film produce only microcrystals and that the drying process does not produce a polymer skin on the surface of the casting. These initial experiments permitted us to determine the optimum casting thickness and solution viscosity for homogeneous composite preparation.

Two castings containing labeled drug were prepared. One contained 20% by weight of labeled disulfiram and the other 50% by weight. These films were vacuum dried prior to characterization with respect to residual solvent content and to specific activity.

Table 3 gives data relevant to composite preparation. Note that excess polymer has been indicated in Table 3. This is needed to compensate for loss during filtering.

The recovered films were then vacuum dried to reduce residual solvent. Residual solvent was determined by baking an aliquot sample of the casting in an evacuated gas sampling bottle. The concentration of solvent in the vapor is measured by gas chromatography. Results, computed as weight percent of solvent in the composite, are presented in Table 4.

The final dose form was prepared by extruding these composites as cylindrical rods through a 1/8-in. die at minimum temperature and pressure. Composites containing 20% by weight

Table 3
COMPOSITE PREPARATION

	20 wt % composite	50 wt % composite
Polymer no.	013973-A	013973-A
Polymer weight (g)	16.00	9.00
^{14}C-disulfiram, weight (g)	3.7490	5.0160
Volume $MeCl_2$ (mℓ)	28	11
Casting thickness (in.)	0.025	0.025
Drying time (days)	~14	~14
Drying temperature (°C)	45	45

Table 4
COMPOSITE CHARACTERIZATION

Material	Pure drug	20% composite	50% composite
Residual solvent[a]	—	0.008	0.004
		0.005	0.006
Mean		0.007 ± 0.002	0.005 ± 0.001
Specific activity[b]	328.14[c]	70.78[d]	—
	342.34	53.13	
		59.54	
		68.24	
Mean	335.24	62.92	—
	±10.04	±8.11	

[a] Measured by GC, reported as wt % of methylene chloride in composite.
[b] Specific activity in μCi/g.
[c] Sample 014747-1.
[d] Sample 014747-3.

of disulfiram were difficult to extrude because of the low melting point of the drug (70°C). At 80°C and 40 psig, extruded material exhibits considerable die swell, indicative of partial melting or excessive softening of the composite. Reasonably homogeneous rods were obtained between 70 and 80°C at pressures up to 140 psig.

All attempts to extrude the 50% composite were unsuccessful. At sufficiently high temperatures, die swell and melting resulted in nonhomogeneity. At lower temperatures the extruded material lacked cohesiveness. No further work was done with this.

Specific activities of the pure drug and of the 20% composite were measured by dissolving each in dioxane and counting an aliquot sample of this in Aquasol® (New England Nuclear, Boston) in a Beckman® LS-230 liquid scintillation counter. Specific activities are also given in Table 4.

III. RESULTS OF IN VIVO EXPERIMENTS

A. Implantation Data

Five Wistar CD-1 male rats each weighing between 100 and 120 g received implants of the composite containing 20% by weight of ^{14}C-disulfiram (sample nos. 014745-1,2,3,4,5). Each rat was anesthetized with Penthrane® (Abbot Laboratories). A slit was made in the skin of the scapular region and a small subcutaneous pocket was opened large enough for introduction of the 1/8-in. diameter rods. Each rat received 500 mg of rod. The wound was closed with wound clips. Each rat was thereafter housed separately in a metabolism cage to facilitate separate collection of urine and feces.

Table 5
IMPLANTATION DATA

Sample no.	Sample weight (g)	Rat no.
Group 1 experimental[a]		
014745-1	0.5060	1
014745-2	0.4975	2
014745-3	0.4988	3
014745-4	0.5011	4
014745-5	0.5011	5
Group 2 controls[a]		
014746-1	0.0998	6
014746-2	0.1003	7
014746-3	0.0998	8
014746-4	0.1004	9
014746-5	0.0994	10

Samples for determination of specific activities

Sample no.	Sample weight (g)	Description
014747-1	0.1220	^{14}C-disulfiram
014747-3	0.1355	Extruded rod

[a] All rats implanted May 17, 1982.

A second similar group of rats (male Wistar DC-1 between 100 and 120 g each) served as controls. Each of these received a 100-mg subcutaneous implant of uncompounded ^{14}C-disulfiram.

This work was conducted at SISA Inc., Cambridge, Mass. under the supervision of Dr. John F. Howes, Director of Pharmacology. A record of samples delivered to SISA and of rats receiving these samples is given in Table 5. Several samples were also sent to SISA for confirmation of specific activities. A record of these is also included in Table 5.

B. Collection Protocol

Rats were individually housed in metabolism cages to facilitate separate collection of urine and feces. Water and food were provided ad libitum.

Prior to implantation, three fecal samples were collected to provide background counts. Urine samples were also collected. The first samples were collected on the day after implantation. A total of 19 collections of urine and 19 of feces were collected from each animal according to the schedule presented in Table 6.

Feces and urine from each rat were collected routinely between assays. Collections for each day were frozen. Prior to the assay the pool for each rat was blended to assure homogeneity.

Following completion of this 13-week (3-month) evaluation, tissue and residual drug at each implantation site of selected animals were excised. Tissue from two animals in each group will be reserved for pathological examination. The excised rods from all group 1 (experimental) animals were analyzed for residual drug.

C. Excretion of ^{14}C-Labeled Metabolites by Rats

Comparison of the quantity of ^{14}C-labeled materials appearing in excreta of each group

Table 6
COLLECTION SCHEDULE FOR URINE AND FECES

Preimplantation: 3 samples for background
Implantation: Monday, May 17, 1982

Week 1	Two collections: May 18, 20 (days 1, 3)
Week 2	Three collections: May 24, 26, 28 (days 7, 9, 11)
Week 3	Two collections: June 1, 4 (days 15, 18)
Week 4	Two collections: June 8, 11 (days 22, 25)
Week 5	Two collections: June 15, 18 (days 29, 32)
Weeks 6—13	One collection weekly: June 25; July 2, 9, 16, 23, 30; August 6, 13 (days 39, 46, 53, 60, 67, 74, 81, 88)

Note: Total number of collections per animal: 19 urine, 19 feces.

as a function of time clearly demonstrates that sample no. 014745 provides sustained release of disulfiram.

Controls exhibited a conventional excretion pattern; very rapid initial release quickly diminished to vanishingly small values. By day 10, controls (group 2) had released a mean about 55% of the implanted disulfiram and by day 20, about 73%. Total recovery from urine and feces was 80%.

One rat of the control group (rat no. 10) died on day 63 of the experiment. The cause of death was unknown. Because excretion data for this rat did not reveal statistically significant differences from the other rats of this group, this animal was included in calculations of mean quantities of disulfiram-derived materials in excreta.

Almost all ^{14}C activity appeared in the urine of the controls. By day 88, 75.83 mg had been recovered from urine and an additional 4.71 mg from feces. Thus 94.2% of the recovered material appeared in the urine.

Animals given the slow release formulation (group 1) excreted disulfiram-derived materials much more slowly. To day 25, only about 2.3 mg had been recovered in urine plus feces. The mean rate of excretion to this time was 0.065 $\pm$ 0.029 (S.D.) mg/day, omitting results for day 1 postimplantation. Between days 25 and 88 the mean rate was 0.24 $\pm$ 0.08 (S.D.) mg/day. In this period the rate rose from ~0.10 to 0.36 mg/day by day 32, and then fell slowly to 0.13 mg/day at the end of this period. The overall mean excretion rate to day 88, but excluding day 1, was 0.16 $\pm$ 0.11 (S.D.) mg/day.

Mean values for group 1 exclude rat number 4 because excretion data were significantly different from the other four animals in the group. On sacrifice, a large pus-filled infection at the implantation site was discovered. No rods remained. Cumulative recovery is presented graphically in Figure 1. Release rates averaged over time intervals between analyses are tabulated in Table 7 and presented in Figure 2.

D. Material Balance

Recovery of ^{14}C-loaded materials from group 2 (controls) rats accounted for 80.54 $\pm$ 9.56% (S.D.). No attempt was made to recover disulfiram remaining at the injection site or expired as $^{14}CO_2$. Percent recovery from both urine and feces varied from 69.0% (rat no. 9) to 95.45% (rat no. 6).

Recovery from urine and feces of group 1 (experimentals) rats accounted for 17.41 $\pm$ 2.27% (S.D.) of the implanted dose. Rods were excised at day 88 and residual disulfiram was determined by oxidation to $^{14}CO_2$ for liquid scintillation counting. The quantity remaining in the rods accounted for an additional 55.53 $\pm$ 14.83% (S.D.). Thus total recovery was 72.95 $\pm$ 14.49% (S.D.). These means omit rat no. 4.

Recoveries for all rats are presented in Table 8.

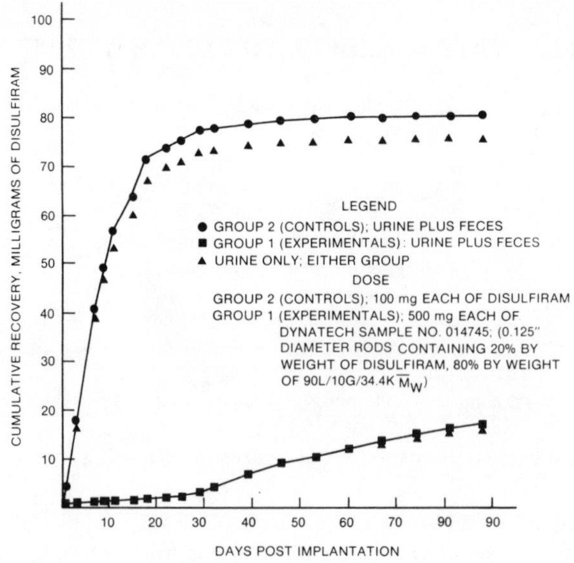

FIGURE 1. Cumulative recovery of ^{14}C-labeled materials expressed as milligrams of disulfiram.

Table 7
DAILY RATE OF EXCRETION OF DISULFIRAM IN URINE PLUS FECES OF RATS IMPLANTED WITH SAMPLE 014745 AND WITH PURE DRUG

Time interval (days)	Excretion rate (mg/day)	
	Experimentals	Controls
0—1	0.95	4.57
1—3	0.10	8.95
3—7	0.05	5.67
7—9	0.09	4.30
9—11	0.04	3.69
11—15	0.04	1.85
15—18	0.03	2.47
18—22	0.07	0.62
22—25	0.10	0.53

Mean ± S.D.[a] 0.065 ± 0.029

Time interval (days)	Excretion rate (mg/day)	
	Experimentals	Controls
25—29	0.23	0.44
29—32	0.36	0.18
32—39	0.35	0.14
39—46	0.32	0.09
46—53	0.22	0.06
53—60	0.26	0.06
60—67	0.16	0.03
67—74	0.19	0.02
74—81	0.18	<0.01
81—88	0.13	<0.01

Mean ± S.D.[b] 0.24 ± 0.08

Note: Overall mean ± S.D.[c] 0.16 ± 0.11

[a] Mean ± S.D. excluding first day, to day 25.
[b] Mean ± S.D. for days 25—88.
[c] Overall mean ± S.D. for days 2—88, excluding first day.

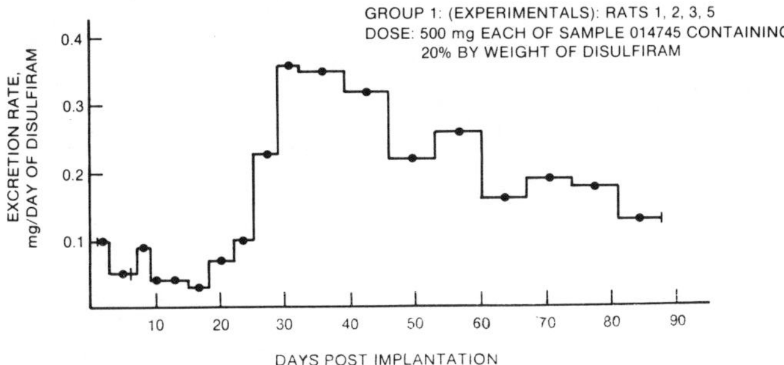

FIGURE 2. Mean daily rates of excretion of disulfiram-derived materials by rats implanted with sample 014745.

Table 8
RECOVERY OF DISULFIRAM

Group 1 (experimentals)

Rat no.	Recovered from excreta (%)	Recovered from rods (%)	Total recovered (%)
1	15.25	63.97	79.22
2	17.46	33.92	51.38
3	16.40	66.27	82.67
4	44.32	—	44.32
5	20.54	57.97	78.51
Mean ± S.D.[a]	17.41 ± 2.27	55.53 ± 14.83	72.95 ± 14.49

Group 2 (controls)

Rat no.	Recovered from excreta (%)
6	95.45
7	80.27
8	77.56
9	68.96
10	80.48
	80.54 ± 9.56

[a] Omitting rat no. 4.

ACKNOWLEDGMENT

This material was prepared from Dynatech Technical Report No. 2223 and submitted to Michael Phillips, M.D., Division of Internal Medicine, Georgetown University Hospital, Washington, D.C. Dr. Phillips and Dr. Gresser are working together on a grant from the National Institute for Alcohol and Alcohol Abuse.

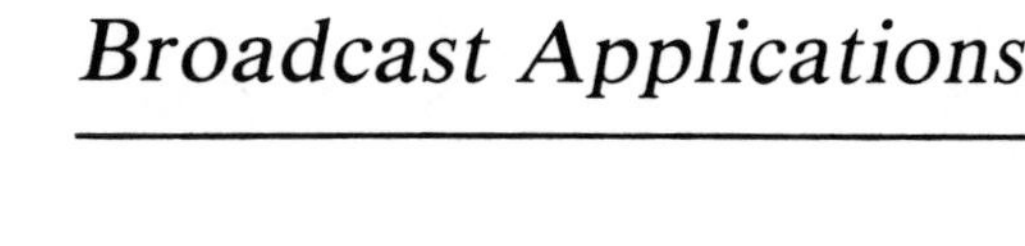

Broadcast Applications

Chapter 6

DEVELOPMENT AND TESTING OF BIODEGRADABLE PROTEIN EXCIPIENTS FOR THE SUSTAINED RELEASE OF MOLLUSCICIDES FOR CONTROL OF SCHISTOSOMIASIS VECTORS

Joseph D. Gresser

TABLE OF CONTENTS

I. INTRODUCTION

A. Program Objectives

The purpose of this work was to develop systems for the sustained release of molluscicides for control of schistosomiasis vectors. These systems should deliver the active agent for periods of up to 6 months.

Compounding of matrix components into a final product should be rapid and should not involve the use of complex equipment, i.e., composites should be formable on location if necessary. Matrix materials should be inexpensive. Matrix materials must, in addition, be biodegradable but must degrade slowly enough so that duration of effective activity meets program goals.

These objectives have been met. Matrices containing Bayluscide® have been prepared from the readily available and inexpensive modified protein colloids currently used as adhesives. These Bayluscide®/protein composites display the characteristics of slow release and slow biodegradability required by program objectives. Also, preparation is rapid, requiring no expensive or complex equipment.

B. Experimental Program

Initial phases of the work concentrated on development of compounding methods for mixing system components, i.e., molluscicides and protein dispersions, and for rendering these water resistant by addition of aldehydic cross-linking agents. Molluscicides included both copper sulfate and Bayluscide® (Bayer), although much more work was done with the latter agent.

Studies were performed to measure the following:

1. Rate of Bayluscide® release from composites of varying Bayluscide® content and composition
2. Rate of degradation of the matrix components in aqueous media of varying pH
3. Rate of degradation of the matrix components in aqueous media supporting bacterial growth
4. Long-range storability of various formulations under warm and humid conditions

Studies were also undertaken at the New England Aquarium (NEA), Boston, to observe the effect of Bayluscide® release from the matrices on mollusc vectors of schistosomiasis. Vectors chosen were *Biomphalaria glabrata, Bulinus truncatus,* and *Oncomelania hupensis quadrasi*.

C. Results of Release Rate Experiment

Results are summarized as follows for the work outlined above. Samples prepared with up to 25 pph* Bayluscide® were hardened with 2 pph formaldehyde. These released between 20 and 40% of their initial Bayluscide® content in 84 days. Samples containing 5, 10, and 25 pph Bayluscide® released 10, 20, and 30%, respectively. Projected lifetimes are between 200 and 420 days, thus meeting program goals.

1. Bayluscide® Release Rates

These results may be compared with release of Bayluscide® from samples hardened with 2 pph formaldehyde and then washed with glutaraldehyde. This process increased water resistance. Release is also a fairly linear function of time and of Bayluscide® content, although slower than observed for those without glutaraldehyde. Samples containing between 10 and 50 pph (parts per hundred of dry protein) released between 8 and 11% of their initial Bayluscide® content in 62 days of immersion in tap water. Glutaraldehyde apparently increases the extent of cross-linking and increases the resistance to diffusion of the active agent. Projected lifetime is up to 775 days assuming the lower release rate. This projection does not take degradation into account.

Experiments were performed with samples containing 20 pph BRL-1100, a synthetic phenolic resin from Union Carbide, New York. These were hardened with 4.0 pph formaldehyde and posttreated with glutaraldehyde. As expected, release was much slower than for materials not containing this resin. Analyses were performed on water in which 1, 2, or 3 such samples had been immersed. After 62 days, mean release was, respectively, 1.0, 0.9, and 0.6%.

D. Results of Degradation Experiments

Samples of fish protein were prepared and hardened with 2 pph formaldehyde. These contained varying additives of Bayluscide® at either 0.0 or 5.0 pph or the fungicide Dowicide® at 0.05 pph level. Half of the samples of each type were postreated with glutaraldehyde and then immersed for 8 weeks in pond water containing normal bacterial populations.

Samples which had not been exposed to a postgelation wash with glutaraldehyde showed degradative weight losses of between 50 and 75%. A clear difference was observed between these samples and those subjected to a postgelation glutaraldehyde wash. The washed samples had lost only between 17 and 29% in the 8-week period. Samples hardened with 6.2 pph HCHO and washed with glutaraldehyde showed no significant improvement over those prepared with 2 pph HCHO, and similarly washed. The projected lifetime of the treated group is therefore between 200 and 330 days, thus meeting program specifications.

E. Long-Term Storability

Samples were placed in storage for over 6 months. Storage conditions were either warm (37°C) and dry or warm and humid. All samples retained their physical integrity and strength. Those stored under humid conditions showed slight color changes but no gross deterioration.

F. Exposure of Molluscs to Bayluscide® Sustained Release Preparations

The species *Marisa cornu ariesta* were exposed to preparations containing 0, 5, 10, and 25 pph Bayluscide®. All preparations contained 0.05 pph Dowicide®. No deaths were observed in tanks containing the controls (0 pph Bayluscide®, 0.05 pph Dowicide®). The most rapid rate of death occurred at Bayluscide® concentration, between 0.40 and 0.50 pph. Deaths occurred sooner among snails exposed to the more highly loaded preparations.

* Throughout the text the abbreviation pph — parts per hundred — indicates parts by weight of the designated material per hundred parts by weight of the dry adhesive grade protein.

Samples have also been tested for activity in a more extensive series of tests at NEA. Species used are *Biomphalaria glabrata* and *Bulinus truncatus*. Tests on *Oncomelania hupensis quadrasi* are scheduled to begin in November. Tests are conducted in triplicate on populations of ten snails each. Each exposure is scheduled to last for 2 weeks at the most or to the death of all snails. Samples are retested at intervals of a minimum of 2 weeks. Between tests samples are stored in running water. Tests on various preparations conducted over periods of 6 to 18 weeks have all resulted in rapid snail kills. No samples have lost their activity after long immersion in water.

G. Recommendations

Based on results of release rate studies, degradation studies, and the exposure experiments at NEA, we recommend for field trials a formula designated herein as B-3. This contains a high loading of Bayluscide® (50 pph), has been crossed-linked with formaldehyde, and has received a postgelation wash with glutaraldehyde. It contains no synthetic resin and does not require addition of a fungicide or bactericide to insure long-term storability or resistance to degradation in water.

II. RATE OF BAYLUSCIDE® RELEASE FROM PROTEIN MATRICES

A. Matrices Hardened with Formaldehyde

1. Formulations and Compounding Methods

Preparations based on fish-derived protein (Lepage's) were made with Bayluscide® wettable powder.* Loadings of the active agent varied from 0 (controls) to 25 pph (parts per hundred of protein, dry weight; Bayluscide® loadings are reported on the basis of the dry weight of modified protein in the commercial preparation). Samples were hardened with 0.32 mℓ of 37% aqueous formaldehyde per 6 g, dry weight, of protein. This corresponds to 2 pph formaldehyde. After the material had gelled, discs were cut from each casting with a no. 12 cork borer. Samples were allowed to air dry to constant weight prior to testing.

Castings were made as follows. Twelve grams (12 g) of the liquid protein dispersion, 50% solids, were weighed into aluminum weighing dishes. The Bayluscide® was added at room temperature with continuous stirring until it was evenly dispersed in the protein suspension. For the 1 pph formula this required about 20 sec; for the 5 pph formula, about 1 min; for the 10 pph formula, about 1 1/2 min and for the 25 pph formula, about 2 1/2 min. The formaldehyde solution was added drop by drop with continuous stirring. Addition required about 15 sec.

After the samples had set for 30 min, no flow was observed in any sample although all samples were sticky. After 1 1/2 hr, samples were no longer tacky. Discs were then cut from each casting as previously described.

Table 1 gives weights and loadings of samples used in the following release rate measurements.

2. Experimental Procedures

Duplicate samples of each composition, each supported in a wire screen, were suspended in 3.5 ℓ of tap water contained in 1-gal plastic jars. Each jar was stirred twice daily. The water was changed once, on day 49 following that analysis for Bayluscide®. This was done to avoid concentrations of Bayluscide® approaching saturation. Measurement of the aqueous solubility of Bayluscide® is described in Section II.D.

The spectrophotometric assay for Bayluscide® using Safranin-O dye has been reported in Dynatech Report No. 1977. Samples 06431-3 and -4 (0 pph Bayluscide®) were used as

* Bayluscide® WP 70 Sr 73 70 wp 2743, Prod. 283290 (Bayer).

Table 1
BAYLUSCIDE® CONTENT OF FISH PROTEIN COMPOSITES

Sample no.	Sample weight (mg)	Bayluscide® (pph)	Bayluscide® (weight %)
06431-3	487	0	0
06431-4	520	0	0
06431-7	569	1	0.99
06431-8	597	1	0.99
06431-11	554	5	4.8
06431-12	559	5	4.8
06431-15	558	10	9.1
06431-16	551	10	9.1
06431-19	585	25	20
06431-20	605	25	20

controls; the mean value of absorbance measured for these controls was subtracted from absorbances measured for samples containing Bayluscide®.

Compounding methods and procedures for measuring release rates will not be described for experiments presented in the following sections as they are quite similar. Where details differ, these will be reported.

3. Results

Results presented in Table 2 give total release of Bayluscide® as a function of time in the leaching bath. Bayluscide® release is reported as the percent of the initial Bayluscide® content of the pellets. Results are corrected for control samples 06431-3 and -4. Mean values for each preparation except for samples 06431-7 and -8 are displayed in Figure 1.

Analyses for samples 06431-7 and -8, those containing 1 pph Bayluscide®, are subject to the greatest error. Measured absorbance for water samples exposed to these samples is, of course, lower than for water samples exposed to the 5-, 10-, and 25-pph samples. Mean values for the corrected absorbance of samples 06431-7 and -8 were greater than 0.2 only on days 45, 49, and 77. (Note: water was changed after sampling on day 49.) Mean values of absorbance for water exposed to the controls which contained no Bayluscide® (samples 06431-3 and -4) usually varied between ~0.04 and ~0.09, but on three occasions fell outside this range. Thus, the corrected values of absorbance (observed absorbance minus control absorbance) are subject to errors, the relative magnitude of which becomes greater the lower the observed absorbance. Results for samples 06431-7 and -8 are reported in Table 2 but are not included in either Figure 1 or in the following discussion of results.

Between day 0 and day 10 Bayluscide® concentration was too low to measure accurately. Mean data for the 5 and 25 pph samples show a decrease in concentration between days 40 and 49. The 10-pph sample shows no change during this time. A similar observation is made for the 5-pph mean between days 77 and 84. At this time the 10-pph sample value increases only slightly.

The observed decrease is attributed to aging of the Safranin-O solution. Usually analyses are performed with fresh or near-fresh solution. The Safranin-O/Bayluscide® complex forms less readily in aged solutions. In addition, as Bayluscide® concentration in the aqueous phase increases, the driving force for release diminishes. This driving force is the concentration gradient of Bayluscide® between the interior of the cake and the water phase; the reduction in observed release becomes more pronounced as the aqueous phase approaches saturation. Thus improved results might have been obtained with more frequent changes of water. In Section II.D, the results of measurements of Bayluscide® solubility are presented.

Table 2
CUMULATIVE PERCENT BAYLUSCIDE® RELEASE AS A FUNCTION OF IMMERSION TIME

	Day															
Sample no.	**1**	**3**	**6**	**10**	**16**	**22**	**24**	**30**	**36**	**45**	**49**[a]	**56**	**63**	**70**	**77**	**84**
06341-7	0	0	0	1.8	5.0	6.6	8.2	12.0	11.8	16.3	15.2	23.4	25.9	30.1	45.2	46.5
06431-8	0	0	0	0	7.1	7.1	8.5	10.7	13.4	15.4	12.4	22.2	27.1	27.8	36.4	33.7
Mean	0	0	0	0.90	6.05	6.85	8.35	11.35	12.60	15.85	13.00	22.80	26.50	28.95	40.80	40.10
				∓0.90	∓1.05	∓0.25	∓0.15	∓0.65	∓0.80	∓0.45	1.40	∓0.60	0.60	∓1.15	4.40	∓6.40
06431-11	0	0	0	0.9	2.1	3.3	4.3	6.5	7.5	8.1	8.4	15.0	17.3	18.1	19.4	18.7
06431-12	0	0	0	0.4	1.8	4.5	4.3	5.2	7.4	6.8	6.4	13.0	15.5	17.1	19.6	19.8
Mean	0	0	0	0.65	1.95	3.90	4.30	5.85	7.45	7.45	7.40	14.00	16.40	17.60	19.50	19.25
				∓0.25	∓0.15	∓0.60		∓0.6	∓0.05	0.65	∓1.00	∓1.00	∓0.90	∓0.50	∓0.10	∓0.55
06431-15	0	0	0	0.1	2.0	3.0	4.0	4.1	8.9	7.5	5.0	16.1	17.4	20.0	19.3	19.9
06431-16	0	0	0	0	1.4	2.4	3.0	4.8	5.6	8.9	(15.1)[b]	14.7	15.6	17.9	20.3	20.4
Mean	0	0	0	0.05	1.70	2.70	3.50	4.45	7.25	8.20	10.05	15.40	16.50	18.95	19.80	20.15
				∓0.05	∓0.30	∓0.30	∓0.50	∓0.35	∓1.65	∓0.70	∓5.05	∓0.70	∓0.90	∓1.05	∓0.50	∓0.25
06431-19	0	0	0.1	0.4	3.1	2.4	4.1	7.8	10.4	12.2	8.2	20.8	22.4	27.0	32.2	30.0
06431-20	0	0	0.2	0.4	2.5	3.8	5.1	5.4	(14.7)[b]	11.3	10.3	21.0	21.7	24.7	24.4	30.1
Mean	0	0	0.15	0.40	2.80	3.10	4.60	6.60	12.55	11.75	9.25	20.90	22.05	25.85	28.30	30.05
			∓0.05		∓0.30	∓0.70	∓0.50	∓1.20	∓2.15	0.45	∓1.05	∓0.10	∓0.35	∓1.15	∓3.90	∓0.05

[a] Water was changed on day 49. Values calculated for day 56 through 84 were added to the higher of the values for days 36, 45, or 49.
[b] Values in parentheses may be spuriously high. Cumulative values for days 56 through 84 are not based on these.

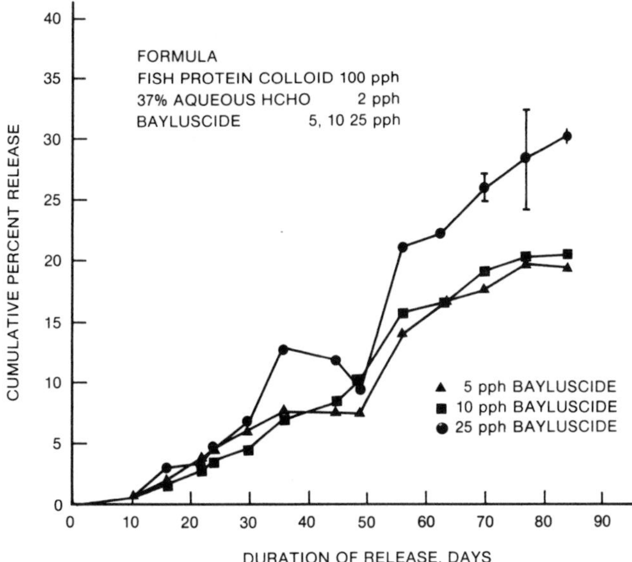

FIGURE 1. Release of Bayluscide® from fish protein matrices.

This was done to estimate the approach to saturation for use in the other release rate experiments described herein.

The cumulative percent release for each formulation is plotted in Figure 1. Cakes containing 5 and 10 pph Bayluscide® have very similar release profiles. The samples containing 25 pph show somewhat more rapid release on a percentage basis. By day 84 the 5-, 10-, and 25-pph samples have released between 20 to 30% of their initial Bayluscide® content. Thus the projected lifetime of these systems, based on linear release until system exhaustion, is 280 to 420 days.

As mentioned, the mean values of percent release for the samples of lower loading are quite similar throughout 84 days of measurements. To day 36, the 5-pph preparations have released a slightly larger mean percent of the initial Bayluscide® than have the 10-pph samples. Thereafter the mean percent release of the 10-pph samples remains slightly in advance. The 25-pph mean percent release is consistently greatest except for several analyses performed during the first 3 weeks.

The conclusion is that percent release as a function of time follows the order 5 pph $\simeq$ 10 pph $<$ 25 pph. The release for the 5- and 10-pph systems is ~0.24%/day, and for the 25 pph, ~0.36%/day.

B. Effect of Bayluscide® Loading on Release Rates from Glutaraldehyde-Washed Samples

Evidence is presented in Section III which shows that resistance to degradation in water is improved if formaldehyde-hardened samples are washed with glutaraldehyde, a difunctional aldehyde. It is important, therefore, to compare release rates obtained for samples prepared with and without the glutaraldehyde treatment.

Fish protein cakes, hardened with 2 pph of formaldehyde, and containing 0, 10, 25, and 50 pph of Bayluscide®, were washed with an aqueous solution containing 30% glutaraldehyde after gelation. Use of this dialdehyde as the primary hardening agent is not possible since the hardening (cross-linking) reaction is too rapid to allow thorough mixing. After drying to constant weight, individual cakes weighed between 6.4 and 8.9 g, depending on Bayluscide® content. Cakes were suspended in 10-gal aquaria containing 35 ℓ of tap water on April 24, 1980. Tanks were lined with polyethylene sheets to prevent Bayluscide® absorption.

Table 3
COMPOSITION OF SAMPLES TREATED WITH GLUTARALDEHYDE AFTER GELATION[a]

Sample[b] no.	Bayluscide® pph	Bayluscide® weight (g)	Dry weight of sample (g)
07730-1	0	0	6.42
07730-2	10	0.542	7.20
07730-3	35	1.356	7.66
07730-4	50	2.710	8.88

[a] Sample composition based on 12 g Lepage's protein dispersion, hardened with 0.32 mℓ of 37% HCHO (2 pph).

[b] See also Dynatech Sample No. 08228 (April 24, 1980).

Table 4
CUMULATIVE PERCENT RELEASE AS A FUNCTION OF BAYLUSCIDE® LOADING

Sample no.	Bayluscide® content (pph)	Immersion (days) 5	11	18	25	35	40	47	56	62
07730-2	10	0	0.1	1.1	1.9	3.6	4.8	7.8	7.8	8.6
07730-3	25	0	0.6	1.6	1.6	3.4	4.0	6.1	6.9	8.4
07730-4	50	0.2	0.5	0.8	1.7	3.6	3.8	7.6	7.5	10.7

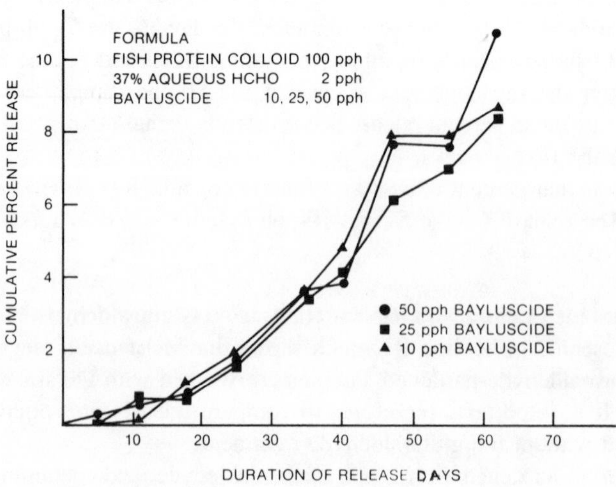

FIGURE 2. Cumulative release of Bayluscide® from fish protein matrices washed with glutaraldehyde.

Sample composition and dry weight is given in Table 3.

Bayluscide® analyses were made regularly over 9 weeks. Results are reported in Table 4 as cumulative percent release.

These data are graphically presented in Figure 2. Release rate is apparently a reasonably linear function of loading; thus, the percent released in a given time interval remains relatively constant for the three loadings.

Also, release is significantly slower than for samples not treated with glutaraldehyde. Linear release rates for untreated samples were in the range of 0.24 to 0.36%/day for loadings of 5 to 25 pph. Glutaraldehyde-treated samples release only 0.14 to 0.16%/day for loadings to 10 to 50 pph.

C. Effect of BRL-1100 on Release of Bayluscide® from Glutaraldehyde-Washed Samples

BRL-1100 is a synthetic phenolic resin made by Union Carbide. This material, infinitely miscible with water prior to polymerization, forms water-insoluble, nonbiodegradable polymers on heating. It is also compatible with water-dispersed protein gels. Several experiments were conducted which included BRL-1100 into the formulations in order to determine the effect of this addition on Bayluscide® release.

Cakes were made of Lepage's protein colloid containing 20 pph BRL-1100 and 50 pph Bayluscide®. These were hardened with 4.6 pph formaldehyde. After gelation, cakes were washed with glutaraldehyde (30% aqueous solution) for 1/2 hr, then heated for ~5 hr at 95°C to promote cross with BRL-1100.

Six 10-gal aquaria, lined with polyethylene, contained 35 ℓ of tap water each. Two tanks contained one cake each, two contained two cakes each, and two contained three cakes each. Appropriate controls of similar cakes but without Bayluscide® provide baseline absorption for the assay. Thus, tanks containing one, two, or three cakes contained 2.71, 5.42, and 8.13 g, respectively, of Bayluscide®.

Bayluscide concentration was monitored periodically for 9 weeks. Results, presented as cumulative percent release, are given in Table 5 and presented graphically in Figure 3.

Over the 9-week interval, samples released only about 1.0% or less of their initial Bayluscide® content. Tanks containing 1, 2, or 3 cakes showed mean release of 1.0, 0.9, and 0.6%. Although the projected duration of release is greater than the longevity of the system as reported in Section III, several formulations were tested at NEA to determine if such slow release is effective against *Bulinus* and *Biomphalaria*.

D. Aqueous Solubility of Bayluscide® Wettable Powder

The kinetics of the release of an active agent from a matrix into an aqueous phase depend in part on the partition coefficient of the agent between the matrix and the aqueous phase as well as on the concentration gradient existing at any moment between the two phases. As the aqueous phase approaches saturation, release per unit time from the matrix decreases. In order to minimize this effect, the water should be changed periodically. The frequency of this change should depend on the saturation concentration of the active agent. Therefore it was necessary to determine the solubility of the Bayluscide®.

Approximately 0.5 g of Bayluscide® wettable powder was placed in each of two jars containing ~250 mℓ of distilled water. The suspensions were ball milled with porcelain balls for 5 days and then filtered through a Whatman® No. 1 filter.

Filtrate was diluted 25 times and assayed for Bayluscide®. Concentration was calculated for the equation C_{ppm} (A − 0.058)/1.20. Results for two samples are given in Table 6.

Concentrations obtained in the release experiments described in Section II.A for the period 40 to 45 days and again between 78 to 84 days were measured to be between ~3.3 to 4.0 ppm and 4.4 and 5.0 pph for the 25-pph sample. Thus the aqueous phase reduced from 23 to 34% of saturation. Although this will not stop release, it is probably sufficient to slow it. Henceforth, water will be changed when concentration is ~15% of saturation.

Table 5
CUMULATIVE PERCENT RELEASE OF BAYLUSCIDE® FROM SAMPLES PREPARED WITH BRL-1100[a]

Sample no.	Number of cakes in tank	Days 5	11	18	25	35	40	47	50	62	62-day mean
08225-1	1	0.1	0.1	0.2	0	0.4	0.3	0.6	0.7	0.9	1.0 ± 0.10
08225-2	1	0.1	0.1	0.2	0.1	0.5	0.5	0.9	1.0	1.1	
08225-3	2	0.1	0.1	0.1	0.1	0.4	0.3	0.4	0.5	0.9	0.9 ± 0.10
08225-4	2	0.1	0.1	0.2	0.1	0.4	0.3	0.6	0.6	0.9	
08225-5	3	0	0.1	0.1	0.1	0.3	0.3	0.4	0.4	0.5	0.6 ± 0.05
08225-6	3	0.1	0.1	0.2	0.2	0.3	0.3	0.4	0.5	0.6	

[a] See 08229 (April 24, 1980).

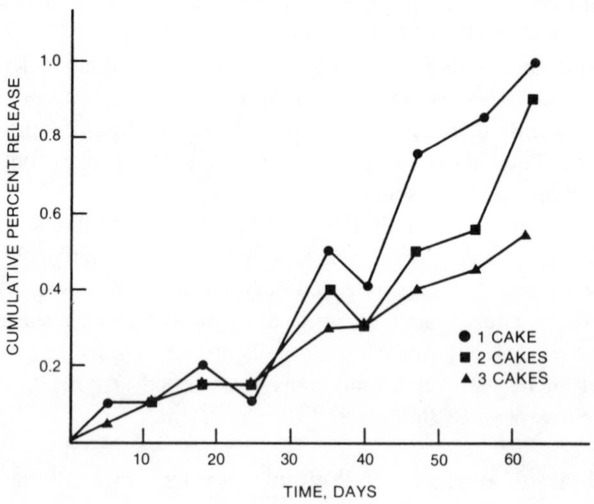

FIGURE 3. Release of Bayluscide® from matrices prepared with BRL-1100.

Table 6
SOLUBILITY OF BAYLUSCIDE® IN DISTILLED WATER

Sample no.	Dilution factor	Absorbance	Concentration (pph)
07281A	25	0.739	14.2
07281B	25	0.775	14.9

Table 7
ANALYSIS OF POND[a] WATER

Temperature (°C)		Phosphate[b]	
Color		Ortho as P	0.01
Turbidity (NTU)		Total as P	
Alkalinity[b]		Oil (grease)[b]	
Phenolphthalein	0.0	Phenol[b]	
Total	7.4	pH	5.7
Chloride[b]		Carbon dioxide[b]	
Chlorine (total)[b]		Oxygen (dissolved)[b]	
Hardness total[b]		Oxygen demand,	
Metal[b]		biochemical (BOD)[b]	
Cadmium		Oxygen demand	
Chromium		Chemical (COD)[b]	22.1
Copper		Solids[b]	
Iron (total)	0.09	Total	
Lead		Suspended	
Manganese		Dissolved	
Mercury (μg/ℓ)	<0.02	Sulfate[b]	
Nickel		Sulfide[b]	
Sodium	1.7	Conductivity	
Zinc		(MICRO MHOS/CM)	
Nitrogen[b]		Bacteria[c]	
Ammonia as N		Total coliform	68,800
Nitrite as N		Fecal coliform	ND[d]
Nitrate as N	0.01	Fecal streptococci	20
Total Kjeldahl as N		Total bacteria	20

[a] Source: Long Pond, Henniker, N.H.
[b] In mg/ℓ.
[c] Count per 100 mℓ of sample (MF).
[d] None detected.

III. BIODEGRADATION OF BAYLUSCIDE®/PROTEIN COMPOSITES

A. Degradation of Formaldehyde-Hardened Animal Gels in Media of Varying pH and Bacterial Content

Animal glue gels, hardened with 1% formaldehyde, were exposed to water buffered to pH 4, 7, and 10 and to water carrying bacterial populations. Buffers were as follows: pH 4 (potassium acid phthalate), pH 7 (monobasic potassium phosphate plus sodium hydroxide), pH 10 (boric acid plus sodium and potassium chlorides). Samples exposed to these environments were protected from bacterial or fungal attack by 0.1% w/v Dowicide® added to the water.

Bacterially contaminated water was obtained by preparing a growth medium,[1] and exposing this to airborne microorganisms. Bacterial growth in this medium was rapid.

The last bath consisted of fresh pond water, pH 5.7, obtained from Long Pond, Henniker, N.H. This water contains a normal population of aquatic flora and fauna. Analysis of this water performed by Water Quality Laboratory, Waltham, Mass., is presented in Table 7. Note that the total coliform count is 68,800/100 mℓ, no fecal coliform detected. Fecal streptococci were measured at 20/100 mℓ as were total bacteria.

Samples were immersed in baths after drying to constant weight. At intervals two samples were removed from each bath, and again dried to constant weight. Percent weight loss as a function of immersion time is given in Table 8 and displayed graphically in Figure 4.

Table 8
PERCENT WEIGHT LOSS OF ANIMAL GLUE GELS ON EXPOSURE TO AQUEOUS ENVIRONMENTS

	Exposure time (weeks)					
Bath	**1**	**2**	**3**	**4**	**5**	**6**
pH 4[a]	10.6 ± 0.6	13.2 ± 0.9	13.0 ± 1.6	15.4 ± 0.3	16.9 ± 0.2	21.8 ± 1.3
pH 7[a]	8.3 ± 0.5	11.8 ± 1.1	12.5 ± 1.9	14.1 ± 0.2	17.5 ± 2.3	21.6 ± 1.7
pH 10[a]	8.2 ± 0.2	10.2 ± 0.1	9.4 ± 0.1	11.5 ± 0.3	5.4 ± 0.7	8.0 ± 0.6
Pond water	12.4 ± 0.8	20.5 ± 7.4	22.3 ± 5.2	31.0 ± 3.2	—	—
Bacterial culture	9.2 ± 0.5	16.9 ± 0.4	44.5 ± 1.2	100%	—	—

[a] 0.1% w/v Dowicide® added to water.

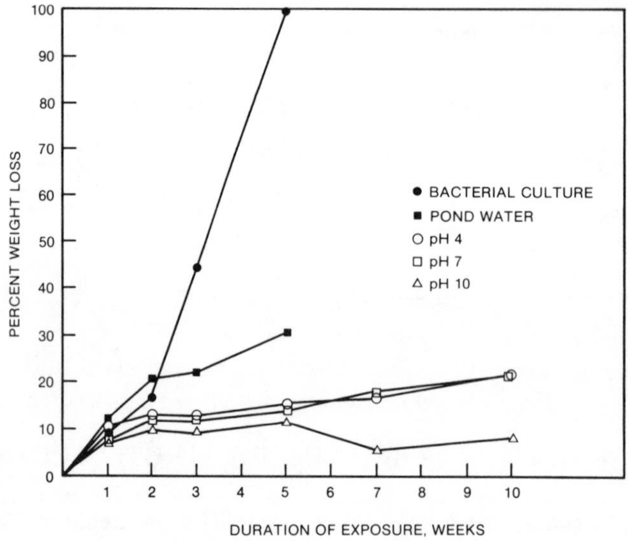

FIGURE 4. Weight loss of animal protein gels on exposure to aqueous media.

At pH 4 and 7 samples show 10% weight loss during the first week. Thereafter weight loss is slow and constant to week 10 (current data) at which the weight loss is ~22%. Thus, in the period between weeks 1 to 10 the average weight loss was ~1.3%/week.

The samples placed in pH 10 buffer showed some growth of mold from week 5. Weight loss computed for these samples was less at weeks 3, 7, and 10 than at week 5. At week 5, weight loss was about that recorded for week 2. Growth of mold would compensate for weight lost by hydrolytic or bacterial degradation.

Rates of bacterial degradation were comparable to those at week 2. About 20% weight loss of samples in pond water and 15% loss of samples exposed to a sewage inoculum were observed at this time. At week 3 the pond water samples had lost only an additional 2%. Samples in inoculum degraded rapidly; by week 5 degradation was complete.

B. Degradation of Formaldehyde-Hardened Fish Gels in Natural Pond Water

Composites containing 5 pph of Bayluscide® wettable powder in fish protein (Lepage's)

Table 9
COMPOSITION OF FISH PROTEIN COMPOSITES FOR DEGRADATION MEASUREMENTS

Type	Sample no.	Lepage's fish protein	Formaldehyde pph[a]	Bayluscide® (pph)	Dowicide® (pph)	Glutaraldehyde[b]
06967-A	1—12	100[c]	2	—	—	No
06967-B	1—12	100	2	—	—	Yes
06967-C	1—12	100	2	—	0.05	No
06967-D	1—12	100	2	—	0.05	Yes
06967-E	1—12	100	2	5	—	No
06967-F	1—12	100	2	5	—	Yes

[a] This (2 pph formaldehyde) corresponds to 0.32 mℓ of 32% aqueous HCHO.
[b] Samples indicated by "Yes" were bathed in 25% aqueous glutaraldehyde for 30 min. Samples indicated by "No" were not so treated.
[c] Used here was 6 g (dry weight). All samples cast in cindicethete aluminum weighting dishes.

were made to test the effect of fungicide and glutaraldehyde wash on rates of degradation. Sample recipes are given in Table 9.

Twelve samples of each of the six formulations were prepared and dried at room temperature to constant weight before testing. All samples were washed for 3 days in running tap water to remove traces of formaldehyde and/or glutaraldehyde.

The twelve samples of each formulation were placed in 2 ℓ of pond water (see Section III.A) contained in small plastic tanks. Water was changed twice each week. At intervals of 1, 2, 3, 4, 6, and 8 weeks, two samples of each formulation were removed and again dried to constant weight. Sample types will be referenced by their letter designations. Sample numbers and formulae are given in Table 9.

Weight loss for each sample is reported in Table 10. Mean percent weight loss calculated from these data is given in Table 11 and is displayed graphically in Figure 5. All samples show rapid weight loss during the first week. It is interesting to observe that during the first week loss is less for samples not treated with glutaraldehyde than for those given this treatment. Groups A, C, and E, not treated with glutaraldehyde, lost between 5.9 and 7.1% of their original weight. Groups B, D, and F, which were treated, lost between 10.9 and 13.9% of their original weight. Initial weights of groups B, D, and F are greater than those of the groups of similar composition but without glutaraldehyde: A, C, and E. This may reflect extensive cross-linking which traps water in the matrix. This water is retained until immersion for 1 week. After 1 week sufficient hydrolysis may have occurred to allow escape of the excess water on drying.

Between weeks 1 and 4, all groups are quite stable showing only 3 to 4% additional weight loss.

Thereafter, differences due to treatment with glutaraldehyde became apparent. Groups A, C, and E (untreated) began to degrade rapidly; by week 6 additional or incremental weight loss for groups A, C, and E was between 12 and 29%, but for groups B, D, and F (treated) it was only between 1 and 2%.

The experiment was concluded in week 8. By this time untreated samples had shown weight losses between 50 and 75%, the treated between 17 and 29%.

Samples A and C may be compared for the effect of Dowicide®. With 0.05 pph of the fungicide, the 8-week mean weight loss was 50% compared to 69% without it. However, comparison of B and D, both treated with glutaraldehyde, reveals a slightly greater 8-week weight loss for D, which contains Dowicide®, than for B (29% compared with 23%). Further, the smallest weight loss at 8 weeks (17%) was shown by group F. This group, treated with glutaraldehyde, contained Bayluscide® but not Dowicide®.

Table 10
DEGRADATION OF FISH PROTEIN COMPOSITES IN POND WATER

		Exposure time (weeks)											
		1		2		3		4		6		8	
Type	Sample no. 06967-	Original Wt. (g)	Final Wt. (g)	Original Wt. (g)	Final Wt. (g)	Original Wt. (g)	Final Wt. (g)	Original Wt. (g)	Final Wt. (g)	Original Wt. (g)	Final Wt. (g)	Original Wt. (g)	Final Wt. (g)
A	1, 3, 5, 7, 9, 11	6.07	5.67	5.99	5.61	6.02	5.53	6.23	5.06	6.00	3.37	6.01	1.72
A	2, 4, 6, 8, 10	6.09	5.62	6.05	5.04	6.02	5.61	5.99	5.37	5.98	3.63	6.04	2.01
B	As above	6.72	5.89	6.62	5.88	6.79	5.98	6.61	5.68	6.72	5.72	6.68	5.11
B	As above	6.71	5.92	6.60	5.98	6.69	5.94	6.70	5.75	6.74	5.68	6.64	5.13
C	As above	6.09	5.67	6.06	5.71	6.05	5.61	6.12	5.56	6.15	4.64	6.13	3.23
C	As above	6.11	5.68	6.11	5.74	6.11	5.65	6.16	5.53	6.12	4.44	6.11	2.95
D	As above	6.67	5.81	6.52	5.73	6.71	5.84	6.56	5.56	6.58	5.42	6.61	4.65
D	As above	6.64	5.73	6.56	5.77	5.70	5.01	6.58	5.61	6.66	5.54	6.72	4.88
E	As above	6.20	5.83	6.16	5.80	6.30	5.81	6.26	5.59	6.28	4.78	6.26	1.50
E	As above	6.26	5.90	6.29	5.92	6.27	5.81	6.29	5.67	6.23	4.95	6.17	1.58
F	As above	6.88	6.14	6.86	6.19	6.87	6.13	7.02	6.12	6.94	5.94	6.89	5.75
F	As above	6.96	6.20	6.82	6.19	6.98	6.20	6.88	6.07	6.90	5.98	6.91	5.69

Note: D = Dowicide® (0.05%); B = Bayluscide® (5%); F = 1/2 hr bath in 25% glutaraldehyde.

Table 11
MEAN PERCENT WEIGHT LOSS OF FISH PROTEIN COMPOSITES AFTER IMMERSION IN POND WATER

Composite type	Exposure time (weeks) 1	2	3	4	6	8
A	7.1 ∓ 0.6[a]	11.5 ∓ 5.2	7.5 ∓ 0.6	13.0 ∓ 2.6	41.6 ∓ 2.2	69.1 ∓ 2.3
B	12.1 ∓ 0.3	10.3 ∓ 0.9	11.6 ∓ 0.4	14.2 ∓ 0.1	15.3 ∓ 0.4	23.1 ∓ 0.4
C	7.0 ∓ 0.1	6.0 ∓ 0.2	7.4 ∓ 0.1	9.7 ∓ 0.5	26.1 ∓ 0.44	49.5 ∓ 2.3
D	13.9 ∓ 0.2	12.1 ∓ 0.1	12.6 ∓ 0.5	15.0 ∓ 0.3	17.2 ∓ 0.4	28.6 ∓ 1.2
E	5.9 ∓ 0.1	5.9 ∓ 0.1	7.6 ∓ 0.3	10.3 ∓ 0.4	22.2 ∓ 1.7	75.2 ∓ 0.8
F	10.9 ∓ 0.1	9.5 ∓ 0.3	11.0 ∓ 0.2	12.3 ∓ 0.5	13.9 ∓ 0.6	17.1 ∓ 0.6

[a] Average deviations.

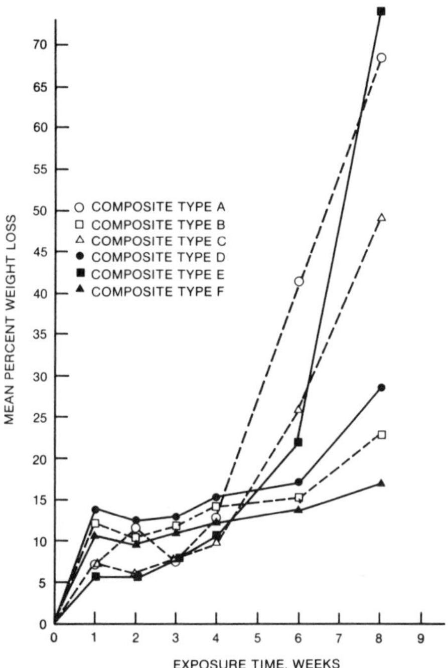

FIGURE 5. Weight loss of fish protein gels on exposure to pond water.

C. Degradation of Formulations Containing BRL-1100

Eight cakes were prepared recently to determine the effect of a phenol formaldehyde additive on longevity in pond water. This additive, BRL-1100 (Union Carbide), is a low viscosity liquid phenolic resin that can be infinitely diluted with water. It is commonly used as a binder in the manufacture of glass wool insulating material and as an impregnant for densified wood. On heating the resin solidifies to a water-resistant solid.

Table 12
COMPOSITION OF SAMPLES CONTAINING BRL-1100

	Composition (pph)			
Cake no.	Protein colloid[a]	HCHO[b]	BRL-1100	Glutaraldehyde wash
08208-1	100	—	5	No
08208-2	100	—	20	No
08208-3	100	2.0	5	Yes
08208-4	100	2.0	20	Yes
08208-5	—	—	100	No
08208-6	—	1.2	100	No
08208-7	100	6.2	—	Yes
08208-8	100	6.2	20	Yes

[a] Lepage's, 12 g total weight.
[b] 37% aqueous.

Table 13
COMPARISON LONGEVITY OF SAMPLES CONTAINING BRL-1100

Sample no.	Initial dry weight (g)	Observations after 4 weeks immersion	Dry weight after 67 days	Weight loss (%)
08208-1	6.10	Nearly complete degradation	—	100
08208-2	6.93	Intact, small apparent loss	4.08	41
08208-3	6.55	Broken into small large pieces, but small apparent loss	5.15	21
08208-4	7.23	Intact, small apparent loss	6.07	16
08208-5	4.43	No apparent change	4.46	0
08208-6	4.57	No apparent change	4.59	0
08208-7	6.44	Broken into large pieces, no apparent loss	5.11	21
08208-8	7.48	Small broken off, otherwise intact with no apparent loss	6.23	17

BRL-1100 is completely compatible with protein colloids; it may be added as a liquid and cross-linked by heating. Cakes were made by the usual methods. In some cases, cakes were washed with glutaraldehyde for 1/2 hr. Cakes containing BRL-1100 were placed in a warming oven for 7 hr at ~95°C for curing.

All cakes were allowed to come to constant weight then washed for 1 day in running water before they were placed in 1 ℓ of pond water.

Formulae are indicated in Table 12. Observations taken 4 weeks after immersion and weight loss after 67 days are presented in Table 13.

After 4 weeks the following comparisons may be offered:

1. BRL-1100 with or without formaldehyde hardens to a vitreous solid with no apparent change after 4 weeks (cakes 5, 6).
2. BRL-1100 added to protein colloid increased degradation lifetime at 20 pph but not at 5 pph (cakes 1, 2).
3. Cakes with 20 pph BRL-1100 appear to resist cracking as well as solubilization by degradative processes (cakes 2, 4, 8). Cakes with ≤2.0 pph HCHO (cakes 2, 4) may resist cracking better than those with 6.2 pph (cake 8).

Table 14
RECIPES[a] AND STORAGE CONDITIONS OF COMPOSITES TESTED FOR STORABILITY

Sample no.	Dowicide® (pph)	Glutaraldehyde wash	Initial weight (g)	Storage
07729-1a	0.05	Yes	7.92	Dry
07729-2b	0.05	Yes	7.82	Dry
07729-3b	0.05	Yes	7.79	Moist
07729-4b	0.05	Yes	7.65	Moist
07729-5a	—	Yes	7.86	Dry
07729-6b	—	Yes	7.86	Dry
07729-7a	—	Yes	7.80	Moist
07729-8b	—	Yes	7.75	Moist
07729-9a	0.05	No	7.22	Dry
07729-10b	0.05	No	7.30	Dry
07729-11a	0.05	No	7.26	Moist
07729-12b	0.05	No	7.20	Moist
07729-13a	—	No	7.32	Dry
07729-14b	—	No	7.32	Dry
07729-15a	—	No	7.15	Moist
07729-16b	—	No	7.26	Moist

[a] All recipes are based on 100 pph Lepage's fish protein adhesive (dry weight), 2 pph HCHO, and 25 pph Bayluscide®.

4. The protein cake which shows least change either degradative or by cracking is cake no. 4. This one has received a glutaraldehyde wash and appears in better condition than the others receiving the wash. Its appearance is similar to cake no. 2 which was prepared with only protein colloid and 20 pph BRL-1100.

When the cakes had been exposed for 4 weeks we tentatively concluded that addition of BRL-1100 protects against degradative weight loss and reduces loss by cracking.

Samples were removed 67 days after preparation and dried to constant weight. Samples were weighed and degradation reported as percent weight loss. Table 13 summarizes observation at 4 weeks and degradation at 67 days (9 weeks).

Data in Table 13 show that polymerized BRL-1100 does not degrade in water. Samples 08208-1 and -2 were most degraded indicating that even with 20 pph BRL-1100, HCHO is necessary for cross-linking the protein. Although 20 pph BRL-1100 apparently aids in maintaining the physical integrity of the cake, i.e., in resistance development of cracks, total degradation of cakes containing 20 pph as compared to other is not markedly greater. Samples 08208-4 and -8 degraded by 16 to 17% in 9 weeks as compared to 21% for samples 08208-3 and -7 which contained, respectively, 5 and 0 pph resin.

Our conclusion is that addition of phenolic resin BRL-1100 offers minimal improvement in water resistance. Several formulations containing BRL-1100 have been tested at NEA against molluscs.

IV. LONG-TERM STORAGE OF BAYLUSCIDE®/PROTEIN COMPOSITES

Storage of protein-based sustained release systems in hot, humid, tropical climates for extended periods may be necessary. If this is so, the Bayluscide®/protein composites must retain their physical integrity, and be resistant to fungal or bacterial degradation.

Four formulations are being tested for storability. These are listed in Table 14. Each contains 25 pph of Bayluscide® wettable powder and was gelled with 2 pph of formaldehyde.

Table 15
COMPOSITION OF COMPOSITES USED IN MOLLUSC TESTS AT DYNATECH R/D COMPANY

Ingredients	A	B	C	D
Lepage's fish protein	100[a]	100	100	100
Formaldehyde (pph)	2[b]	2	2	2
Dowicide® (pph)	0.05	0.05	0.05	0.05
Bayluscide® WP (pph)	0	5	10	25

[a] 100 parts based on dry weight of Lepage's adhesives.
[b] 0.32 mℓ of 37% aqueous HCHO per 12 g Lepage's.

Samples 07729:1-4 and 9-12 contain, in addition, 0.05 pph of Dowicide® (sodium pentachlorophenate). After gelling, samples 07729:1-8 were hardened further with a wash of 25% aqueous glutaraldehyde for 30 min.

The four samples of each preparation were placed, two to a bag, in heat-sealed polyethylene containers. Each bag contained paper towels, one dry and one thoroughly wet with water. One bag containing only a wet paper towel was also included in the experiment. All bags have been in storage at 85 to 90°F (29.5 to 32.2°C) since March 20, 1980.

By May 9, all of the samples stored dry showed no changes. All were hard and inflexible; none showed growth of fungus, or gave evidence of decomposition.

Samples stored with the wet paper were flexible and softer than initially, but otherwise maintained their integrity. They did not show any tendency to crumble when handled, nor were they tacky. The two cakes in each bag when passed together were easily separable; they would not stick together. No growth of fungus was observed.

The wet paper towel in the bag with no samples did support the growth of many small colonies of a gray green mold. The absence of such mold in all other samples suggests that an antifungal agent such as Dowicide® is not necessary for protection, and that such protection may be conferred by Bayluscide®.

Samples have been held in storage until October 1, 1980. At this time, they are less flexible and drier. Otherwise, no changes are apparent.

No decomposition or growth of mold is apparent on any sample stored dry. The color of these is yellow amber.

Samples stored with wet paper show slight changes. Those treated with glutaraldehyde are darker brown. All of those stored wet show a grayish film except the two which were both treated by addition of Dowicide® and glutaraldehyde wash.

V. EFFECT OF SUSTAINED RELEASE OF BAYLUSCIDE® ON *MARISA CORNU ARIESTA*

Composites were made of the compositions indicated in Table 15 according to previously described methods.

After drying to constant weight and washing for 3 days in running water, each type was tested in duplicate. One cake weighing approximately 6 to 7 g was placed in each of eight 10-gal aquaria. Aquaria were lined with plastic.

Six or seven snails, *Marisa cornu ariesta,* had been previously acclimated to the aquaria for several weeks. The aquaria were each filled with tap water filtered through Barnstead Cartridges Nos. D8902 and D8904 for ion exchange and for removal of organic materials. Aquaria were held at 75 to 77°F and continuously aerated.

Table 16
RECORD OF SNAIL DEATHS

Tank	Day 1[a]	2	3	4	5	6	7	8	9	10	Number of snails placed in tank
A1				No deaths among controls							6
A2											6
B1				1			4	1[b]		1	6
B2		1	6								7
C1			1	3[c] 2[d]				2[d]		3	6
C2			1	5 1							7
D1		1	3	2							6
D2		1	5	1							7

[a] Cakes entered February 16, 1980 (day 0). Day 1 is February 12, 1980. Morning observations on left-hand side of column, evening observations on right-hand side.
[b] Appeared dead but recovered.
[c] One appeared dead but recovered.
[d] Both appeared dead but recovered.

Table 17
BAYLUSCIDE® CONCENTRATION[a] AS A FUNCTION OF TIME

Samples no.	Bayluscide® concentration (pph)	Tank no.	Time (days) 1[b]	3	4	8	16
07300:A-1	0	A-1	0	0	0	0	0
07300:A-2	(controls)	A-2	0	0	0	0	0
07300:B-1	5	B-1	0	0.03	0.15	0.38	0.49
07300:B-2		B-2	0	0.40	0.85	1.35	0.81
07300:C-1	10	C-1	0	0.19	0.44	1.26	2.71
07300:C-2		C-2	0	0.11	0.56	1.22	2.17
0700:D-1	25	D-1	0	0.81	1.18	1.26	2.75
0700:D-2		D-2	0	0.71	1.12	1.49	2.63

[a] Concentration in ppm.
[b] Cakes entered February 11, 1980 (day 0).

Observations were taken twice daily on snail mortality. Snails appearing dead were placed in a holding tank. Those which recovered within 24 hr were returned to the tank containing the Bayluscide® source. A record of snail deaths is given in Table 16. All snails exposed to cakes containing Bayluscide® died within 9 days. Snails exposed to controls did not die, indicating that the Dowicide® release was not sufficient to kill snails and that the protein preparations are not toxic to snails.

Water was assayed periodically for Bayluscide® concentration. Table 17 gives initial weights of all samples and concentration of Bayluscide® in tank water as a function of time.

Bayluscide® assays taken on days 3, 4, 8, and 16 are plotted for each tank in Figure 6. Assays for tanks C_1 and C_2 and D_1 and D_2 agree well. Tanks B_1 and B_2 give divergent results. Between days 8 and 16 concentrations observed in tanks C_1, C_2, D_1 and D_2 were quite similar. A mean maximum concentration of 2.69 ppm was reached in 16 days (tanks D_1 and D_2); in 8 days the mean concentration in those tanks was 1.37, about half as great.

Snail kill as a function of concentration is shown in Figure 7. Beneath the concentration axis is given the mortality observed in each tank as a function of concentration. The solid

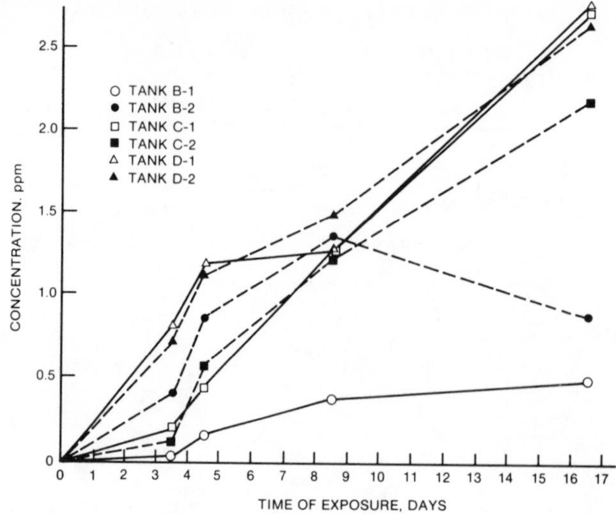

FIGURE 6. Bayluscide® concentration in aquaria containing *Marisa cornu ariesta*.

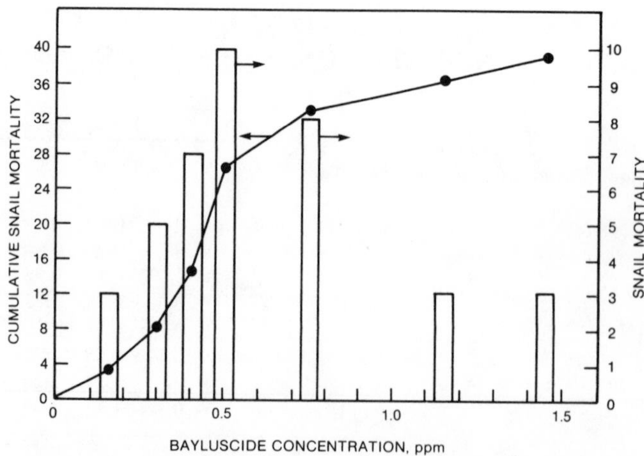

FIGURE 7. Mortality of snails *(Marisa cornu ariesta)* as a function of Bayluscide® concentration.

line gives cumulative kill (left vertical axis). The vertical bars give kills observed at the indicated concentrations (right vertical axis).

Figure 7 does not indicate time to reach effective concentrations. This can be judged from Table 16. The majority of deaths in tanks D_1 and D_2 (cakes 07300-D) occur on day 3, before those in tanks C_1 and C_2 (cakes 07300C), day 4. The majority of deaths in tank B_1 occur between days 5 through 8. This is in accord with the Bayluscide® content of cakes 07300-B, -C, and -D ($B < C < D$). Tank B_2 reached killing doses early because this cake releases Bayluscide® more rapidly.

The maximum kill rate occurs at Bayluscide® concentrations between 0.40 to 0.50 ppm, suggesting that for this species a higher concentration would not be required.

VI. RESULTS OF TESTING AT NEW ENGLAND AQUARIUM

A. Description of Test Procedures

The activity of various preparations is being tested on three species of schistosomiasis vectors. These molluscs are *Biomphalaria glabrata, Bulinus truncatus,* and *Oncomelania hupensis quadrasi.* All snails were bred and raised under the direction of Drs. Harold L. Asch and Yung-San Liang of the Lowell Research Foundation, Lowell, Mass., and were shipped directly to the New England Aquarium (NEA), Boston, Mass. Tests at NEA were conducted by Mr. Al Barker and Mr. Guy McCleod, Director of Research at NEA.

On receipt at NEA the snails were placed in new, 1-gal plastic buckets with filter Boston city water to remove organic matter and inorganic impurities. Snails were acclimatized in these, and if no unusual mortality was observed within 24 hr, experiments were begun. New buckets were required for each test because it was found that Bayluscide® was reversibly absorbed by the plastic and would leach out in clean water. This was discovered shortly after the program was begun; snails acclimatized in previously used buckets died rapidly. Analysis of the water confirmed the presence of Bayluscide® leachate. Buckets were also aerated because degradation of the protein matrices depleted the oxygen content of the water.

Each preparation was tested in triplicate; each of three identical samples was placed in separate 1-gal buckets 24 hr after the introduction of 10 snails into each bucket.

Usually several preparations were tested simultaneously. Testing schedules are given in Tables 18 and 19. Each test was scheduled to run for a maximum of 2 weeks. If all snails died before this time, the test was discontinued. Buckets were checked daily for dead snails. Those whose deaths were in question were allowed a 24-hr period for recuperation. If they revived, the snail was again placed in the test bucket.

Each group of simultaneous tests was accompanied by a control of 30 snails; 3 groups of 10 snails were held in the 1-gal plastic buckets, but were not exposed to any preparation. These controls served as a check on the effect of factors other than preparation toxicity such as water temperature variation, water quality, etc. No unexpected mortality has been observed in these controls.

The purpose of these tests is to evaluate the toxic effect of these preparations as well as the duration of the effect. To determine the latter the following procedure was used. After each exposure of snails to samples, samples were removed and stored in running tap water for a minimum of 2 weeks prior to retesting. Procedures for retesting were identical with those used for the initial tests.

Multiple testing of each sample was conducted with mollusc populations classified as either juvenile or adult. This was done in order to determine if these age groups displayed different sensitivity to the active agent.

Several experiments were conducted with water constantly flowing through the buckets. All others were static. Finally, in one case for each species, autoclaved Wisconsin silt was added to the bucket to observe whether Bayluscide® would be strongly absorbed.

Tables 18 and 19 summarize experimental design and results for *Biomphalaria* and *Bulinus*. The first column in each table is a code designation for compositions tested. Compositions C1 to C4 are controls, protein matrices containing no active agent. Compositions B1 to B6 are matrices containing Bayluscide®, and composition M1 is the only composition containing copper sulfate.

The second column gives the number of cakes of each composition added to each bucket.

Entries in the third column indicate whether the test was conducted under static conditions, indicated as S, or under flow through conditions, F. The one experiment with each species performed under static conditions with silt added to the bucket is indicated by the entry S/S.

The following columns are headed by the dates on which experiments were initiated or terminated. The entries are horizontal bars indicating the duration. Bars are broken by the

Table 18
BIOMPHILARIA TEST SCHEDULE AND RESULTS

Formula	No. of cakes	Test	5/19 6/2	6/16[a] 6/30	7/14 7/28	8/11 8/25	9/8 9/22	10/6 10/20	11/3 11/17
B4	1	S	3—4 days —J—	1 day —A—		1 day —J—	1 day —A—		
B4	4	S	1—2 days —J—		1 day —A—		1 day —A—		
B1	1	S	2—3 days —J—	1 day —A—	1 day —A—				
B3	1	S	3 days —J—	1 day —A—	1 day —J—				
M1	1	S	2 days —J—	2 days —A—	2 days —J—				
B6	4	S/S	2 days —J—	1 day —A—					
C1	1	S	3 dead in 2 weeks —J—						
B6	1	S		1—2 days —A—		1 day —J—	1 day —A—		
B4	4	F		1—2 days —A—		1 day —J—		1 day —J—	
B6	4	F			1 day —J—		1 day —A—		1 day —A—
B5	1	S			1 day —J—	1 day —A—	1 day —A—		

Note: A, adult; J, juvenile; F, flow through; S, static; S/S, static with silt.

[a] Tests scheduled for 6/16 were run on 7/28.

Table 19
BULINUS TEST SCHEDULE AND RESULTS

Formula	No. of cakes	Test	6/2 6/16	6/30 7/14	7/28 8/11	8/25 9/8	9/22 10/6	10/20 11/3
B3	1	S	1 day —J—	1 day —J—	1 day —A—			
B2	1	S	1 day —J—	1 day —A—	1 day —A—			
M1	1	S	1 day —J—	1 day —A—	6 days —J—			
B6	4	S	1 day —J—		1 day —A—		1 day —J—	
C2	1	S		1—2 dead in 14 days —J—				
B6	4	S/S		1 day —A—		1 day —J—		
B4	1	S			1 day —A—	1 day —J—		1 day —A—
B5	1	S			1 day —A—	1 day —J—	1 day —A—	
B4	4	F			1 day —A—	1 day —J—		1 day —A—
B6	4	F				1 day —J—		1 day —A—
C4	1	S					4 dead in 14 days —A—	

Note: A, adult; J, juvenile; F, flow through; S, static; S/S, static with silt.

Table 20
COMPOSITION OF SAMPLES TESTED AT NEW ENGLAND AQUARIUM

Code designation[a]	Fish protein[b]	Formaldehyde[c]	Glutaraldehyde wash[d]	BRL-1100[e]	Hydrated copper sulfate	Bayluscide® 70% wettable powder
C-1	100	1.0	No	—	—	—
C-2	100	1.0	Yes	—	—	—
C-3	100	1.0	No	20	—	—
C-4	100	1.0	Yes	20	—	—
M-1	100	1.0	Yes	20	50	—
B-1	100	1.0	No	—	—	50
B-2	100	1.0	Yes	—	—	25
B-3	100	1.0	Yes	—	—	50
B-4	100	1.0	No	20	—	50
B-5	100	1.0	Yes	5	—	50
B-6	100	1.0	Yes	20	—	50

[a] C, control samples; m, copper sulfate; B, Bayluscide®.
[b] All compositions are based on 100 parts of modified fish protein (Lepage's) measured as dry weight.
[c] Values (mℓ) of 37% aqueous formaldehyde.
[d] Refers to treatment of formaldehyde-gelled samples with a wash of 20% aqueous glutaraldehyde.
[e] Phenolic plastic resin (Union Carbide) to increase water resistance.

letters J or A which indicate whether experiments were conducted with juveniles or adults of the species. Entries over each bar summarize results to date. These will be discussed in Section VI.C.

B. Sample Composition

Samples were prepared as follows. Lepage's fish-derived protein (12 g) (~50% solids) was weighed into aluminum weighing dishes of ~2 in. diameter. The dry weight of protein, 6 g is used as the basis for reporting composition in Table 20; i.e., 6 g of protein, dry weight, is indicated as 100 parts.

In some cases a phenolic resin, BRL-1100, supplied by Union Carbide, was added. After polymerization, BRL-1100 is insoluble in water. The purpose of adding the resin was to increase water resistance.

The active agent was added next. Six formulas incorporating Bayluscide®, 70% wettable powder (Bayer), were prepared. One formula included hydrated copper sulfate instead of Bayluscide®. In each case the active agent was added dry and stirred into the protein dispersion until evenly mixed.

Four control samples were prepared omitting the active agents. Two of these contained BRL-1100.

After compounding, 1.0 mℓ of 37% aqueous formaldehyde was added with stirring. Samples were then allowed to gel for at least an hour. Water resistance was increased in some cases by washing the gelled cakes with 20% aqueous glutaraldehyde. This treatment was given to two of the four controls as well as to five of the seven preparations containing active agents. Sample compositions are listed in Table 20.

C. Results

Daily observations of conditions including pH, temperature, and dissolved oxygen (DO) are kept on separate sheets. Records of snail mortality are summarized in Tables 18 and 19. Above each bar is indicated the time in days required for all snails in each of the three replicates to die.

Samples can be classified as those which contain Bayluscide®, those with copper sulfate, and controls containing neither agent. Effectiveness of preparations as judged by the time required to kill is in the order: Bayluscide® > copper sulfate ≫ control. Note that in no case did significant deaths occur among snails exposed to controls. Deaths occurring in 2 weeks were 3, 2, and 5 out of 30 for snails exposed to controls C1, C2, and C3.

After 8 weeks in water, M1 samples required 2 days to kill 30 juvenile *Biomphalaria* and 6 days to kill 30 juvenile *Bulinus*.

Bayluscide®-containing preparations kept in water for an equal time required only 1 day for total kill.

D. Recommendation

The testing program is now complete for *Biomphalaria* and *Bulinus*. Results to date indicate that biodegradable protein matrices incorporating high loadings of Bayluscide® are a feasible means for controlling fresh water molluscs.

Duration of toxic effect and longevity of the preparations are the parameters by which to select a preparation for field testing. Thus, for duration of toxicity all Bayluscide® preparations studied thus far may be considered greater than the following times: B1 > 10 weeks; B2 > 10 weeks; B3 > 10 weeks; B4 > 18 weeks; B5 > 10 weeks; and B6 > 18 weeks. There is no reason to suppose that all preparations would not last as long as B4; the times indicated are simply the period of observation.

Based on rates of degradation reported earlier, samples washed with glutaraldehyde following the gelation reaction degrade more slowly. Glutaraldehyde treatment is more effective in retarding degradation than is addition of phenolic resin.

We therefore recommend for field trial formula B3. This contains a high loading of Bayluscide® (50 weight percent) and has a postgelation treatment with glutaraldehyde.

VII. RELEASE RATES AND DEGRADATION RATES EXHIBITED BY SAMPLES HELD IN LONG-TERM STORAGE

A. Degradation

Samples described earlier were held in storage at 30°C under both dry and moist conditions. These were removed after 7 months; no visible deterioration was observed. These samples were then subjected to measurement of Bayluscide® release rates and extent of degradation. Each cake was placed in 3.5 ℓ of distilled water. Bayluscide® concentration was measured periodically over a 50-day exposure period. Cakes were weighed prior to these measurements, and then afterward brought to constant weight to determine total weight loss. Results are reported in Table 21.

After removal from storage but before testing, all samples showed a slight weight loss over the 7 months. Nos. 07729:1-8 had lost an average of 3.3% and nos. 07729:9-16 a mean of 4.1%. Nos. 1-8 had been washed with glutaraldehyde.

Total mean weight loss after 50 days immersion for samples washed with glutaraldehyde was 11.53%, which when calculated as a daily rate is 0.23%/day. This agrees with the degradation rate calculated for the samples prepared immediately before testing. Again, the slightly slower rate observed in this series of tests reflects the lower bacterial population in the water bath.

Samples not washed with glutaraldehyde (nos. 07729:9-12 and 13-16) degraded somewhat more rapidly, as would be expected. Nos. 9-12, containing 0.05 pph Dowicide®, lost a mean of 14.70% in 50 days, a rate of 0.29%/day. Those not containing Dowicide® (nos. 13-16) lost a mean of 19.5%, a rate of 0.39%/day. Because both groups exhibited rather large standard deviations from the mean; these differences are probably not significant.

Table 21
DEGRADATION OF STORED SAMPLES

Sample[a]	Initial weight[b]	Weight before testing[c]	Weight after testing	Weight loss (%)[d]	Mean weight loss ± S.D. (%)
07729-1	7.92	7.6716	6.7670	11.8	11.53 ± 0.85
07729-2	7.82	7.5697	6.6132	12.6	
07729-3	7.79	7.5780	6.7550	10.9	
07729-4	7.65	7.4414	6.6399	10.8	
07729-5	7.86	7.5920	6.7102	11.6	11.53 ± 0.38
07729-6	7.86	7.5781	6.6972	11.6	
07729-7	7.80	7.4481	6.6673	11.0	
07729-8	7.75	7.4845	6.5920	11.9	
07729-9	7.22	6.0972	5.4340	10.9	14.70 ± 4.04
07729-10	7.30	7.0877	5.6448	20.4	
07729-11	7.26	7.0898	6.1371	13.4	
07729-12	7.20	7.0103	6.0195	14.1	
07729-13	7.32	7.1500	5.4560	23.7	19.58 ± 3.57
07729-14	7.32	7.1133	5.7590	19.0	
07729-15	7.15	6.9690	5.9156	15.1	
07729-16	7.26	7.0608	5.6104	20.5	

[a] Samples 1 to 8 were washed with glutaraldehyde. Samples 1 to 4 and 9 to 12 contained 0.05 pph Dowicide®. Samples 1, 2, 5, 6, 9, 10, 13, and 14 were stored dry, the remainder moist. All samples contained 25 pph Bayluscide® 70% WP.

[b] Weights before storage. All weights reported in grams.

[c] Weights after removal from storage, before testing.

[d] Calculated on basis of weights before testing.

B. Release Rate Experiments

Release of Bayluscide® was followed by high performance liquid chromatography (HPLC). Bayluscide® concentrations over the 50-day period are reported in Table 22. Mean values for each of the four formulations represented in Table 22 are plotted in Figures 8 through 11. Formulae are given in Table 21 of report no. 2068. Samples washed with glutaraldehyde (nos. 07729:1-8) released 9.99 ± 0.36% in 50 days (0.20%/day). Since each sample contained 25 pph of Bayluscide®, the weight of Bayluscide® in each cake is 1.56 g. Thus, the weight of Bayluscide® lost in the 50 days is 1.56 g × 0.0999 = 0.156 g. The mean total weight loss for samples 07729:1-8, the glutaraldehyde-washed samples, is 0.8202 ± 0.078 (S.D.) g. This release of Bayluscide® accounts for 156/820 or ~19% of the total weight loss.

VIII. CONFIRMATION OF RELEASE RATES AND DEGRADATION RATES EXHIBITED BY FORMULA B3G

A. Degradation Rates

Three samples of formula B3 were prepared for confirmation of both release and degradation rates. Formula B3 is the preparation recommended for field trials, and therefore it was judged necessary to demonstrate reproducibility of the results previously reported. In common with the other formulae tested, B3 has a specific gravity between 1.1 and 1.3 when dry, and in some cases tends to float when swollen with water. To overcome this problem, aquarium gravel was added while processing. The weight of gravel was approximately 30% of the total dry weight of final product. This recipe will be referred to as B3G. Formula B3G has the following composition: 12.0 g Lepage's Fish Glue, 50 weight percent solids; 3.0 Bayluscide® 70 WP (50 pph); 1.0 mℓ 35° aqueous HCHO; and 4.0 g gravel, followed by 30-min wash in 20% aqueous glutaraldehyde after gelation.

Table 22
CUMULATIVE PERCENT RELEASE OF BAYLUSCIDE® FROM STORED CAKES

Sample	Days exposure to distilled water							Mean % release
no.	4	7	14	21	30	42	50	± S.D. at day 50
07729-1	<0.1	0.1	0.7	1.5	2.7	6.8	9.7	x = 9.75
07729-2	<0.1	0.2	0.6	1.6	2.8	6.7	10.1	S = ±0.29
07729-3	<0.1	0.1	0.6	1.4	2.8	6.6	9.8	Rate = 0.20%/day
07729-4	<0.1	0.1	0.6	1.3	2.7	7.1	9.4	
07729-5	<0.1	0.1	0.7	1.3	2.8	6.9	10.2	x = 10.23
07729-6	<0.1	0.1	0.7	1.7	2.9	6.9	10.5	S = ±0.29
07729-7	<0.1	0.2	0.7	1.6	2.7	7.0	9.9	Rate = 0.21%/day
07729-8	<0.1	0.1	0.6	1.6	2.8	6.8	10.3	
07729-9	<0.1	0.1	0.8	1.5	2.9	6.9	11.1	x = 11.58
07729-10	<0.1	0.2	0.7	1.4	2.8	6.9	11.7	S = ±0.55
07729-11	<0.1	0.2	0.7	1.6	2.8	7.2	11.2	Rate = 0.23%/day
07729-12	<0.1	0.2	0.7	1.5	3.0	7.4	12.3	
07729-13	<0.1	0.3	0.8	1.5	3.1	7.4	11.5	x = 11.8
07729-14	<0.1	0.2	0.8	1.6	2.7	7.3	12.1	S = ±0.29
07729-15	<0.1	0.2	0.7	1.5	2.9	7.7	12.0	Rate = 0.24%/day
07729-16	<0.1	0.1	0.6	1.7	2.8	6.9	11.6	

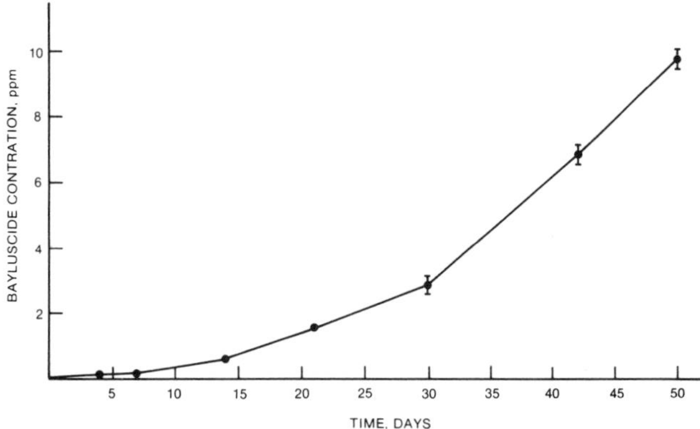

FIGURE 8. Bayluscide® release from samples 07729:1-4.

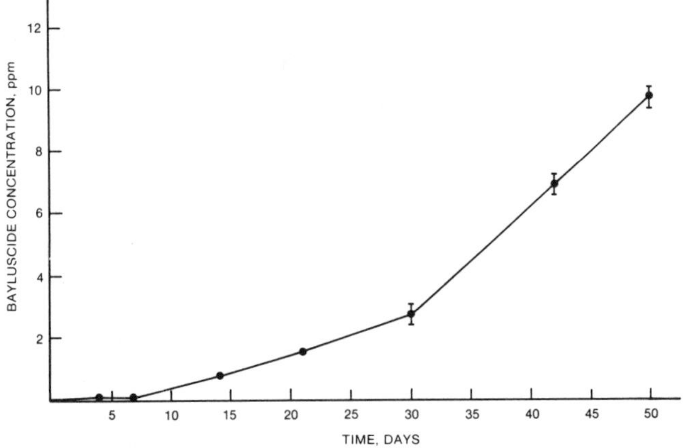

FIGURE 9. Bayluscide® release from samples 07729:5-8.

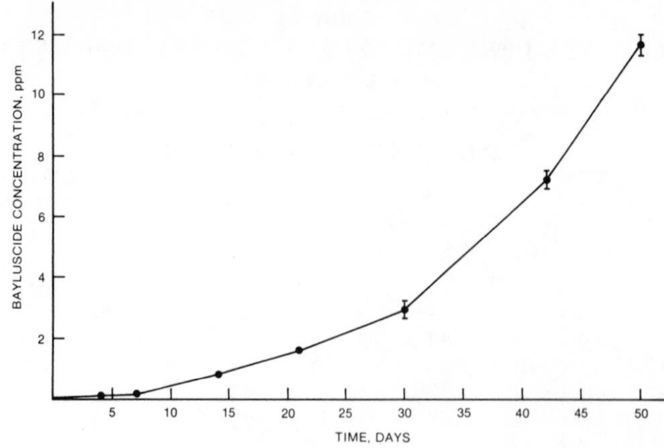

FIGURE 10. Bayluscide® release from samples 07729:9-12.

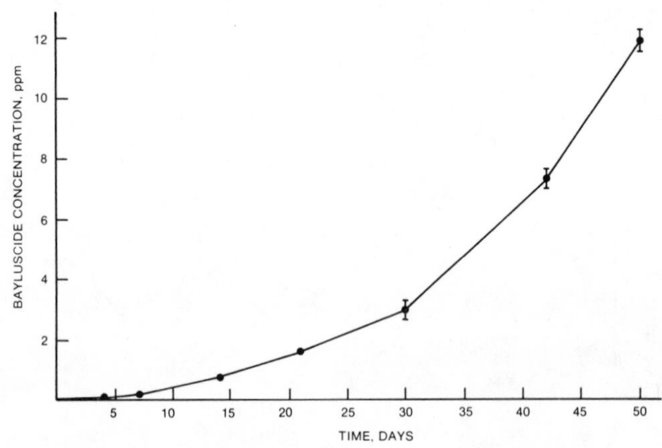

FIGURE 11. Bayluscide® release from samples 07729:13-16.

Each of the samples of B3G was placed in 3.5 ℓ of distilled water. Analyses were made by HPLC of Bayluscide® release over a period of 50 days. After 50 days, the samples were removed and brought to constant weight for measurement of degradative loss. Results are as indicated in Table 23.

The calculated weight loss includes loss of both matrix material and Bayluscide®. Mean weight loss is 1.0733 g as shown in Section VIII.B. Bayluscide® loss is 10.1% of the initial loading or 0.3 g. Thus, Bayluscide® weight loss accounts for ~28% of the total weight loss.

The rate of weight loss over the 50-day test period is based on weights excluding gravel. This weight loss is 11.6/50 = 0.23 ± 0.01%/day in distilled water. This is somewhat slower than those reported for the glutaraldehyde-washed samples in Dynatech Report No. 2068. Those samples were exposed to pond water containing a bacterial population; over an 8-week period, mean degradation weight losses for three types of glutaraldehyde-washed samples were 17.1, 23.1 and 28.6%. The mean daily rate of degradation is therefore 0.41%/day. The slightly slower rate observed in the current tests is due to the use of distilled rather than pond water.

Table 23
DEGRADATION OF FORMULATION B3G

Sample no.	Initial weight (g)	Final weight (g)	Weight loss (g)	Loss (%)[a]	Loss (%)[b]
07750-21/6	13.2773	12.1440	1.1333	8.5	12.2
07750-22/7	13.2916	12.1981	1.0935	8.2	11.8
07750-23/8	13.1342	12.1410	0.9932	7.6	10.9
Mean values	13.2344 ± 0.0870	12.1610 ± 0.0321	1.0733 ± 0.0722	8.1 ± 0.5	11.6 ± 0.7

[a] Percent loss calculated in total dry weight including gravel.
[b] Percent loss calculated in dry weight excluding gravel.

Table 24
RELEASE OF BAYLUSCIDE® FROM FORMULATION B3G

Sample no.	Cumulative percent release of Bayluscide®: day 4	7	14	21	30	42	50	Mean percent release at 50 days ± S.D.
07750-21/6	<0.1	0.2	0.8	1.8	2.9	7.7	9.8	x = 10.1
07750-22/7	<0.1	0.2	0.8	1.9	3.2	7.8	10.1	S = ±0.25
07750-23/8	<0.1	0.3	0.9	1.8	3.0	7.7	10.3	Rate = 0.2%/day
				Controls				
07750-17	<0.1	<0.1	<0.1	<0.1	<0.1	<0.1	<0.1	Control
07705-18	<0.1	<0.1	<0.1	<0.1	<0.1	<0.1	<0.1	Control

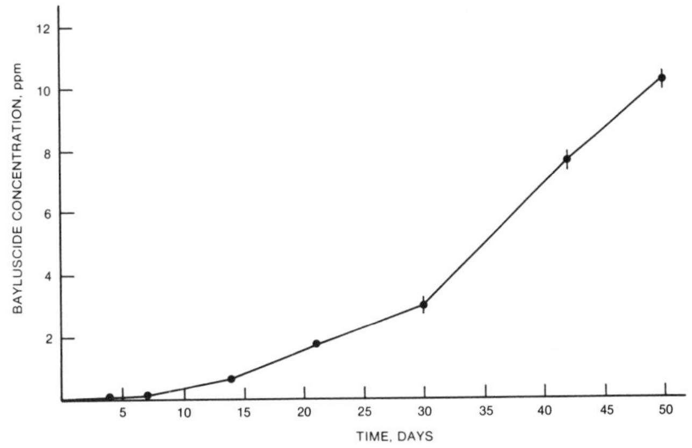

FIGURE 12. Confirmation of release rate for formulation B3G.

B. Rate of Bayluscide® Release From B3G

Weekly measurements of Bayluscide® release from samples 07750-21/6, -22/7, and -23/8 were performed by the HPLC analysis described previously. Over the 50-day interval, the three samples had released 10.1 ± 0.25% (S.D.) of the initial Bayluscide®. Mean daily release is therefore 0.20%/day which agrees closely with results presented in Report No. 2068. Data are given in Table 24 and illustrated in Figure 12.

Table 25
BAYLUSCIDE® CONCENTRATION AS A FUNCTION OF TIME IN STATIC AND FLOW-THROUGH TESTS AT NEW ENGLAND AQUARIUM

I. Flow-Through Tests (New Cakes, Formula B3)

	Concentration (pph)			
Time (hr)	**Tank 1**	**Tank 2**	**Tank 3**	**Control**
2	<0.05	<0.05	<0.05	<0.05
4	<0.05	<0.05	<0.05	<0.05
8	<0.05	<0.05	<0.05	<0.05
24	0.3	0.1	0.1	<0.05
48	6.6	0.7	1.2	<0.05
72	4.2	2.1	2.1	<0.05

II. Static Tests, Formula B3; Cakes Immersed in Water for 36 Days Prior to Tests

	Concentration (pph)			
Time (hr)	**Tank 3**	**Tank 4**	**Tank 5**	**Control**
24	6.3	5.6	6.8	<0.05
58	6.5	6.5	7.9	<0.05
72	8.5	7.5	6.8	13.7
168	13.7	10.2	11.6	<0.05

The calculated weight loss includes loss of both matrix material and Bayluscide®. The mean total weight loss is 1.07 g. As shown in Section VIII.B, Bayluscide® loss is 10.1% of the initial loading or 0.30 g. Thus, Bayluscide® weight loss accounts for approximately 28% of the total weight loss.

IX. LABORATORY TESTS OF SUSTAINED RELEASE PREPARATION B3 (B3G) ON *ONCOMELANIA*

A. HPLC Analysis of Bayluscide® Concentration as a Function of Time in *Oncomelania* Tests

Tests using cakes of formulation B3 were conducted on *Oncomelania hupensis* as described earlier. One cake containing 3.0 g of Bayluscide® was used in each test. Test were conducted in 4.0-ℓ tanks.

Bayluscide® concentration was monitored by HPLC under both static and flow-through conditions. Cakes used in static tests (both containing Bayluscide® and controls) had been continuously immersed for 36 days prior to tests and had been tested on *Oncomelania*.

Cakes used in flow-through experiments had not been previously used and had received only the usual 3-day pretrial wash. Data are presented in Table 25 for convenience (these data have been previously reported in Section II, Tables 2 and 4).

Release rates may be calculated for the cakes used in the static experiments. In 168 hr (7 days) concentration in these tanks increased to 13.7, 10.2, and 11.6 ppm giving a mean of 11.83 ± 1.76 (S.D.) ppm. Since each cake contains 3.0 g of Bayluscide®, and tank volumes are 3.79 ℓ, the mean daily percent release may be calculated as follows:

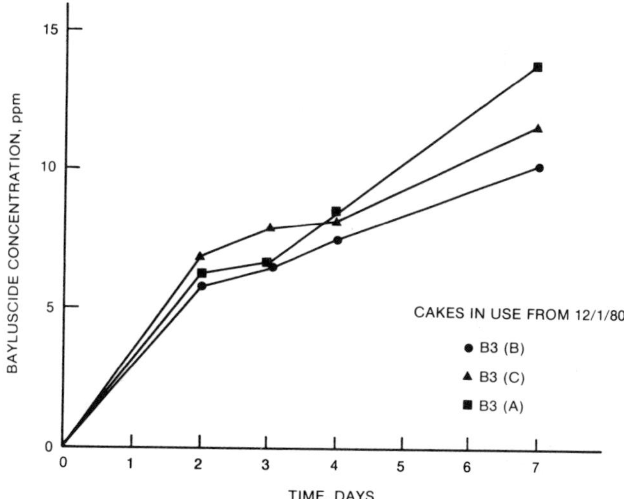

FIGURE 13. Bayluscide® concentration in static tests with used cakes on *Oncomelania hupensis quadrasi* (1/5/81).

$$\text{Mean percent release/day} = \frac{(11.83\ \text{ppm})\left(0.001\ \dfrac{\text{g}/\ell}{\text{ppm}}\right)(4.0\ \ell)}{(7\ \text{days})\ (3.0\ \text{g})} \times 100$$

$$= 0.23\%/\text{day}$$

This agrees very well with previously reported release rates of ~2.0%/day for glutaraldehyde-washed preparations. Reproducibility of release rates is thus clearly demonstrated.

Flow-through tests were also conducted in 4.0-ℓ tanks. Flow rate was maintained at ~40 ℓ/day (i.e., 10 turnovers per day). Release rates in tanks 2 and 3 are not measurable due to flow conditions; concentrations are seen to build up more slowly than in the static tests. This is due not only to constant removal of Bayluscide®, but also to the initially slow release generally exhibited by new samples during the first several days of exposure.

Concentrations may be correlated with snail kill. All snails subject to static tests died within 1 day of exposure to the cakes. The measured mean concentration after 24 hr in the three tanks was 6.2 ± 0.6 (S.D.) ppm. Thus, this represents an upper limit to the required concentration. Snails subject to flow-through conditions died within 2 to 3 days after exposure. Measured concentrations in the three flow-through tanks were 0.7, 1.2, and 6.6 ppm. Thus, concentrations as low as 0.7 ppm may be sufficient for control.

Figures 13 and 14 reproduce the data for the static and flow-through tests.

B. Results of Laboratory Tests on *Oncomelania*

Test methods for determining the effectiveness of the Bayluscide®/protein matrices on *Oncomelania* were conducted as previously reported except that screens were placed just under the water surface to prevent the snails from leaving the water. Formula B3 was lethal to both juvenile and adults within 1 day. Control cakes, containing no Bayluscide®, resulted in no deaths over the 2-week period of observation.

Tests on B3 under flow conditions (10 turnover volumes per day) also were successful; both juveniles and adults died in 2 to 3 days of exposure.

Care was taken to insure that snails were dead. Loss of opercula and decomposition of the body were obvious signs. When death was uncertain, snails were gently prodded to

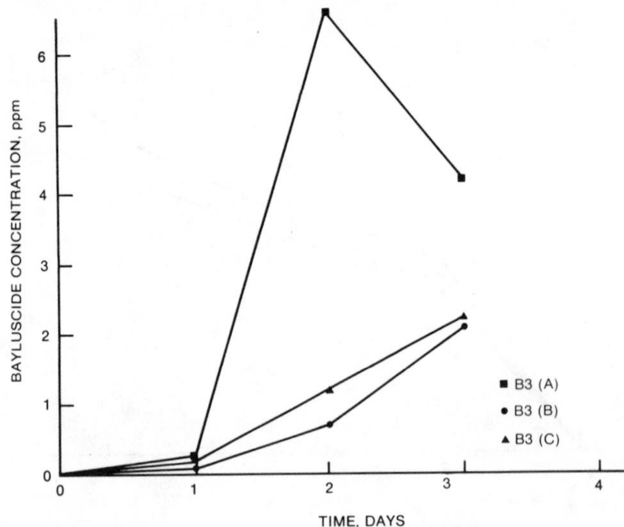

FIGURE 14. Bayluscide® concentration in flow-through tests with new cakes (12/16/80) on *Oncomelania hupensis quadrasi.*

stimulate motion. These were also restored to fresh water for recovery. No recoveries were observed.

Table 26 summarizes results of *Oncomelania* tests to date. A second round of testing on *Oncomelania* was conducted with two changes in protocol. First, each tank was equipped with a plastic board, one end of which was immersed in the water. A strip of filter paper was laid on this, its lower end immersed so that it remained moist. This device permitted snails to leave the water if the environment became intolerable.

The second change involved addition of some gravel to the B3 formula. This increased the density of the cake so that when water swollen they will not float. Table 26 summarizes the tests and their results. In these tables the formulation is indicated as B3G (G = gravel included in B3 formula).

Tests were also conducted on *Oncomelania* restricted to an environment of mud. The mud had been sterilized prior to use as described in the report of the New England Aquarium. Pellets of B3G were placed in petri dishes containing the autoclaved mud so that either 2.5 or 12.8% of the total surface was occupied by the pellets.

From the results presented in Table 26, it is evident that preparations B3 and B3G demonstrated continued efficacy against *Oncomelania* at both life stages (juvenile, adult) even after long exposure to water.

ACKNOWLEDGMENTS

This work was carried out under the sponsorship of the World Health Organization (WHO Contract Reference T16-181-B2-57 and Dynatech Report No. 2068 and Addendum). The guidance of Dr. Kenneth E. Mott, Secretary, Steering Committee of the Scientific Working Group on Schistosomiasis, is acknowledged with appreciation.

Table 26
SUMMARY OF LABORATORY TESTS ON *ONCOMELANIA*

Formulation	Conditions	Age	12/1	12/15	1/5	1/19	2/2	2/23	3/9
B3	1S caged	J	1 day[a]		1 day				
B3	1S caged	A	1 day		1 day				
—	0S caged	J	No deaths		No deaths				
—	0S caged	A	No deaths		No deaths				
B3	1F caged	J		2 days		2 days			
B3	1F caged	A		3 days		2 days			
—	0F caged	J		No deaths		No deaths			
—	0F caged	A		No deaths		No deaths			
C2	1S caged	J			No deaths 1st 4 days				
C2	1S caged	A			No deaths 1st 4 days				
B3G	1S escape	J					2 days		
B3G	1S escape	A					No deaths		
—	0S escape	J					No deaths		
—	0S escape	A					2 days		
—	MUD (0)[b]	J						2 dead — 9 days	5 dead — 2 days
B3G	MUD (12.8)	J						9 days	
—	MUD (0)	A						No deaths	1 dead — 4 days
B3G	MUD (12.8)	A						4 days	
B3G	MUD (2.5)	J							2 days
B3G	MUD (2.5)	A							4 days

[a] Each entry indicates the days to 100% mortality or as otherwide indicated.
[b] Numbers refer to percent of mud surface occupied by pellets of B3G.

REFERENCE

1. **Khan and Trothier,** *Appl. Environ. Microbiol.*, 35, 6, 1978.

Chapter 7

SUSTAINED RELEASE HERBICIDES

Donald L. Wise

TABLE OF CONTENTS

I. BACKGROUND

There has been continued success in developing new and more effective herbicides since World War II. As this technology has become more sophisticated, development costs have risen, making these vital chemicals more expensive. At the same time the progressive development of increasingly more complex and toxic chemical herbicides has raised concern about the impact of these active substances on the environment. An increase in regulations with respect to government use has resulted. With rising costs and increasingly restrictive regulations regarding the application of herbicides there arose a need for more effective systems for delivery of herbicides to meet government needs. The significance of an effective, long-term, environmentally acceptable herbicide system is clearly recognized.

A. Background on Sustained Release Herbicide Systems

The concept of integrating a biologically active herbicide into a carrier was originated with experimental studies on herbicides impregnated in clay granules by Danielson of the U.S. Department of Agriculture (USDA). The object of impregnating an inert carrier with a herbicide was to achieve physical selectivity such that postemergence application on growing crops could be carried out rather than solely by preemergence spray applications on the soil. This granular application of herbicide was shown to have essentially the same weed-killing potency obtained with spray applications. It is clear that the mechanism for herbicide release to the soil was by extraction with soil moisture and rainwater. The inert material used initially was granular Fuller's earth (Attaclay), and later trials were made with activated charcoal, perlite, vermiculite, pyrophyllite, and tobacco pulp.

Steward has pointed out[2] that research by the U.S. Department of Agriculture at Fort Lauderdale on the use of herbicide carrier materials for control of aquatic plants has been in progress since 1964. Basically, there have been two main types of sustained release granular herbicides: either sinking granules which release the herbicide near the bottom for the control of submerged plants, or floating granules which release the herbicide at the water surface for control of floating and emerged vegetation. A comprehensive review of this work and other novel approaches to aquatic plant control has been prepared by Guscio and Gangstad.[3]

The work of the Office of the Chief of Engineers, Department of the U.S. Army, is summarized through 1971.[3] Here aquatic plant control is the objective. Work has been directed towards biological or integrated systems of aquatic plant control.[4] Work has been with both chemical herbicides[5] and plant pathogens.[6] Since the water hyacinth, the aquatic plant most needing control, provides a suitable breeding ground for mosquitoes, it may be practical to consider controlled release of both a mosquito larvicide and an aquatic plant herbicide. A synergistic effect may be noted with such coupled control.

B. Background on Related Controlled Release Systems — Larvicides

The concept of integrating a larvicide into a carrier was initiated by Raley and Davis[7] with experimental studies on larvicides impregnated into a mixture of casting plaster and sawdust. This combination was cast as briquettes in a perforated metal can and used to control mosquito larvae in ponds and streams in the San Joaquin Valley of California. Later, Elliot[8] demonstrated that briquettes made of sand, cement, and larvicide provided effective larvae control for only 150 days. On the other hand, Laird[9] found larvicide-impregnated cement briquettes retained larvicidal properties after almost 5 years in the field but, by chromatographic analysis, found that 40 to 50% of the initial available larvicide remained in the briquettes after these 5 years in the field. More recently Barnes et al.[10] used three different types of briquettes to evaluate Abate® and Malathion®; these were commercial charcoal briquettes, casting plaster, and a commercial brand of ready-mix concrete and casting plaster.

Recently, attention has been directed towards polymeric formulations to provide slow release or controlled release of larvicides in water. Miles and Woehst[11] used both rigid and expanded (foamed) polyvinyl chloride (PVC) impregnated with abate. These workers thus demonstrated controlled release or diffusion of larvicide from a polymer. The formulations produced lethal concentrations to mosquito larvae in reservoirs for a period of 20 weeks. This work was followed very shortly by the laboratory evaluations of Whitlaw and Evans[12] using polymer pellets of PVC, polyurethane foam, and polyamide. Granular foam pellets, rigid pellets, and also emulsions were evaluated.

Later, experiments were carried out by Wilkinson et al.[13] using pellets of PVC, polyethylene, and charcoal granules containing a polymeric binder. This work[12,13] was the initial part of a continuing series of experiments carried out at the U.S. Army Environmental Hygiene Agency at Edgewood Arsenal, Aberdeen Proving Ground, Md. Further extensive work was carried out using the mosquito larvicides Dursban® and Abate® with the polymers PVC, polyethylene, and chlorinated polyethylene[14-16] While clearly demonstrating the potential of sustained release it was found that the nonbiodegradable polymers used did remain in the environment containing substantial portions of residual larvicide. This work of Wilkinson et al.[13] in addition to polymer evaluation, also considered the larvicide Abate®, Dursban®, Fenthion®, and Naled®.

Later Nelson and Whitlaw carried out experiments with ^{14}C labeled larvicides[17] in PVC pellets. Interestingly, Nelson and Miller[18] earlier found that concentration of larvicide in the PVC pellets had little effect on release rate. Miller et al.[19] also reported on microencapsulated formulations using a proprietary polymer.

Most significantly perhaps, the work of Miller at al.[20] showed that single applications of a slow release system maintained average residues above 0.9 ppb, the mosquito larvicidal level for a LC_{90} for 18 months.

Overall, the most significant design parameter was found by Nelson et al.[21] and also confirmed by Lawson et al.[22] to be surface-to-volume ratio. This work was carried out with chlorinated polyethylene pellets. On this basis trials were carried out in New Jersey and Arkansas.[23]

An alternative approach to the use of nonbiodegradable polymers for controlled release of larvicides is to dissolve the larvicide in a natural or synthetic rubber. This approach, part of a continuing program by Prof. N. F. Cardarelli of the University of Akron, Ohio has found application for specific larvicides,[24] herbicides to control aquatic plants,[25] and an array of pesticides.[26,27] Of particular interest is the stated reduction in required amounts of active chemical when released slowly.[26] A summary of Cardarelli's work has been presented.[27] Since the mechanism of this release system is also based on extraction by water of the active material dissolved in the rubber, the rubber particles will necessarily remain. Also, on the basis of this mechanism and following the work at Edgewood, substantial amounts of active chemical will in all probability therefore remain in the environment. Systems described by Cardarelli are based on rubbers having lifetimes on outdoor exposure of 4 to 10 years.

C. Need for Design of a Release System

In all of the above-cited work directly or indirectly related to sustained aquatic herbicide/algaecide release systems there is little, if any, flexibility for *designing* a specific dissolution rate. To be sure, a cement composition and physical configuration may be found to yield a particular release rate, and commercial nonbiodegradable plastics or rubbers can be tailored somewhat to yield a given release of dissolved material. What is most suitable is to have the flexibility to quite specifically design the herbicide delivery system. Moreover, this delivery system must be innocuous to the environment. Use of available equipment for manufacture and broadcasting is essential. The following describes a system for sustained release of aquatic herbicide. This system of compositions permits the design of the delivery rate with biodegradable polymer.

II. BASIS FOR BIODEGRADABLE POLYMER SELECTION

The technical basis which makes possible the proposal to prepare biodegradable polymer matrices capable of slowly releasing herbicides/larvicides is found in recent work on absorbable sutures. Long-standing dissatisfaction with catgut and other suture materials stimulated investigation of synthetic replacements, particularly materials which may be absorbed by the body without tissue reaction. Success in this search has been attained through utilization of polyglycolic acid for this purpose. A chemically similar material, polylactic acid, has found acceptance for use as a surgical repair material. The qualities which suit these materials for sutures and implants, namely absorbability and innocuousness, recommend them particularly as vehicles for other biologically active agents to be released. Here ready at hand, then, are thermoplastic polymers which will lend themselves to additive incorporation and which will dissipate acceptably in the environment. The following discussion outlines the nature of these materials.

Polyglycolic acid and polylactic acid are aliphatic polyesters formed from the two initial members of the family of α-hydroxy carboxylic acids. The polymerization is dependent on first forming the cyclic dimer, lactide or glycolide, of these materials. In the case of glycolic acid:

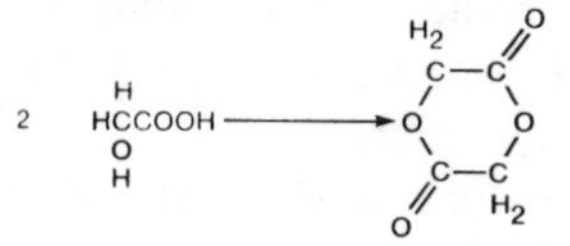

```
                           H2   O
                            C—C//
       H                   /    \
2    HCCOOH ————————————→ O      O
       O                   \    /
       H                    C—C
                          O//   H2
```

and with lactic acid:

```
                            CH3  O
                             C—C//
       H                    /    \
2  CH3CCOOH ————————————→  O      O
       O                    \    /
       H                     C—C
                           O//   CH3
```

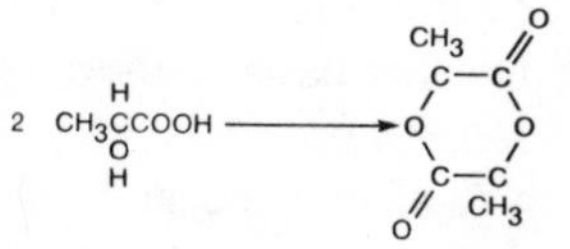

The lactide may be converted to the polymer through heating in the presence of a catalyst either in solution or in bulk. For example, the effectiveness of various catalysts and kinetics of glycolide polymerization has been summarized by Chujo et al.[28,29] Copolymers of glycolic acid and lactic acid may be prepared readily. These copolymers are linear polyesters which may be characterized by the general formula:

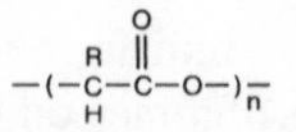

$$-(-\overset{R}{\underset{H}{C}}-\overset{O}{\overset{\|}{C}}-O-)_n-$$

Since lactic acid is optically active it is possible to prepare polylactic acid from both the DL- and L(+) forms. Kulkarni and co-workers[30,31] prepared both forms of polylactic acid for evaluation as surgical repair materials. Poly (DL-lactic acid) melts at 60°C and is amorphous. The L(+) polymer, on the other hand, is crystalline and melts at 170°C. In keeping with these qualities the L(+) polymer was observed to be dissolved more slowly by tissue fluids than the DL-polymer. Both lactic acid polymers were found to be free of tissue reaction upon implantation. In use as pins for fracture repair, poly(DL-lactic acid) functioned satisfactorily and had virtually disappeared from the fracture site after 8 months.[31] The D(−) form of lactic acid has been little studied in such applications because of the difficulty of obtaining the acid in this form.

Polyglycolic acid has found high favor as a suture material. From the standpoint of manufacturers, the material is easy to form as filaments, and surgeons have been enthusiastic about both its functional characteristics and the lack of interaction with tissue.[32-35] The polyglycolic acid is a crystalline polymer melting at about 225°C. In early animal studies, using isotopically labeled polyglycolic acid, it was shown[32] that the material is completely absorbed within 9 months following implantation. Upon further development it was found[35] that satisfactory sutures can be prepared from polyglycolic acid which is absorbed by animal tissues within 2 to 3 months.

The most probable mode of absorption of these polymers by tissue fluids is hydrolysis to the monomer acid, although it has been suggested[33] that esterase enzymes play a role. Since both lactic and glycolic acids are naturally present in the tissues mechanisms for their disposition are at hand, a factor which undoubtedly accounts in large degree for the lack of tissue reactivity. Indeed, the studies of polyglycolic acid sutures showed that the ultimate products of metabolism were excreted principally in the urine and as expired carbon dioxide, virtually none remaining in the tissues.

The chemistry of this family of polymers is not restricted to these two initial members of the α-hydroxy carboxylic acids. Higher acids also undergo the biomolecular esterification described above to form lactides. These in turn may be converted to the linear polyesters. It has been claimed that polymers may be prepared from acids as large as α-hydroxy stearic acid. It is also possible to prepare polyesters from β-hydroxy carboxylic acids. In this case the intermediate is the β-lactone. Both poly-β-hydroxy butyric acid and poly-β-hydroxy propionic acid have been evaluated as suture materials. In addition it will be appreciated that various substituents might be placed on side chains of the polyester in order to alter properties. Many copolymers are obviously possible. Thus, unexplored avenues for tailoring to obtain desired dissolution rates or physical nature appear available.

The experimental work of Walter Reed researchers with polylactic acid for surgical applications has emphasized the achieving of high mechanical strength with this polymer. The experimental work of Dynatech engineers (Dynatech R/D Company, Cambridge, Mass.), on the other hand, has been oriented toward design of a specific polymer dissolution rate when used as a matrix for biologically active material. Specifically, Dynatech engineers have made polylactic acid polymer starting from both the L(+) and DL forms of lactic acid. Proceeding by converting lactic acid to lactide and then to the polymer, significant differences in ultimate physical properties are noted with these two forms of lactic acid. Polyglycolic acid polymer has also been prepared starting from glycolic acid, and again converting to the glycolide before polymerization. Several catalysts as well as a range of catalyst concentrations have been used in preparation of these polymers. Techniques have been established for purification of the polymer and evaluation of physical properties. Moreover, practical molding techniques have been developed for preparation of conventional physical forms of the polymer. A technique for integrating the active agent into the polymer with loadings as high as 70 parts by weight of biologically active agent to 30 parts by weight polymer has been achieved. Evaluations of the release rates of these systems are achieved using H^3-labeled polymer and C^{14}-labeled active agent.

III. SUMMARY OF EXPERIMENTS AT USDA

Further support for the feasibility of a sustained release herbicide system based on a polylactic acid delivery system is given by recent experimental results with this technology. For this purpose the sodium salt of 2,4-D and the acid form of 2,4-D were incorporated into polylactic acid in several physical forms. These test samples were evaluated by the Agricultural Research Service, USDA, Beltsville, Md. This work was carried out on Project 4-5-72-D under the direction of Dr. L. L. Danielson of the USDA.

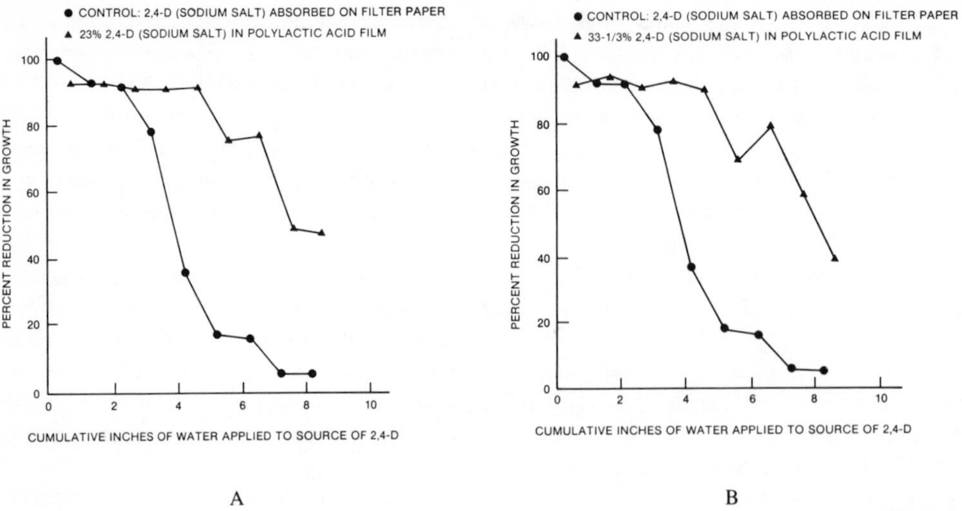

FIGURE 1. Extended provision of herbicide from a polylactic acid source. (A) 23% herbicide. (B) 33 1/3% herbicide.

A. Bioassay Test Procedure

In the initial feasibility tests, 2,4-D was incorporated into polylactic acid and cast into thin films of approximately 5-μm thickness. The thin film of herbicide/polymer was placed in a test tube between granular packing to maintain a continually moist environment. The test tube has a small opening cut in the bottom to permit throughput of water. Data were obtained by percolating successive portions of water, twice weekly, through the test tubes containing the herbicide source and then applying the extract to petri dishes in which mustard seedlings were cultured. The amount of water passing through the herbicide/polymer system and through the control (herbicide absorbed on filter paper was used) was calculated to be equivalent to that of approximately 4 in. of irrigation per week. The degree of growth reduction in the mustard seedlings served as a measurement of the effectiveness of the supply of herbicide. Specifically, the stem lengths of the then longest of 50 seedlings were measured. On the basis of this test it is seen that the polylactic acid/herbicide source prolonged herbicide delivery significantly.

B. Initial Experiments Using the Soluble 2,4-D Salt Form

Figure 1 shows how the polylactic acid/herbicide source prolonged the release of even the soluble sodium salt form of 2,4-D. In Figure 1A the herbicide is 23% by weight of the total sample (or 30 parts by weight herbicide to 100 parts by weight polymer), while in Figure 1B the herbicide is 33 1/3% by weight of the total sample (or 50 parts by weight herbicide to 100 parts by weight polymer). The experiments were conducted over a period of about 5 to 6 weeks, indicating that at this level of extractive exposure, effective lifetime is substantially enhanced beyond that of the control. The purpose of using the more water-soluble sodium salt form of 2,4-D was to establish as quickly as possible the feasibility of this sustained release concept.

C. Experiments Using the Acid Form of 2,4-D

Additional experiments were carried out using films of polymer/herbicide in which was incorporated the acid form of 2,4-D. It is of interest to note that the acid form of 2,4-D is completely soluble in polylactic acid at the concentrations used, forming a clear film of polymer/herbicide. By forming a solution, the acid form of 2,4-D may be considered to be

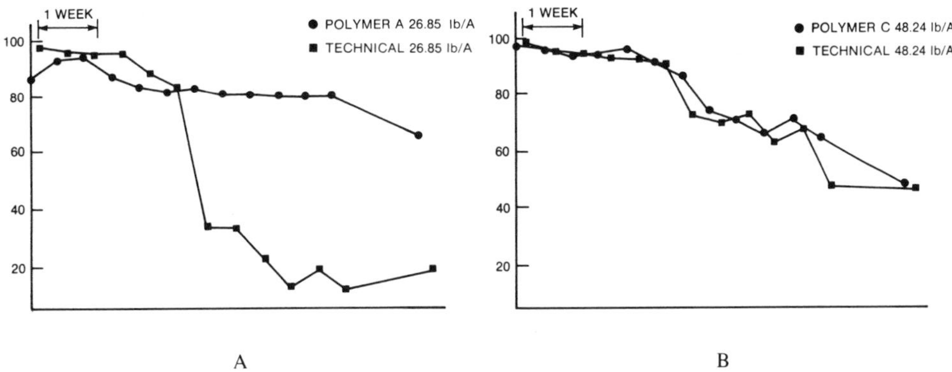

FIGURE 2. Sustained release of 2,4-D (acid) from films of a biodegradable polymer matrix. (A) Ratio of 10PHR (9.1% by weight) herbicide/polymer. (B) Ratio of 20PHR (16.7% by weight) herbicide/polymer.

molecularly dispersed in the polymer/herbicide matrix. On the other hand, the sodium salt of 2,4-D remained a finely divided dispersion of particles within the polymer/herbicide matrix. In Figure 2A is shown the release of the acid form of 2,4-D compared with the control over a period of about 8 weeks. It is interesting to note that after about 6 weeks the polymer/herbicide system was 80% effective, while the control had dropped to below 20% effectiveness. For this test (results in Figure 2A), the herbicide was 9.1% by weight of the total polymer/herbicide film (10 parts of herbicide to 100 parts of polymer). In Figure 2B is presented the results of a similar system releasing the acid form of 2,4-D with a herbicidal loading of 16.7% (20 parts herbicide to 100 parts of polymer). For this higher loading the herbicide release from the polymer/herbicide system follows that of the control. That is, release drops rather steadily and at the end of about 7 weeks the system is only 50% effective. Greater release rates are known to occur as the chemical loading of the polymer/chemical system is increased. It is surprising, however, that the control test in this experiment has such persistence; in all other tests the control had much less persistence than is shown in this experiment.

D. Experiments with Granular Clay

Based on the success of the feasibility tests using films of herbicide/polymer, samples of polymer and 2,4-D on granular clay were prepared and tested. The overall object of preparing the clay/polymer/herbicide system was that such a system is immediately suitable for conventional broadcast application techniques. These samples were prepared as follows. A weighed amount of polymer, herbicide, and 24- to 48-mesh clay granules was blended together with a solvent (acetone). The solvent was flashed off as the system was gently turned to permit uniform penetration and coating of the clay by the polymer/herbicide matrix. For these particular tests a given ratio of polymer/herbicide was added to three different amounts of clay granules. Specifically, the samples were as follows:

24- to 48-mesh clay (g)	Polymer (g)	2,4-D (acid) (g)
5	1	0.2
10	1	0.2
20	1	0.2

The results of these tests in a similar percolation test tube experiment as described earlier are presented in Figure 3. No control is available. It is interesting to note that the release

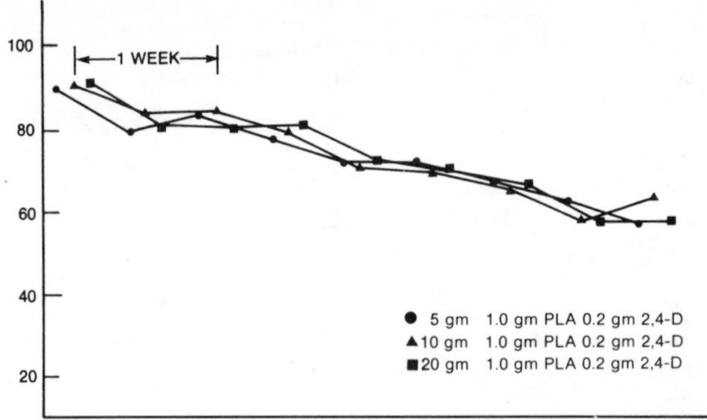

FIGURE 3. Sustained release of 2,4-D (acid) from a biodegradable polymer matrix on/in clay granules.

of herbicide was independent of the ratio of herbicide/polymer to clay over the range studied. Overall, these results demonstrate the sustained release of herbicide from a practical conventional clay carrier when incorporated into a biodegradable polymer. It appears that extension of this work to an array of herbicides appears.

IV. ENGINEERING DESIGN

The object of a sustained release herbicide system is the zero-order release of herbicide over a 24- or more month period coupled with the biodegradation of the carrier material. Here zero-order release is defined as in chemical kinetics and means that a constant release of active agent with time is obtained. For nonbiodegradable materials the release mechanism is by pure diffusion and the release from monolithic spheres or cylinders of carrier/active agent cannot, on a theoretical basis, be zero ordered.[36] A detailed description of the mathematics involved in diffusion controlled release from various geometrics has been presented by both Harris[37] and Collins,[36] for example.

For a biodegradable carrier, on the other hand, where the release mechanism is by both diffusion of the active agent and by hydrolysis of the carrier, zero-order controlled release may be experimentally obtained. Engineers at Dynatech have developed systems for straight-line or zero-order release from both spheres and cylinders. For example, in vivo results from a system of small spherical particles resulted in a zero-order release over the full design period and until all of the active agent was released. Also at this time the polylactic acid carrier material was noted to be completely exhausted. While no definitive theoretical basis is yet available for *a priori* design of a new system, these impressive results demonstrate that other similar systems may be designed. Selection of particular polymer characteristics is largely by experience. On this basis, then, the design requirements for an aquatic herbicide system based on a similar biodegradable carrier may be stated.

A. Engineering Calculations

For purposes of calculation, it will be assumed that broadcast application will be by means of finely divided particles of polylactic acid/herbicide. It will further be assumed that these particles are slurried into an aqueous medium prior to being sprayed into the infected area. Broadcasting will be assumed to be by conventional nozzle sprayers using a backpack cannister of the slurry. Again, for purposes of calculation, the following will be assumed for the herbicide/polymer matrix:

1. The particles of herbicide/polymer are perfect spheres.
2. The particles are all of uniform size.
3. The particles are the mean size of a 24- to 48-Tyler® mesh sieve, and are uniform spheres of 0.02 in. diameter (0.05 cm).
4. It is to be noted that obtaining an effective herbicide level is dependent upon the amount of material broadcast, pool size, flow conditions, and other field conditions. Design of the actual release system for a 24-month period is therefore seen to be somewhat independent of the dosage levels defined here.

On this basis the particular release rate required for polymer design may be calculated. For zero-order release, the herbicide released from a given area of the sphere, assuming that the diffusion/hydrolysis release moves from the surface of the sphere into the center, is

$$(1/A)\ dN/dt = \rho/2\ (dV/dt) \tag{1}$$

where (1/A) dN/dt = rate of herbicide release per unit surface area, the mass transfer rate; A = area of surface "front" of herbicide — viewed as a sphere decreasing in volume with respect to time; N = mass of herbicide in granule; V = volume of spherical particle; and ρ = density of spherical particle. Since the area of a spherical particle of diameter D is πD^2 and the volume is $(\pi/6)\ D^3$, then becomes

$$(1/A)\ (dN/dt) = (\rho/\pi D^2)\ d\ (\pi D^3/6)/dt \tag{2}$$

Upon taking the derivative, this becomes

$$(1/A)\ (dN/dt) = (\rho/2)\ (dD/dt) \tag{3}$$

For an incremental or specific zero-order release period it may be assumed that

$$(1/A)\ (dN/dt) = \rho/2\ \Delta D/\Delta t \tag{4}$$

i.e., herbicide release rate, mg/day · cm^2 = $\rho/2\ \Delta D/\Delta t$. For design conditions of a 0.05-cm diameter spherical particle and a 24-month sustained release period the term $\Delta D/\Delta t$ = 7.0×10^{-5} cm/day. The density term, ρ, for a typical polymer, is 1.4×10^3 mg/cm^3. Thus the zero-order release from the exposed surface area on which to select the polymer is 0.05 mg/day · cm^2.

Experiments at Dynatech have resulted in polylactic acid controlled release systems with release rates of from 0.001 to 1 mg/day · cm^2 controlled release for periods of greater than 12 months. Since the design objective for herbicide release is similar to background work it appears that the design goal of 2 years controlled release using an herbicide/polymer matrix suitable for broadcast application as 24- to 48-mesh particles sprayed from an aqueous slurry is entirely feasible.

B. Available Techniques for Preparation of the Herbicide/Polymer Matrix

Techniques are available to vary processing conditions of the herbicide/polymer matrix. A number of techniques have been successfully applied at Dynatech to prepare the active agent/polymer systems. One is a high temperature vacuum melt system through which the active ingredient is blended in heat-softened polymer. Another technique is to dissolve both the polymer and the active ingredient in a common solvent and then flash off the solvent. A further technique is to dissolve only the polymer in a solvent and then uniformly disperse the active ingredient in the solution, following which the solvent is removed. Ball milling is used to reduce particle size. The objective of investigating polymer/herbicide blending techniques is to insure that the most intimate blending of active ingredient in the matrix structure is achieved in order to prevent leaching of any one of the components while still maintaining biological activity of the larvicide. It is especially significant to note the significant preliminary preparation of a 2,4-D-polylactic acid combination made at Dynatech. Specifically, a solution or molecular dispersion of 2,4-D was readily combined with polylactic acid. In summary, conventional preparation techniques are available and no equipment development appears to be required.

C. Large-Scale Processing

Once the polymer solubility characteristics, the herbicide content of the matrix, and technique for preparing the herbicide/polymer matrix have been established, a method of inexpensively mass producing the system is needed. There are a number of available approaches for practical large-scale processing depending on the manner in which the blending of the herbicide and polymer is carried out. If formation of the herbicide/polymer matrix is by the hot-melt vacuum technique, then size reduction by conventional crushing and grinding equipment will be practical. If a solvent blending technique is used, then spray drying in standard equipment to both remove solvent and to form small granular particles is practical. Overall, it is clear that no major engineering innovations will be required to produce economically on large scale the proposed larvicide system.

D. Estimate of Production Economics

The economics of the larvicide/polymer matrix system are of interest. The current selling price of technical-grade lactic acid is approximately 70¢/lb in tank car quantities, and large-volume application should result in the lowering of this figure. For example, citric acid, a product of fermentation as is lactic acid, is estimated to be reduced from 30¢/lb to perhaps 16¢/lb for large-scale application in detergents. Since only laboratory processing of lactic acid to the lactide and then to the polymer has been carried out, conversion efficiency and production costs are not available. Work at Dynatech indicates no particular processing problems for synthesis of the polymer or formation of the polymer/chemical matrix. It is typical, however, that polymer costs are double the monomer costs. Even on a more conservative basis, large-scale production costs of polylactic acid are not expected to exceed $4.00/lb.

E. Longer-Term Development Potential

It has been emphasized that the polymer biodegradability should be tailored to any particular herbicide and the information gained as a result of working with one herbicide such as 2,4-D should be directly applicable in the design of other herbicide/polymer matrix systems. Once the practicality of sustained release herbicide using a biodegradable polymer has been demonstrated, confidence will be built up in the broader use of the polymer/herbicide sustained release concept. Therefore, as new herbicides are developed, their full potential can be utilized by providing for them this polymer/herbicide concept. Further application of such a system can be extended to ''natural'' or biological herbicides.

ACKNOWLEDGMENT

This work was carried out at Dynatech R/D Company, Cambridge, Mass., and the U.S. Department of Agriculture, Beltsville, Md.

REFERENCES

1. **Danielson, L. L.,** Experimental use of herbicides impregnated on clay granules for control of weeds in certain vegetable crops, *Weeds*, 7, 418, 1959.
2. **Steward, K. K. and Nelson, L. L.,** Evaluations of Controlled Release PVC Formulations of 2,4-D on Watermilfoil, Aquatic Plant Control Res. Plan. Conf., December 1971.
3. **Guscio, F. J. and Gangstad, E. O.,** Aquatic Plant Control Res. Plan. Conf., Office of the Chief of Engineers, Department of the U.S. Army, December 1971.
4. Proc. Res. Plan. Conf. Integrated Systems of Aquatic Plant Control, Waterways Experimental Station, Vicksburg, Miss., October 20 to 29, 1973.
5. Tech. Rep. No. 7, Aquatic Plant Control Program, Office of the Chief of Engineers, Department of the U.S. Army, November 1974.
6. Tech. Rep. No. 8, Aquatic Plant Control Program, Office of the Chief of Engineers Department of the U.S. Army, November 1974.
7. **Raley, T. G. and Davis, E. D.,** *Mosquito News*, 9, 68, 1949.
8. **Elliot, R.,** *Trans. R. Soc. Trop. Med. Hyg.*, 49, 528, 1955.
9. **Laird, M.,** *WHO Chron.*, 21, 18, 1967.
10. **Barnes, W. W., Webb, A. N., and Savage, L. B.,** *Mosquito News*, 27, 488, 1967.
11. **Miles, J. W. and Woehst, J. E.,** *Pest. Formul. Res.*, p. 183, 1967.
12. **Whitlaw, J. T. and Evans, E. S.,** *J. Econ. Entomol.*, 61, 889, 1968.
13. **Wilkinson, R. N., Barnes, W., Gillagly, A. R., and Minnemeyer, C. D.,** *J. Econ. Entomol.*, 64, 1, 1971.
14. Entomol. Spec. Study No. 31-004-71, AD 729342, 1970.
15. Entomol. Spec. Study No. 31-006-71, AD 729343, 1970.
16. Entomol. Spec. Study No. 31-014-71, AD 729344, 1970.
17. **Nelson, L. L. and Whitlaw, J. T.,** USAEHA Spec. Study No. 31-019-71/72, 1972.
18. **Nelson, L. L. and Miller, T. A.,** USAEHA Spec. Study No. 31-008-72, 1971.
19. **Miller, T. A., Lawson, M. A., Nelson, L. L., and Young, W. W.,** *Mosquito News*, 33(3), 413, 1973.
20. **Miller, T. A., Nelson, L. L., and Young, W. W.,** *Mosquito News*, 33(2), 172, 1973.
21. **Nelson, L. L., Miller, T. A., and Young, W. W.,** *Mosquito News*, 33(3), 396, 1973.
22. **Lawson, M. A., Miller, T. A., Oakleaf, R. J., and Young, W. W.,** *Mosquito News*, 33(4), 561, 1973.
23. **Nelson, J. H., Evans, E. S., Pennington, N. E., and Young, W. W.,** Controlled Release Pesticide Symp., University of Akron, Akron, Ohio, September 1974.
24. **Cardarelli, N. F.,** U.S. Patent #3,417,181, 1968.
25. **Bille, S., Mansdorf, S. Z., and Cardarelli, N. S.,** Final Report: Development of Slow Release Herbicide Materials for Controlling Aquatic Plants, Contract No. DACW73-70-C-0030, Office of the Chief of Engineers, Department of the U.S. Army, 1971.
26. **Cardarelli, N. F.,** Presentation to the Am. Chem. Soc., Jt. Symp., Fertilizer/Pesticides Combination, Washington, D.C., September 1971.
27. **Cardarelli, N. F.,** Presentation to the Annu. Meet. North Central Mosquito Control Association.
28. **Chujo, K., Kobayashi, H., Suzuki, J., Tokuhara, S., and Tanabe, M.,** *Makromol. Chem.*, 100, 262, 1967.
29. **Chujo, K., Kobayashi, H., Suzuki, J., and Tokuhara, S.,** *Makromol. Chem.*, 100, 267, 1967.
30. **Kulkarni, R. K., Pani, K. C., Neuman, C., and Leonard, F.,** *Arch. Surg.*, 93, 839, 1966.
31. **Kulkarni, R. K., Moore, E. G., Hegyeli, A. F., and Leonard, F.,** *J. Biomed. Mater. Res.*, 5, 169, 1971.
32. **Morgan, M. N.,** *Br. Med. J.*, 2, 308, 1969.
33. **Kelly, R. J.,** *Rev. Surg.*, March/April, 142, 1970.
34. **Herrmann, J. B., Kelly, R. J., and Higgins, G. A.,** *Arch. Surg.*, 100, 468, 1970.
35. **Frazza, E. J. and Schmitt, E. E.,** *J. Biomed. Mater. Res. Symp.*, 1, 43, 1972.
36. **Collins, R. L.,** A Theoretical Foundation for Controlled Release, paper presented at Controlled Release Pesticide Symp., University of Akron, Akron, Ohio, September 1974.
37. **Harris, F. W.,** Theoretical Aspects of Controlled Release, paper presented at Controlled Release Pesticide Symp., University of Akron, Akron, Ohio, September 1974.

Mechanisms

Chapter 8

BASIS FOR DESIGN OF BIODEGRADABLE POLYMERS FOR SUSTAINED RELEASE OF BIOLOGICALLY ACTIVE AGENTS

Joseph D. Gresser and John E. Sanderson

TABLE OF CONTENTS

I. TECHNICAL DISCUSSION

A. Introduction

Release of drug from a biodegradable matrix system is governed by a number of factors. Both the rate and duration of release from PLGA have been shown, by work carried out at Dynatech R/D Company, Cambridge, Mass. to depend on the nature of the matrix, the drug, and the interaction of the drug/polymer composite with components of the in vitro environment. Identifiable parameters upon which these time factors depend include

1. Polymer composition
2. Drug content of the composite
3. Solubility of the drug in water or tissue fluid
4. Total dose delivered to the recipient
5. Dose form (i.e., injectable powder or implant)

The purpose of this section is to discuss these dependencies and to illustrate them with data generated by Dynatech scientists as well as with results reported in the literature.

B. Choice of Sustained Release Mode

Choice of a method to control the rate at which a drug becomes available to a recipient depends, of course, on program requirements. Available techniques include the following:

1. Direct injections of drug forms of low solubility. Release depends on slow dissolution of the depot. The method is inflexible if varying rates of release are required: varying the release rate must be achieved by having available several different forms such as salts, or complexes.
2. Reservoir devices. Slow release of many drugs has been achieved by enclosing them as saturated solutions in silicone rubber. Release is controlled by the diffusion of drug through the silicone; rate control is achieved by varying the wall thickness. Silicone devices are implantable, not injectable, and silicone is not biodegradable. On exhaustion of the device, the implant must be surgically removed. Since diffusion of the active agent occurs from solution, these devices allow prolonged contact of the active agent with fluids. Stability may be adversely affected.
3. Microencapsulated particles. Microencapsulation may be achieved by several techniques, including spray drying and coacervation. The membrane formed around the drug core may or may not be biodegradable. If slow release is to be achieved, it may be by diffusion of the drug through the membrane which obviously must remain intact for the duration of release. This requirement is difficult to realize for long-lasting systems, especially biodegradable ones. Both biodegradable and nonbiodegradable membranes may swell or rupture due to osmotic pressure increase in the interior of the microcapsule. When this occurs, the drug is rapidly "dumped" into the surrounding environments. Processing techniques, such as spray drying, frequently leave porous structures; intact membranes of uniform thickness are difficult to achieve. Coacervation and *in situ* polymerization expose the active agent to conditions which may result in denaturation and which may also leave significant quantities of components other than drug and encapsulating polymer.
4. Monolithic or matrix devices. These devices are characterized by a homogeneous distribution of drug in a polymeric matrix which itself may be either biodegradable or not. If the matrix is biodegradable, the mechanism of drug release is bioerosion of the matrix as well as by diffusion of the drug through the polymer lattice.

Matrix systems are flexible and among the simplest to prepare. Advantages of matrix systems for sustained drug release are listed below:

1. Drug loading may be as high as 75 wt % and may be precisely controlled. This gives a means for adjusting the rate of release.
2. Porosity of the matrix may be controlled and minimized by extrusion of the matrix as part of the dose fabrication process.
3. The matrix system is flexible. The extruded composite, formed with cylindrical symmetry or molded as spherical beads, may be used as an implant. Cryogenic grinding techniques easily convert the extruded matrix device into an injectable powder.
4. Matrix systems are among the simplest to prepare and therefore fabrication costs are low.
5. No *in situ* polymerization is required which thereby eliminates many chemical residues such as polymerization catalysts.

It is the considered judgment of Dynatech engineers that the matrix approach is the most reasonable method for development of a sustained release system. The following discussions describe the empirical and theoretical background assembled, mostly at Dynatech, on matrix systems using the tissue-compatible and biodegradable copolymers of lactic and glycolic acids (PLGAs). Following the extended discussion of drug release from PLGA, results of more recent work with polypropylene fumarate (PPF) will be given. Experimental data for PPF systems indicate that slow release can now be achieved with very soluble drugs more easily than with PLGA.

C. Biological Half-Life of PLGA as a Function of Polymer Composition

In vivo degradation rates of copolymers of lactic and glycolic acids have been shown to depend strongly on the mole ratio of the monomers.[20] These workers implanted rats with ^{14}C-labeled polymers of varying composition and at times up to 11 months postimplantation analyzed the excised implants for residual ^{14}C. They found that homopolymers, polylactic and slow-cured polyglycolic acids had, respectively, in vivo half-lives of 6.1 and 5.0 months. Half-lives of copolymers reached a minimum of 1 week for that copolymer with an equimolar ratio of the two monomers.

Polymer composition can therefore be used to control the rate of drug release. If drug release depends entirely on polymer degradation, it will be a first-order process, as found for PLGAs by the authors.*

D. Dependence of Release Rates on Total Dose Delivered

The relation between release rate and dose delivered is exemplified by the drug norethisterone. In a series of experiments conducted by Dynatech for the World Health Organization (WHO), this fertility control steroid was administered as a component of a PLGA composite to rats, dogs, and baboons. Total dose varied from 33 to 56,000 μg, i.e., more than three orders of magnitude. This range demonstrated variations in release rate from ~25 to ~364 μg/day. The following empirical relation between excretion rate and dose is based on a linear regression analysis of the data:

$$R_S = 1.4 \times 10^{-2} D^{0.8} \tag{1}$$

where R_S = total excretion rate (μg/day) and D = dose (mg). This equation predicts that doses differing by a factor of 100 should cause a variation in release rate of about a factor

* With the exception of the work of Miller, Brady, and Cutright, all experimental results were determined at Dynatech R/D Company.

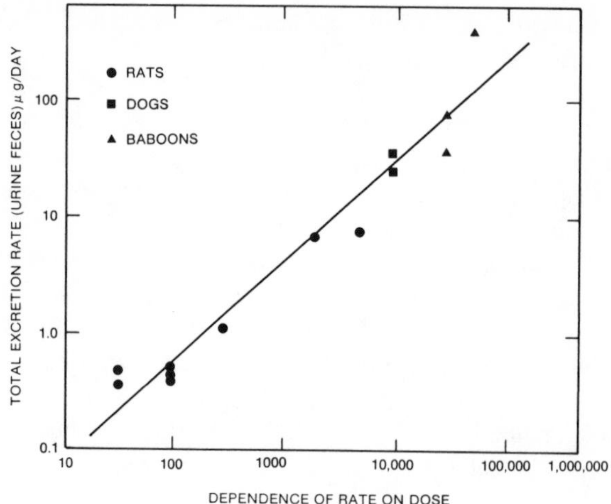

FIGURE 1. Dependence of rate on dose.

of approximately 44. The linear regression is presented graphically in Figure 1. From this, an estimate of system duration was developed using the release profile obtained for each dose. This is given in the following equation:

$$T = \frac{X}{R_I} + \frac{Y}{R_S} D \tag{2}$$

where T = system duration (days); R_I = initial excretion rate; X = fraction of dose used in initial rapid release; R_S = excretion rate during period of sustained release; and Y = fraction of dose used in sustained release.

By substituting Equation 1 into Equation 2 and assuming that $X/R_I \simeq O$ and Y = 1, a simple relation between system duration and dose is obtained for norethisterone:

$$T \simeq 70\ D^{0.2} \tag{3}$$

Thus, increasing the dose by a factor of 100 should increase duration by about 2.3 times.

E. Dependence of System Duration on Drug Solubility

Sustained release systems for many other drugs have been formulated at Dynatech. This has permitted a correlation between system lifetime and the aqueous solubility of the drug to be established. Obviously such a correlation also depends on the absolute dose of the drug delivered as well as on the other factors enumerated previously. However, from the above analysis it will be seen that over the range of doses used, system duration is less sensitive to dose than to solubility.

Figure 2 shows approximate system lifetimes for several sustained-release systems as functions of drug solubility in water (pH 7). Doses range from 40 to 700 mg. If similar duration/dose correlations hold for these drugs as for norethisterone (Equation 1), the over this dose range duration for any specific drug should vary by no more than a factor of 1.7. This range is indicated by the dashed lines parallel to the regression line of Figure 2. Thus, dose will contribute less to duration than will solubility. Solubilities range from 0.02 μg/mℓ for the antimalarial quinazoline derivative, WR-158122, to 4000 μg/mℓ for naltrexone free base. Over this range system duration varies from ~30 days for the latter to ~1600 days for the former.

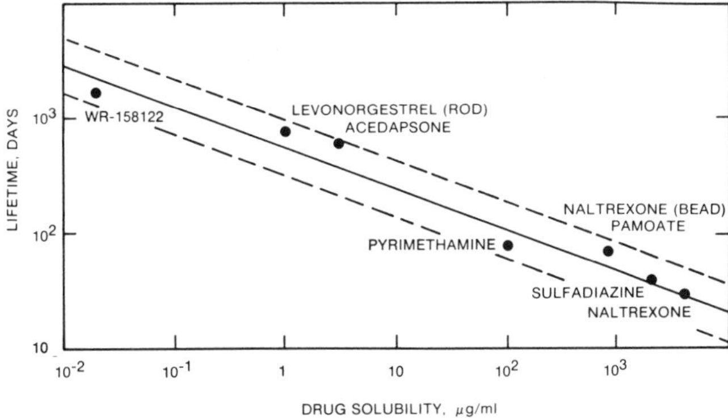

FIGURE 2. Effect of drug solubility on duration of release from PLA/PGA polymers.

Table 1
APPROXIMATE SYSTEM DURATION AS A FUNCTION OF DRUG SOLUBILITY

Drug	Solubility (μg/mℓ)	Approximate system duration (days)
WR-158122[a]	0.02	1600
Levonorgestrel	1.0	750
Acedapsone	3.0	600
Norethisterone	10	50
Pyrimethamine	100	80
Naltrexone pamoate	800	70
Sulfadiazine	2000	40
Naltrexone base	4000	30

[a] An antimalarial drug supplied by Walter Reed Army Institute for Medical Research with this code number.

The empirical relationship obtained from a linear regression analysis of the data in Table 1 is

$$\log T = -0.355 \log S + 2.7625 \tag{4}$$

or approximately

$$T = 578.8\ S^{-0.355}$$
$$T \simeq 5.8 \times 10^2\ S^{-0.4}$$

where T = system duration (days) and S = solubility (μg/mℓ).

System duration is determined by extrapolation from cumulative release profiles for each drug, usually to about 80% exhaustion. For systems of short lifetimes, lifetime is taken as the time over which release of drug is sufficient for therapeutic efficiency.

Except for levonorgestrel, naltrexone and its pamoate, and sulfadiazene, compounds used to develop the Figure 2 correlation were delivered as injectable powders. The levonorgestrel was implanted as 1/32-in. cylindrical rods, and the naltrexones and sulfadiazine as 1.5-mm beads.

The conclusion is that drug solubility is a sufficient parameter by which to gauge system duration.

F. Analysis of Drug Release as a Function of Dose Form

The rate at which norethisterone or its metabolites are excreted in the urine and feces of test animals exhibits the following dose dependency (see Section I.D):

$$\frac{dm}{dt} = 0.014\ m^{0.82} \tag{5}$$

Here dm/dt is the total excretion rate (μg/day) of norethisterone (NET) and m is the total dose of NET (μg). The excretion rate, which is taken to be equivalent to the rate of drug release from the matrix, is not strongly sensitive to excipient molecular weight, weight percent of the drug in the matrix, or the species of test animal. The data on which Equation 5 is based summarize the in vivo work done at Dynatech with rats, dogs, and baboons with doses ranging from 33 to 56,000 μg.

The excretion rates used to construct Figure 1 were determined from the slopes of the midportion of the cumulative release vs. time plots for each of the systems investigated. The midportion of these plots is characteristic of the release profile following the initial release but prior to exhaustion of the drug reservoir.

Sufficient information is subsumed in Equation 5 to suggest a mechanism for the observed rate-dose dependency. Two models will be illustrated which will bind the observed behavior and from these a model will be generated which will predict the experimentally observed exponent of Equation 1. An assumption underlying the following development is that an equilibrium is established so that the rate of drug excretion by the animal is equal to the rate at which drug is released from the matrix.

1. Case I: Drug Release from a Single Erodible Sphere

This model assumes that the mass of injected matrix particles acts as a single sphere which releases drug from its surface as its radius decreases. An increase of dose corresponds to an increase of the radius. This can be applied to the polylactic/glycolic acid copolymer of Dynatech sample 29110-2 which showed concomitant release of both tritium derived from the labeled polymer and ^{14}C from NET. As excretion of both isotopes ceased simultaneously and as tritium appeared mainly in the urine, it is reasonable to conclude that hydrolytic erosion of the polymer proceeded from the particle surface inward, simultaneously releasing NET and monomeric polymer fragments.

A system with these characteristics will release drug at a rate given by:

$$\frac{dm}{dt} = R_o\ (4\pi r^2) \tag{6}$$

where R_0 is an erosion constant giving the release rate per unit area per unit time and r is the effective radius of the agglomerated mass of particles.

It is necessary to express r in terms of m, the dose of NET:

$$m = \frac{4}{3}\ \pi r^3 \rho c \tag{7}$$

where ρ is the matrix density (μg/cm³) and c is the drug concentration in the matrix (μg drug/μg matrix, i.e., the weight fraction of the drug in the matrix).

Solving Equation 7 for r and substituting in Equation 6 yields:

$$\frac{dm}{dt} = [3^{2/3}(4\pi)^{1/3}(c\rho)^{-2/3}R_o]m^{2/3} \tag{8}$$

Equation 8 applies to a system of particles which behaves as a single sphere of radius r which releases drug to the organism from its surface. Drug contained in particles in the interior of the sphere does not become available until the surface has eroded sufficiently. The exponent of m is 0.67, less than the observed value.

A somewhat more realistic approach is based on the assumption that the geometry of the particle distribution is that of a prolate spheroid. Although this will affect the release rate for a given dose, the dependence of rate on dose still exhibits an exponent of 0.67 if the particle agglomeration is sufficient to warrant treatment as a single entity.

For a prolate spheroid the release rate is given by:

$$\frac{dm}{dt} = \left[2\pi b^2 + \frac{2\pi ab}{\epsilon} \sin^{-1} \epsilon\right] R_o \tag{9}$$

where a, b are the lengths of the major and minor axes and ϵ is the eccentricity given by $(a^2 - b^2)^{1/2} a^{-1}$.

The dose, m, is given by:

$$m = \frac{4}{3} \pi ab^2 \rho c \tag{10}$$

Choosing $a = xb$ to maintain generality yields:

$$\frac{dm}{dt} = R_o \left[2\pi + \frac{2\pi x^2}{x^2 - 1} \sin^{-1} \frac{x^2 - 1}{x}\right] \left(\frac{3m}{4\pi x \rho c}\right)^{0.67} \tag{11}$$

or simply:

$$\frac{dm}{dt} = R_o\, K \left(\frac{m}{\rho c}\right)^{0.67} \tag{12}$$

Further, the release rate is not very sensitive to the eccentricity. Values of K calculated for several values of x and the corresponding value for a sphere are as follows:

x	K
2	5.17
4	6.13
6	6.91
Sphere	4.84

Thus changing the distribution from a sphere to a prolate spheroid with a major axis 6 times the length of the minor increases the release rate by a factor of only 1.43.

2. *Case II: Drug Release from Independent Spherical Particles*

If the injected matrix particles behave as totally independent spheres, then an increase in dose results from an increase in the number of particles. The release rate is still a function of surface area, but now:

$$\frac{dm}{dt} = R_o 4\, \pi r_c^2 n \tag{13}$$

where r_c is the constant radius of each particle and n is the number of particles. The dose m is given by:

$$m = \frac{4}{3} \pi r^3 n\rho c \tag{14}$$

Solving for n in Equation 14 and substituting in Equation 13 yields:

$$\frac{dm}{dt} = \left[\frac{3R_o}{r_c \rho c}\right] m \tag{15}$$

It should be noted that the particle radius r_c may be included among the constants as it also remains constant, i.e., the dose depends only on the number of particles, n. The exponent of m is 1.0, larger than the experimental value.

Here, too, it can be shown that if the particle distribution is described by a prolate spheroid with completely independent particles, the dependence of rate on dose is still linear, i.e., the exponent of m = 1.

3. Case III: Particles Partially Agglomerated into Spherical Masses

The experimentally observed exponent of m in the rate equation is 0.82, intermediate between 0.67 calculated for a single sphere and 1.0 for a mass of independent particles. It is therefore reasonable to assume that the injected dose behaves neither as a completely agglomerated spherical mass or as totally independent particles. The model will assume that the dose must be expressed as a function of both r_g, the radius of the massed particles, and n_g, the number of these masses; i.e., m = f(r, n).

The rate, dm/dt, will again depend on the surface area, but this in turn depends both on the radii of the masses and their number:

$$\frac{dm}{dt} = R_o 4 \pi r_g^2 n_g \tag{16}$$

r_g may be further defined in terms of the number of particles in each mass n_p and the radius of each particular r_p:

$$V_g = \frac{4}{3} \pi r_g^3 = n_p \frac{4}{3} \pi r_p 3^* \tag{17}$$

$$r_g = n_p^{1/3} r_p \tag{18}$$

Substituting this value into Equation 12 gives:

$$\frac{dm}{dt} = R_o 4 \pi n_p^{2/3} r_p^2 n_g \tag{19}$$

Since N, the total number of particles is

$$N = n_p \cdot n_g \tag{20}$$

$$\frac{dm}{dt} = R_o 4 \pi r_p^2 N n_p^{-1/3} \tag{21}$$

* Assuming the density of particles and medium are the same. In any case, they are constants and do not influence the functional dependence.

Since interaction between particles is expected to increase with increasing numbers of particles, one would expect a relationship between the number of particles in each mass and the total number of particles of the form:

$$n_p = KN^x \tag{22}$$

Therefore:

$$\frac{dm}{dt} = k_o 4\pi r_p^2 KN(1 - x/3) \qquad 0 \leqslant x \leqslant 1 \tag{23}$$

This expression gives the proper limiting behavior in that when $x = 0$:

$$\frac{\partial m}{\partial t} \simeq N \simeq m \tag{24}$$

i.e., no interaction, as in case II, and when $x = 1$:

$$\frac{dm}{dt} \simeq M^{2/3} \simeq m^{2/3} \tag{25}$$

i.e., complete interaction as presented in case I.

For an intermediate case where $x = 0.5$:

$$\frac{dm}{dt} = k_o 4\pi r_p^2 KN^{0.83} \tag{26}$$

or, since the dose $m = 4/3\pi r_p^3$ NPC:

$$\frac{\partial m}{\partial t} = Kk_o \frac{4\pi^{0.17} r_p^{0.5}}{(\rho c)^{0.83}} m^{0.83}$$

which is very close to the observed exponent of 0.82.

G. Release Rate as a Function of Drug Loading and of Polymer Molecular Weight

The rate of release of a drug from a polymer matrix has frequently been observed to be a function of the drug content of the drug/polymer composite. Such a dependence is clearly demonstrated by release of the narcotic antagonist, naltrexone, from PLGA matrices synthesized to have a lactic-to-glycolic acid mole ratio of 3:2.[8] Four composites containing 50, 60, 70, and 80 wt % naltrexone were prepared as 1/16-in. diameter rods. In vitro release into pH 7 buffer at 37°C indicates that release rates increased with increased loading in the order 2.1, 2.8, 5.0, and 11.0%/day.

The dependence of release rate of molecular weight seems to be more pronounced at lower than at higher molecular weights. Experiments conducted at Dynatech[17] on sustained release of sulfadiazine from polylactic acid indicate a depression of release rate with increase of molecular weight. Data indicate a decrease in release rate from 0.8 to 0.4%/day with an increase in molecular weight from 150,000 to 210,000. However, no further decrease was observed with an increase in polymer molecular weight to 450,000.

H. Extrusion Temperatures

Glass transition temperatures (T_g) have been measured at Dynatech for PLGAs of varying composition. These values, reported in Table 2, were determined by differential thermal analysis; all lie in the range of 44 to 58°C.

Table 2
GLASS TRANSITION TEMPERATURES OF SEVERAL PLGAs

Polymer	T_g°C
Poly-(dl)-lactic	58
90L(−)/10G[a]	57
75L(−)/25G	48
50L(−)/50G	48
25L(−)/75G	48
Polyglycolic	44

[a] Symbol for PLGA synthesized from 90 wt% L(−)-lactide and 10 wt% glycolide.

Table 3
EXTRUSION[a] TEMPERATURES OF DRUG-POLYMER COMPOSITES IN °C AS A FUNCTION OF POLYMER COMPOSITION AND DRUG LOADING FOR TWO DRUGS

Polymer			Levonorgestrel		Bovine serum albumin		
Composition	$\overline{M}_w$	**Pure polymer**	**50%**	**70%**	**5%**	**10%**	**50%**
Poly dl-lactic	**105,000**	**~105°**	**—**	**—**	**85°**	**~60°**	**45°**
90L(−)/10G[b]	40,000	~120°	~130°	170°		—	
90L(−)/10G	165,000	~150°	157°	190°		—	
75L(−)/25G	40,000	~83°	96°	—		—	

[a] Extrusion pressures are 45 to 60 psi.
[b] Symbol for a PLGA synthesized from 90 wt% L(−)-lactide and 10 wt% glycolide.

Experiments have been conducted at Dynatech to investigate the effect of inclusion of protein into poly-(dl)-lactic acid. This polymer can be extruded at temperatures between 100 and 110°C, depending on molecular weight. Inclusion of bovine serum albumin (BSA), a protein with a molecular weight of 50,000, lowered the temperatures required for extrusion dramatically. Table 3 data for BSA show that inclusions of 5, 10, and 50 wt % BSA decreased extrusion temperatures by ~20, 45, and 60°C. Obviously BSA served as a plasticizer.

The temperature at which composites are extruded depends, of course, on composite viscosity which depends in turn on the nature of the active agent as well as its loading. Table 3 illustrates the effect of these variables on extrusion temperature. These data show that the polymer synthesis from 75 wt % L(−)-lactide and 25 wt % glycolide extruded at the lowest temperature (83°C). Inclusion of the high melting steroid levonorgestrel in all cases resulted in a composite which required a high extrusion temperature.

An experiment has been conducted at Dynatech to investigate the feasibility of preparing BSA-polymer matrices by mixing the components in absence of any solvent. A 10 wt % content of BSA reduced the extrusion temperature by only 15 to 25°C, much less than the 45°C indicated above. This is strong evidence that the distribution of BSA in the polymer was not nearly as homogeneous as that achieved in the composites described above which were prepared with the aid of polymer solvents. These results do suggest, however, that dry mixing is feasible. Particle size reduction of both protein and polymer by low temperature grinding may result in better distribution of the protein throughout the polymer.

II. SUMMARY

The mechanism of drug release from PLGA matrices is complex, combining release by hydrolytic degradation of the polymer, lattice diffusion, and pore diffusion. The contribution of each depends on polymer composition and other parameters previously mentioned. Pore diffusion is directly dependent on the porosity of the drug/polymer composite, and porosity, in turn, depends on fabrication techniques. Polymers with lower glass transition temperatures and crystalline melting points will have lower viscosities at a given extrusion temperature and pressure. Increased flow will therefore result in reduced porosity at moderate temperatures and pressures. Evidence indicates that porosity, in one case, may be reduced sufficiently so that release is governed mainly by polymer degradation.

ACKNOWLEDGMENT

This work was carried out in the Chemical Engineering Department at Dynatech R/D Company.

REFERENCES

1. **Anderson, L. C., Wise, D. L., and Howes, J. F.,** An injectable sustained release fertility control system, *Contraception,* 13, 375, 1976.
2. **Benagiano, G. E., Schmitt, D., Wise, D. L., and Goodman, M.,** Sustained release hormonal preparations for the delivery of fertility regulating agents, *J. Polym. Sci. Polym. Symp.,* 66, 129, 1979.
3. **Gresser, J. D., Wise, D. L., Bech, L. R., and Howes, J. F.,** Larger animal testing on an injectable sustained-release fertility control system, *Contraception,* 17, 253, 1978.
4. **Jackanicz, T. M., Nash, H. A., Wise, D. L., and Gregory, J. B.,** Polylactic acid as a biodegradable carrier for contraceptive steroids, *Contraception,* 8, 227, 1973.
5. **Sadek, S. E.,** Methods of improving control of release rates and products useful in same, U.S. Patent 3, 976, 071, 1976.
6. **Schwope, A. D., Wise, D. L., Sell, K. W., Skornick, W. A., and Dressler, D. P.,** Development of a synthetic burn covering, *Trans. Am. Soc. Artif. Intern. Organs,* 20, 103, 1974.
7. **Schwope, A. D., Wise, D. L., and Howes, J. F.,** National Institute on Drug Abuse, Development of polylactic/glycolic acid delivery systems for use in treatment of narcotic addiction, *Res. Monogr.* 4, 13, 1976.
8. **Schwope, A. D., Wise, D. L., and Howes, J. F.,** Lactic/glycolic acid polymers as narcotic antagonist delivery systems, *Life Sci.,* 17, 1877, 1975.
9. **Schwope, A. D., Sell, K. W., Dressler, D. P., Skornick, W. A., and Wise, D. L.,** Evaluation of wound-covering materials, *J. Biomed. Mater. Res.,* 11, 489, 1977.
10. **Sharon, A. C. and Wise, D. L.,** Development of drug delivery systems for use in treatment of narcotic addiction, Natl. Inst. Drug Abuse Monogr. Ser., Willette, R. C., Ed., in press.
11. **Wise, D. L., McCormick, G. V., and Willet, G. P.,** Sustained release of an anti-malarial drug using a copolymer of glycolic/lactic acid, *Life Sci.,* 19, 867, 1976.
12. **Wise, D. L.,** Sustained release of pharmaceuticals from polyester matrices, U.S. Patent 3,978,203, 1976.
13. **Wise, D. L., Schwope, A. D., and Sell, K. W.,** Wound covering and method of application, U.S. Patent 3,395,308, 1976.
14. **Wise, D. L., Fellman, T. D., Sanderson, J. E., and Wentworth, R. L.,** Lactic/glycolic acid polymers, in *Drug Carriers in Biology and Medicine,* Academic Press, 1979, 237.
15. **Wise, D. L., Gregory, J. B., Newborne, P. M., Bartholomew, L. C., and Stanbury, J. B.,** Results on biodegradable cylindrical subdermal implants for fertility control, in *Polymeric Delivery Systems,* Vol. 5, Kostelnik, R. J., Ed., Gordon & Breach Science Publishers, New York, 1978, 121.

16. **Wise, D. L., Schwope, A. D., Harrigan, S. E., and McCarty, S. E.,** *Polymeric Delivery Systems,* Vol. 5, Kostelnik, R. J., Ed., Gordan & Breach Science Publishers, New York, 1978, 75.
17. **Wise, D. L., Gresser, J. D., and McCormick, G. J.,** Sustained release of a dual anti-malarial system, *J. Pharm. Pharmacol.,* 31, 204, 1979.
18. **Wise, D. L., McCormick, G. J., Willet, G. P., Anderson, L. C., and Howes, J. F.,** Sustained released of sulfadiazine, *J. Pharm. Pharmacol.,* 30, 686, 1978.
19. **Wise, D. L., Rosekrantz, H., Gregory, J. B., and Esbr, H. J.,** Long term controlled delivery of levonorgestrel in rats by means of small biodegradable cylinder, *J. Pharm. Pharmacol.,* 32, 399, 1980.
20. **Miller, R. A., Brady, J. M., and Cutright, D. E.,** *J. Biomed. Mater. Res.,* 11, 711, 1977.

Chapter 9

MECHANISMS FOR THE SUSTAINED RELEASE OF BIOLOGICALLY ACTIVE AGENTS

Shafik E. Sadek

TABLE OF CONTENTS

I. BACKGROUND

The concept of long-term sustained release of medication is an attractive one. Patients whose well being is dependent on constant or frequent administration of medication can be relieved of the need for frequent administering of the medication by qualified personnel; simultaneously these personnel could be relieved of that task thus allowing them to be employed elsewhere where their services can be more beneficial.

One of the first attempts at long-term release of medication was demonstrated by the Population Council which has successfully demonstrated the feasibility of long-term fertility control in women by using contraceptive steroids. When these steroids were released in tiny quantities from subcutaneously implanted capsules of silicone rubber, they became available at a constant rate to the human system until the supply was exhausted.

Although the implantation of the silicone capsule is relatively simple, the removal of the exhausted capsule is obviously much more complex. The idea of a product which would be completely assimilated by the body after the medicament has been exhausted was considered. The first type of sustained release system considered was a product in which the medicament is incorporated into a slowly soluble polymer matrix. When the system is implanted in the body, the polymer will slowly dissolve, and in doing so — it was believed — will release the medicament. At the end of the release period, both chemical and polymer would be gone.

The incorporation of medicaments into tissue-absorbable preparations has been actively studied since the 1940s. The use of gelatin, sodium alginate, and cellulose-glycolic acid-ether are typical of materials currently used. These polymer systems, however, dissolve within 24 hr after incorporation in the body and are consequently unsuitable as matrix materials for sustained release over long periods of time. This search for long-lived polymer materials led to the investigation of the use of synthetic suture materials first as matrices for birth control steroids, then for various other chemicals.

In the early stages of the work carried out, it was believed that the release of the chemical occurred simultaneously with the dissolution of the matrix: the chemical was released from the areas where it was directly exposed to the fluids with which it was in contact. As the polymer slowly dissolved, exposing fresh surface and fresh chemical, the dissolution of chemical proceeded until the polymer was totally dissolved. This "dissolving life-saver" model assumed that only chemical directly exposed to the surrounding fluid could dissolve; any particles of chemical totally encased by the polymer are incapable of dissolution. If this theory is correct, then the ratio of the rates of dissolution of chemical and of matrix will remain constant and equal to the mass ratio of the chemical to polymer in a well-distributed system. Tests carried out showed, however, that the rates of dissolution of chemical and of polymer were not in direct proportion to one another during the release period. Furthermore, the ratio of their averaged rates of dissolution during the release period was not in the same proportion as their ratio in the matrix. It was therefore concluded that the "life-saver" model was inappropriate in describing the mechanism of release. Other mechanisms of release were then postulated. These were based on diffusional processes occurring within the chemical/polymer matrix. This describes an attempt at developing a better understanding of the sustained release mechanism of chemicals within a polymer matrix.

II. DISSOLVING LIFE-SAVER MODEL

Sustained release from a polymer matrix was first visualized as being similar to a dissolving life saver. As the matrix gradually dissolved, it released to the surrounding fluids the chemical with which the dissolved polymer is associated. The release of chemical is therefore directly proportional to the dissolution of the polymer; the ratio of the masses released (or of the

Table 1

Set #1 Steroid Release Data

Ratio of (drug/polymer) present in matrix		Cumulative mass ratio (drug/polymer) released	
PLA-DL	0.30	0.1/1.5	= 0.0667
PLA-DL	0.10	0.04/2.1	= 0.019
PLA-DL	0.30	0.18/2.1	= 0.086
PLA-DL	0.50	1.02/2.2	= 0.046
PLA-DL	0.30	0.06/3.0	= 0.020
PLA-L(+)	0.30	0.16/10.8	= 0.0148
PGA	0.30	0.44/21.2	= 0.0208

Set #2 Naltrexone Base Release Data

$75L^+/25G$	0.50	(1 week)	0.11/0.006	= 18.3
$75L^+25G$	0.50	(2 weeks)	0.20/0.022	= 9.1
$75L^+/25G$	0.50	(3 weeks)	0.24/0.029	= 8.3
$25L^+/75G$	0.50	(1 week)	0.11/0.020	= 5.5
$25L^+/75G$	0.50	(2 weeks)	0.124/0.035	= 3.5
$50L^+/50G$	0.50	(1 week)	0.16/0.080	= 2.0
$50L^+/50G$	0.50	(2 weeks)	0.173/0.114	= 1.5
$50L^+/50G$	0.50	(3 weeks)	0.173/0.120	= 1.4

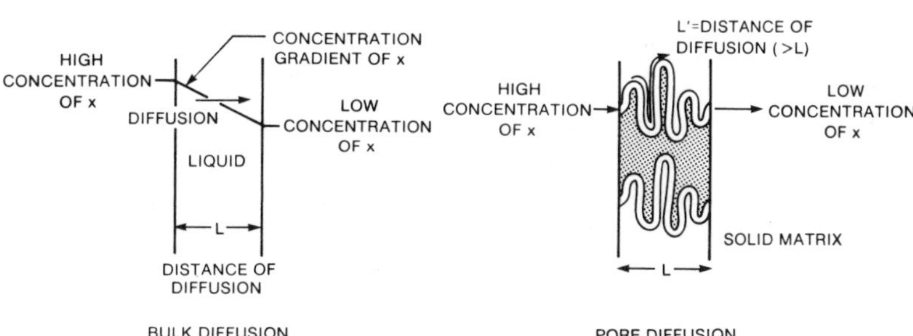

FIGURE 1. Bulk and pore diffusion.

rates of release) of chemical to polymer is then equal to the ratio of chemical to polymer within the matrix. This criterion provides the basic test for verifying the accuracy of the life-saver model in describing sustained release.

Table 1 shows two sets of release data. The first set represents the release of steroid from a polymer matrix. The solubility of the steroid is low and the ratio of steroid released to polymer dissolved is considerably below the ratio of steroid to polymer in the matrix. Had the life-saver model been a true representation of the dissolution process, the release of steroid would have necessarily been considerably higher. The second set of data represents the release of a relatively soluble chemical. It is observed that the drug in this case is released much more rapidly than the polymer in the matrix. Had the life-saver model been truly representative of the dissolution, the release of the chemical could not have been so high. This set of data indicates that the chemical is being leached out from within the matrix. Both these sets of data are shown plotted in Figure 1.

The data show that the chemical is not merely released as a result of the dissolution of the polymer, but its release is governed by other factors.

III. DIFFUSION

A. Background

When a polymeric material lies in between two fluids of different composition, there is a tendency for the components of these fluids to flow through the material in such a manner so as to equalize the compositions on both sides of the material. The rate of movement of each component through the material is governed by either or both of two different mechanisms. One of these may be characterized as a pore or capillary diffusion; the other may be characterized as a ''permeation''. Capillary or pore diffusion rates are independent of the physicochemical properties of the porous material; except for its porosity, other properties do not affect the fluxes of the components. In the case of ''permeation'', the compatibility between the matrix and the permeating material is a strong factor affecting the rate of transfer. When diffusion of liquids is being considered, the capillary or pore diffusion is therefore identical in nature to bulk diffusion with the matrix of the material acting merely as a geometric barrier; this barrier increases the resistance to diffusion by reducing the effective cross-sectional area for diffusion and by the flow into numerous tiny channels instead of allowing it to proceed unhindered across a wide area. A schematic diagram of the pore diffusion of a component through a material is shown in Figure 1. This is compared to the bulk diffusion of that same component in a bulk fluid.

The rate of diffusion of a component X at steady state is directly proportional to the concentration gradient across the diffusional pore path of that component and to the area across which diffusion occurs, i.e., diffusional flow is equal to:

$$\text{diffusion flow } \alpha \text{ area} \times \frac{\text{concentration difference}}{\text{diffusional path length}}$$

If the concentration at the ''high concentration'' face of the material is C_h and the concentration at the ''low concentration'' face of the material is C_∞ then the concentration driving force (ΔC) for diffusion in both cases of bulk diffusion and pore diffusion is

$$\Delta C = C_h - G_\infty$$

The diffusional path in the case of bulk diffusion is the distance L and the area across which diffusion can occur is A. In the case of the restraining matrix the path along which the component X must flow to travel from the high concentration to the low concentration face is L′; this is substantially greater in length than L, and so:

$$L' = \alpha L$$

where α is a geometric factor *greater* than unity. Similarly the diffusional, pore cross-sectional area, a, when a restraining matrix exists, is smaller than the apparent face area A, and therefore:

$$a = \beta A$$

where β is a geometric factor *less* than unity. The bulk diffusional flow may now be expressed as:

$$R_{bd} = \text{bulk diffusion rate of X from a face area A} = DA\,\frac{\Delta C}{L}$$

Here D is a proportionality constant called the diffusion coefficient. It is a property of the diffusing material X in the fluid. Similarly the pore diffusion flow can be expressed as:

$$
\begin{aligned}
R_{pd} &= \text{pore diffusional rate of X from a matrix whose face is A} \\
&= D\,a\,\frac{\Delta C}{L'} \\
&= \left(D\,\frac{\beta}{\alpha}\right) A\,\frac{\Delta C}{L} \\
&= D_e\,A\,\frac{\Delta C}{L}
\end{aligned}
$$

The "effective" diffusion coefficient D_e is lower than the diffusion coefficient of the component in the bulk fluid owing to the effect of the geometric factors α and β.

Permeation differs from pore diffusion in that the diffusing material is physically or chemically attached to the material forming the matrix. The movement of the permeating component X occurs when it moves from one active site to another within the material and *not* by the movement of X along channels within a matrix. In order for this mechanism of diffusion to be the dominant one, it is necessary for the component X and the separating material to have some affinity towards one another. This is evidenced by the solubility of X in the matrix material. The concentration driving force, then is no longer:

$$\Delta C = C_h - C_\infty$$

Because of the equilibrium existing between the concentration of X in the fluids on both sides of the material and the concentrations of X within the matrix, the concentration difference providing the diffusional driving force within the matrix is now:

$$\Delta C' = C_h' - C_\infty'$$

where C_h' and C_∞' represent the concentrations of X within the matrix material in equilibrium with the concentrations C_h and C_∞ in the fluid. The relationship between C_h' and C_h and between C_∞' and C_∞ may be generally approximately expressed in terms of a proportionality constant γ as:

$$C_h' = \gamma C_h$$

and

$$C_\infty' = \gamma C_\infty$$

This is described schematically in Figure 2. The factor γ is a Henry's low constant, relating the concentrations C' and C. The rate of permeation of X through the matrix material is then defined as:

$$R_s = \text{rate of permeation} = D_s A\,\frac{(C_h' - C_\infty')}{L}$$

D_s represents the diffusion coefficient of the component X through the solid matrix material *itself,* and not through its porous structure. Since it is easier to measure C_h and C_∞ rather than C_h' and C_∞', it is convenient to express the fluxes in terms of the driving force $\Delta C =$

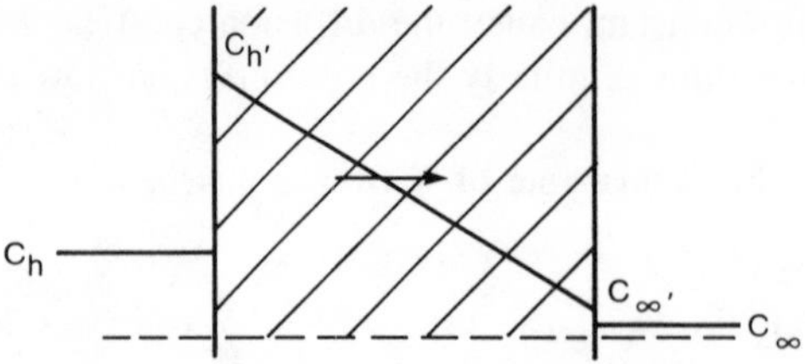

FIGURE 2. Concentration gradients during permeation.

Table 2
WATER VAPOR TRANSMISSION RATES MEASURED AT 28°C AND % R.H.

Sample	Permeability (g/mm 24 hr/m²)
Normal insensible water loss from human body	83[3]
Insensible water loss 11 days postburn (80%)	~1100[3]
Remoistened freeze-dried skin	28
Polylactic acid (#14117-2 and #14139-1)	4
75/25 lactic/glycolic copolymer (14149-7)	4.5
Poly ϵ-caprolactone (#14166)	17.6
Nylon 6	7
Saran Wrap®	0.2
Polyurethane	13
Epigard®	110
Collagen	30
Collagen — poly-ϵ-caprolactone laminate	24

$C_h - C_\infty$ and define a new factor called the ''permeability'', $P = D_s\gamma$. That factor, the product $D_s\gamma$, is the property generally reported as a result of experimental transport tests. In terms of P, the rate of permeation is expressed as:

$$R_s = P\,A\,\frac{\Delta C}{L}$$

When dealing with water the permeability is often expressed in terms of relative humidity or vapor pressure driving forces, and so:

$$R_{sw} = P'_w\,A\,\frac{\rho_w}{L}\left(\frac{p_{hw} - p_{\infty w}}{p_{sat,w}}\right)$$

where ρ_w represents the density of water and $p_{sat,w}$ represents the vapor pressure of water at the temperature of the experiment.

B. Permeation of Water through Polymers

Permeabilities of vapors and liquids through polymers have been studied extensively. Of interest is the permeability of water through various polymers. Table 2 lists some of these values; a standard driving force — that of pure water on one side of the membrane (= 100% relative humidity) with dry air on the other side — is used to express these results. This is a common form of expressing permeability data.

It is observed that permeabilities of materials to water can be very low (as in Saran Wrap®) or they can be very high (as in the case of cellulosic materials). The permeabilities of polylactic and polylactic/polyglycolic polymers fall within an intermediate range. Because of the biocompatibility of these polymers and their hydrolysis products they are used as sutures and are good candidates as sustained release matrices. These polymers are therefore of special interest to us and it is instructive to analyze some of their reported moisture transport data.

It is reported that the permeability of water vapor (or pure water, when both are in equilibrium in an atmosphere of 100% relative humidity) through a 75/25 polylactic/polyglycolic copolymer is about 4.5 g/mm/day/m²), i.e.;

$$P_w = \frac{4.5 \times 0.1}{10^4} \times \left(\frac{1}{1\ g/cm^3}\right) = 4.5 \times 10^{-5}\ cm^2/day$$

Note that here the permeability is calculated based on the polymer/liquid water equilibrium.

Some experiments indicate that the equilibrium moisture content of these polymers in a humid (100% R.H.) atmosphere is approximately 5%. The proportionality constant γ = moisture concentration in polymer/water concentration in pure water $\cong 0.05$. Note that the constant γ is calculated based on polymer/liquid water equilibrium in order to remain consistent with the calculation of the permeability, P.

Under these conditions, then:

$$\begin{aligned} D_{sw} &= P_w/\gamma \\ &= 4.5 \times 10^{-5}/0.05 \\ &= 0.9 \times 10^{-3}\ cm^2/day \end{aligned}$$

Let us now estimate the time required for allowing moisture to diffuse from the surroundings (an aqueous medium or 100% R.H.) into a sheet of polymer. A simple analysis of the water absorption process allows us to estimate — within an order of magnitude — the time required for a sheet to absorb from an initial state of dryness, a certain fraction of its equilibrium moisture from humid surroundings. The rate of absorption may be expressed in terms of the diffusivity or in terms of the rate of moisture picked up by the film as:

$$\text{Rate of absorption of water} \cong \frac{D_{sw}(2A)\,(C'_\infty - \overline{C})}{t/2} \cong At\,\frac{d\overline{C}}{d\theta}$$

where 2A represents the area of the two faces of the sheet of polymer; t represents the thickness of the polymer film; C_∞' represents the equilibrium moisture content of the polymer in contact with water; and $\overline{C}$ represents the average moisture of the film at some time θ. By integrating and rearranging the above equation, we get:

$$4\,\frac{D_{sw}\theta}{t^2} \cong \ln\left(\frac{C'_\infty}{C'_\infty - \overline{C}}\right)$$

If we consider, say 90% of the equilibrium moisture pick up, then:

$$\frac{\overline{C}_\infty}{\overline{C}_\infty - C_f} = \frac{1}{1 - 0.9} = 10$$

and so:

$$\theta = \frac{2.3}{4}\,\frac{t^2}{D_{sw}}$$

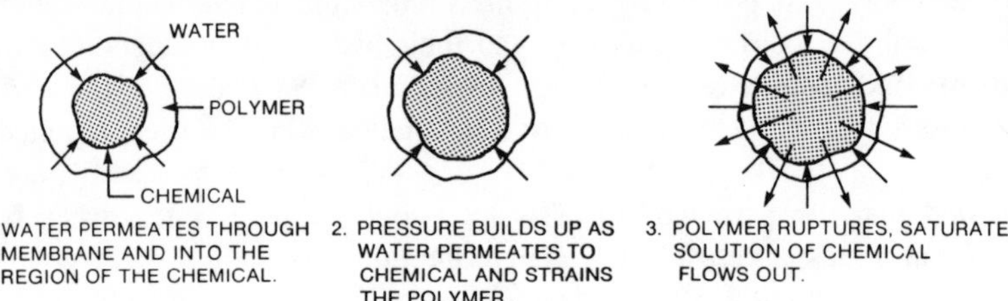

FIGURE 3. The effect of osmotic pressure on rupture of polymer.

For polylactic/polyglycolic copolymers, $D = 0.9 \times 10^{-3}$ cm^2/day. Therefore, for a sheet 2-mil thick ($= 5 \times 10^{-3}$ cm), the time elapsed before the sheet picks up 90% of its average moisture content is approximately equal to:

$$\theta = \frac{2.3}{4} \times \frac{25 \times 10^{-6}}{0.9 \times 10^{-3}} = 0.016 \text{ days}$$

$$= 23 \text{ min}$$

The rate of moisture picked up by the polymer is therefore relatively rapid, and a thin polymer film approaches its equilibrium moisture content readily, within a period of time considerably shorter than the desired period of a sustained release system (1 week to 1 year).

IV. SUSTAINED RELEASE MECHANISMS

A. Transport of Chemicals through Polymeric Membranes

A chemical encapsulated or dispersed within a polymeric material and placed within an aqueous fluid will tend to move by some means of transport mechanism from within the polymer to the external medium.

Similarly to water permeating through a polymer under its own driving force of moisture concentration gradients, a chemical will be transported across a polymer under its own concentration driving forces. When the chemical is a liquid, the mechanisms by which it permeates are similar to the mechanisms by which water permeates. When the chemical is a solid, its transport generally occurs via solution. The chemical first dissolves in the fluid permeating the polymer, then diffuses or flows out in solution. In addition to this diffusional transport mechanism, it is possible for the concentrated solution to flow out of the high concentration region within the polymer to the external aqueous solution by the bulk flow of a saturated chemical solution flowing under pressure. The pressure is created within the polymer by the unidirectional flow of water from the surroundings, through the polymer, and into the regions where the chemical is dispersed. The water continues flowing from the exterior and into these regions if its thermodynamic activity is higher in the surrounding aqueous layer than it is in the saturated solution of chemical dispersed within the polymer. The water will continue flowing into the system and the solution within it — if unrelieved — may reach its osmotic pressure. If no pores exist, the pressure rises within the material, and the polymer may crack at some weak spot thus creating its own outflowing channels. This process is described schematically in Figure 3. If no ''pores'' are available to relieve the pressure build-up within the cell, it will finally burst at some weak points creating its own outflowing channels.

It is therefore possible to have three different mechanisms causing a chemical to be transported or released from a water-permeable polymer:

1. By diffusional transport, driven by the concentration difference, through the structure of polymer
2. By diffusional transport, driven by the concentration difference along micro- or macropores in the polymeric material
3. By bulk flow, driven by the pressure difference across the polymeric material

Rates of release of chemical by these three mechanisms may be expressed as:

(1) R_s = rate of transport through the polymer structure

$$= (D_{s\gamma})\, A\, \frac{(C_h - C_\infty)}{L}$$

(2) R_p = pore diffusion rate of chemical

$$= (D_e)\, A\, \frac{(C_h - C_\infty)}{L}$$

(3) R_b = bulk flow driven by the pressure difference across the polymer

$$= \frac{R_{sw}}{\rho_w} C_h$$

where ρ_w refers to the density of water; C_h refers to the concentration of chemical in solution at the "high-concentration" region, i.e., its saturation concentration; and R_{sw} = rate of water permeating from the bulk of the surrounding liquid into the region where the chemical lies.

The first two mechanisms, related to diffusional transport, have been described earlier. The third, the bulk flow term, may be directly derived at steady state. At steady state, the rate of water influx is equal to its outflow. The influx of water is governed by its rate of permeation through the polymer and into the region where the chemical lies. At steady state, therefore:

$$R_{sw} = \text{mass rate of water permeating to the chemical}$$
$$= P_w \frac{A\, \rho_w}{L} \left(1 - \frac{p_w}{p_{sat\ w}}\right)$$

Since the outflowing water is saturated with chemical, the rate of release of chemical is therefore equal to:

$$R_b = \text{volumetric rate of water permeation X } C_h$$
$$= \frac{R_{sw}}{\rho_w} C_h$$
$$= P_w \frac{A}{L} \left(1 - \frac{p_w}{p_{sat\ w}}\right) C_h$$

If relatively few pores exist within the material, the major mechanism contributing towards the release of the chemical is bulk flow-saturated solution. If a large number of pores exist, the diffusional flux may exceed the bulk flow release rate.

In general, the total rate of release is the sum of release rates by the three mechanisms expressed above.

B. Pressure Build-Up within the Matrix

The pressure building up within the encapsulated chemical will be dependent on the geometry of the system and on the number of pores leading from the encapsulated material to the surrounding solution. If only a few pores exist with small diameters and a high degree of tortuosity, the pressure with the material will be higher than with a greater number of pores of larger diameter and less tortuosity in order to allow the same efflux of liquid in both cases. When no pores exist within the material the pressure within the material will reach the osmotic pressure of the solution. Since these pressures may be very high, the polymer may rupture before the osmotic pressure is reached and pore flow initiated.

The osmotic pressure (P_0) is defined as the pressure to which a solution must be raised in order to maintain it in equilibrium with the solvent. It is equal to:

$$P_o = -\frac{RT}{V} \ln X$$

where R = universal gas constant; T = temperature (°Absolute); V = specific volume of solution; and X = mole fraction of solvent (water). It is equal to:

$$\frac{(1 - W)/18}{(1 - W)/18 + nw/M}$$

where W = weight fraction of solute in the solution; M = molecular weight of solute; and n = number of ions resulting from the dissociation of the solute in water (n = 1 for nonionic solutes).

The osmotic pressure — for a given solute — increases with an increase in solute concentration. At saturation, therefore, highly soluble solutes will show a higher osmotic pressure than relatively insoluble ones.

A saturated salt solution, e.g., which reaches 25% by weight of sodium chloride has an osmotic pressure of 3500 psi, while a chemical whose molecular weight is 100 and whose solubility is 10% by weight will have an osmotic pressure of only 370 psi.

The tensile strength (σ) of most polymers falls within the range between 1,000 and 10,000 psi. Tests carried out at Dynatech indicate that polylactic acid has a tensile strength of about 7000 psi; lactic/glycolic copolymers have strengths ranging between 2000 and 7000 psi at high rates of deformation. Creep strengths are lower and are probably about one half the values indicated. Based on these values, the conditions of stability of polymer encapsulating a chemical may be calculated.

A spherical capsule of chemical whose diameter is d, surrounded by a polymer film of thickness t will burst if:

$$t/d < \frac{P_o}{4\sigma}$$

Cylindrical capsules will burst if:

$$t/d < \frac{P_o}{2\sigma}$$

Consider, then, a polymer whose tensile strength under creep is about 2000 psi encapsulating a sodium chloride sphere. The capsule will burst if:

$$t/d < \frac{3500}{800}$$

$$= 4.4$$

The wall thickness of a 100 μm-capsule must therefore be on the order of 45 μm or more to resist bursting. If, on the other hand, a chemical whose osmotic pressure at saturation is 370 psi is encapsulated, the capsule will burst if:

$$t/d < \frac{370}{8000}$$

$$= 0.046$$

In this case, the wall thickness of a 0-μm-capsule need only be on the order of 5 μm to resist bursting.

With some soluble, low molecular weight chemicals, it is therefore possible that the pressure may build up sufficiently in a relatively pore-free polymer to rupture the polymer and cause permeation to proceed by the bulk flow of the saturated solution, whereas in others, the likelihood of bursting is remote.

C. Relative Magnitudes of the Various Release Mechanisms

Three different mechanisms contribute to the sustained release of chemicals encapsulated or dispersed in a polymer: (1) diffusion of the chemical through the polymer; (2) diffusion of chemical along the pores of the polymer; and (3) bulk flow of saturated chemical solution through pores of the polymer.

The rates of these three mechanisms have been expressed earlier and defined as:

(1) Rate of transport through polymer structure:

$$R_s = D_s \frac{A}{L} (C_h' - C_\infty') \cong D_{s\gamma} \frac{A}{L} (C_h - C_\infty)$$

(2) Pore diffusion rate:

$$R_p = D_e \left(\frac{A}{L}\right) (C_h - C_\infty)$$

(3) Bulk flow transport:

$$R_b = \frac{R_{sw}}{\rho_w} C_h = P_w \frac{A}{L} \left(1 - \frac{P_w}{P_{sat\ w}}\right) C_h$$

If the material is placed within a large volume of receiving solution such that $C_\infty \ll C$ then, and if $P_w \ll P_{sat,w}$, i.e., the chemical at saturation reduces the vapor pressure of water appreciably, then:

$$R_s{:}R_p{:}R_b = D_s\gamma{:}D_e{:}P_w$$

D_s represents the diffusion coefficient of chemical through solid polymer and γ represents a Henry's low type of constant for the chemical relating its concentration within the aqueous and polymer phases. D_e represents the effective diffusion coefficient of salt in aqueous solution in a porous matrix whose pore volume fraction is ϵ. D_e has been found to be related to the bulk diffusivity D by the geometric relationship $D_e = D\beta/\alpha$. Experiments on porous materials indicate that $\beta/\alpha = \epsilon^2$. If the same relationship holds for the polymer matrixes used, then $D_e = D_\epsilon^{\,2}$. P_w represents the permeability of water through the polymer.

In order to estimate the relative magnitudes of the contribution of each mechanism to the release it is necessary to define the values of the different terms in the above relationship. As an example, a sodium chloride/polymer system was used as one test system. Sodium chloride was selected because most of its properties are known and because it is easy to measure quantitatively.

The aqueous diffusion coefficient:

$$D \equiv 1 \text{ cm}^2/\text{day}$$

The permeability of water through lactic/glycolic copolymers is about:

$$P_w = 4 \times 10^{-5} \text{ cm}^2/\text{day}$$

Some experiments with sodium chloride have indicated that the value of D_γ is less than 1.4×10^{-5} cm²/day. (Run NMH-1-27A.) The ratios of the contributions to the release rate may now be approximately estimated as:

$$R_s{:}R_p{:}R_b = D_{s\gamma}{:}D\,\epsilon^2{:}P_w$$

$$= (\text{less than } 1.4 \times 10^{-5}){:}\epsilon^2{:}4 \times 10^{-5}$$

If the polymer has a pore fraction of say 3.2%, then:

$$R_s{:}R_p{:}R_b = (\text{less than } 1.4 \times 10^{-5}){:}10^{-3}{:}4 \times 10^{-5}$$

The release under these conditions will be predominantly by pore diffusion of the salt. If one now considers relatively pore-free materials (with $\epsilon \sim 0.1\%$ pore volume), the relative contributions are

$$R_s{:}R_p{:}R_b = (\text{less than } 1.4 \times 10^{-5}){:}10^{-5}{:}4 \times 10^{-5}$$

In this case release by bulk flow of saturated solution will predominate via the few pores which may be present. If the sparsity of pores allows the pressure to build up beyond the bursting level, and an excessive porosity develops, the dominant mechanism will naturally shift to pore diffusion. It is clear that the porosity of a sample will have a great bearing on the mechanism of its release. For this reason, some tests were carried out to determine the pore volume of some samples of materials used to encapsulate sodium chloride. Mercury intrusion porosimetry was used to determine the pore size distributions. Sample NMH-1-30-1 was prepared by dissolving dl-lactide in methyl chloride (10 g/100 mℓ), casting a film (0.020-in. thick), and air drying at room temperature. Sample NMH-1-37 was prepared with the intent of creating a porous film. This was done by dissolving dl-lactide in methyl chloride (10.4 g/100 mℓ) and adding water to the solution (5 mℓ/100 mℓ of solution), then stirring vigorously in a blender for 60 sec. A film was then cast (0.02-in. thick) which was left to air dry.

It is observed that the mean pore size of both samples is about 5 μm (based on mercury porosimetry), and that the fine porosity of the sample NMH-1-37 was only about twice that of the other sample (0.09 cc and 0.04 cc void per gram, respectively). Visual inspection of the former sample showed a large number of holes about 1 mm in diameter; these cannot be detected by mercury intrusion porosimetry. These large holes may have contributed as much as 0.3 cc void per gram material in addition to the fine pores. Note that these values of porosities indicate that the main mechanism of release of salt *from such films* must be by pore diffusion. The same conclusion will be true of the release of other chemicals encapsulated within such films and which do not form a solid solution with the polymer (i.e., do not plasticize it).

Referring now to the release experiment mentioned above — which was carried out over a relatively short period of time, (Run NMH-1-27A), and from which a value of D_γ was estimated to be less than 1.4×10^{-5} cm²/day — it is possible to estimate the maximum possible value of the porosity of the polymer used. If the release during this test were totally controlled by pore flow (i.e., if $\gamma = 0$), then the rate measured must be equivalent to an effective diffusion coefficient of:

$$D_e = D\,\epsilon^2 = 1.4 \times 10^{-5} \quad \text{cm}^2/\text{day}$$

Since $D = 1$ cm²/day, then $\epsilon = 0.004$ cm³ void/cm³.

It is clear that over a longer period of time this capsule must burst yielding higher release rates than those measured during the limited initial test period. This behavior was observed in subsequent tests when, after a period of very slow release, a high rate was obtained till the salt was depleted.

V. RATES OF RELEASE

In the previous section, the major mechanisms of sustained release were described. In general, the release of chemical may occur from a matrix within which the chemical is well distributed — dispersed as discrete particles, or in solid solution — or from a capsule with the chemical surrounded by the polymer. In any of these cases, the transport of chemical may occur either by diffusion of chemical through the polymeric structure and/or pores or by bulk flow of the saturated chemical solution under the osmotic pressure buildup within the system. In this section, the formulation of some of the mechanisms of release will be attempted.

A. Rates of Release of a Chemical Uniformly Dispersed throughout a Polymer Matrix

Consider a matrix throughout which a chemical which forms no solid solution with the polymer (i.e., $\gamma = 0$) is uniformly dispersed in the form of individual tiny particles. When the matrix is placed in an aqueous solution, water permeates readily through the matrix; the chemical within the matrix dissolves in the permeating water forming a solution whose concentration reaches saturation near the center of the matrix but falls off gradually as the surface is approached. At the surface, the concentration depends on the stirring rate of the bulk of the solution. Figure 4 shows a schematic diagram of the concentration distribution across such a matrix. Within the matrix a "dissolving front" is observed. On the diagram, to the right of the dissolving front, there exist solid undissolved particles of chemical. In that region the solution within the matrix is saturated with chemical. To the left of the dissolving front, no solid chemical exists and the solution concentration is less than saturation ($C < C_{sat}$). At the matrix surface, the solution concentration (C_i) is somewhat higher than the concentration of chemical in the bulk of the solution (C_b). The difference between these two concentrations depends on the degree of stirring of the solution: the difference decreases with an increase in the degree of stirring and disappears completely (i.e., $C_i = C_b$) when perfect mixing is achieved.

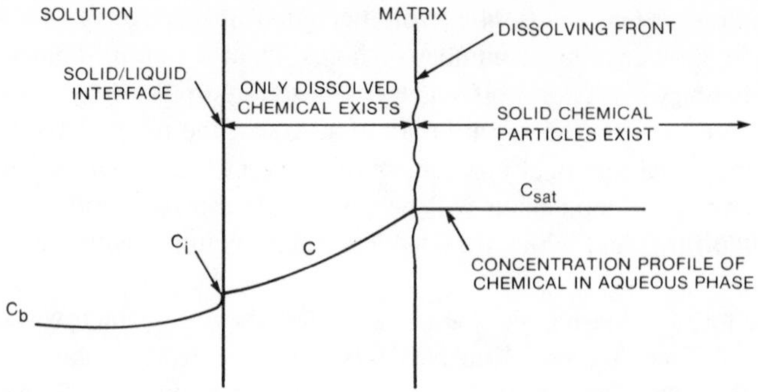

FIGURE 4. Diagram showing concentration distribution across section of matrix during release.

A differential equation may be written to express the rate of change of concentration within the matrix in the left-hand region (unsaturated region). This equation is

$$\frac{\partial}{\partial X}\left(-\ D_e\ A_x\ \frac{\partial C}{\partial X}\right) = A_x\ \frac{\partial C}{\partial \theta}$$

where D_e = effective diffusion coefficient; X = distance within matrix from polymer surface; A = cross-sectional area at some distance x; C = concentration of chemical in the permeating solution; and θ = time.

The dissolving front at any instant θ lies at a distance Z from the surface, and so the initial condition is

$$Z = 0 \text{ when } \theta = 0$$

The boundary conditions for the process are the following:

(1) The rate of release of chemical to the surrounding liquid

$$= +\left(D_e\ A\ \frac{\partial C}{\partial X}\right)_{(x=0)} = k\ A_{x=0}\ (C_i - C_b)$$

(2) The rate at which the dissolving front recedes

$$= \left(D_e\ A\ \frac{\partial C}{\partial X}\right)_{(x=z)} = C_l\ A_{x=z}\left(\frac{dz}{d\theta}\right)$$

where C_l = loading of chemical in mass per unit volume of matrix.
Also,

$$C_{x=z} = C_{sat}$$

In general, the loading level of chemical C_l is considerably greater than the saturation concentration C_s. Also, within the period of release, the effective diffusion coefficient, D_e, may be assumed to remain constant. Based on the assumptions that the accumulation of dissolved chemical within the matrix is negligibly small compared to the total amount of solid chemical loading and that the effective diffusion coefficient, D_e, remains constant during the release period, the differential equation may be solved for various configurations. For flat plates, the equations may be solved and analytic expressions written describing the fraction of chemical (-f) released and the rate of release (R) at any time θ.

1. Release from Flat Plates

For flat plates, the fraction of chemical released is a function of the diffusivity (D_e), the plate thickness (2L), the loading of chemical and its solubility (C_s), as well as the stirring rate. The fraction of chemical released can be expressed as:

$$f = -D_e/kL + \sqrt{(D_e/kL)^2 + 2(D\theta/L^2) \times (C_{sat} - C_b)/C_i}$$

L represents the half thickness of the plate.

The effect of stirring on the fraction released is a result of its effect on the mass transfer coefficient k. It is possible to approximate the value of k if the rate of stirring is expressed as the time taken to sweep the surface of the plate free from the solution and replace it with fresh solution. If that time is expressed as T and the diffusion coefficient of the chemical in bulk solution is D, then:

$$k \cong 2\sqrt{\frac{D}{t}}$$

The term D_e/kL is then equal to:

$$\frac{D_e}{kL} = \frac{D_e}{2L}\sqrt{\frac{T}{D}}$$

In order to get an estimate of the effect of stirring on the release, let us substitute some values in the above term. Let us assume that we are dealing with a film 0.1-cm thick (= 2L), which gives an effective diffusion coefficient of chemical (D_e) equal to 10^{-3} cm^2/day. The true diffusion coefficient in bulk solution (D) may generally be expected to be about 1 cm^2/day. The stirring term is then equal to:

$$\frac{D_e}{kL} = \frac{10^{-3}}{0.1}\sqrt{\frac{T}{1}} = 10^{-2}\sqrt{T}$$

A solution stirred only once a day (T = 1 day) will then show an error equivalent to $D_e/kL \cong 0.01$. This is a small error when about 10% of the chemical has been released (i.e., $f \sim 0.10$). Better stirring will introduce less error.

In relatively well-stirred solutions, the fraction of chemical released as a function of hire may therefore be expressed more simply as

$$f = \sqrt{2(D_e\theta)(C_{sat} - C_b/C_1)/L^2}$$

in well-stirred solutions. It is observed that the rate is initially high but slowly tapers off until the material is all released when:

$$\frac{2D_e\theta}{L^2}\frac{(C_{sat} - C_b)}{C_e} = 1$$

i.e.:

$$\theta_{final} = \frac{L^2}{2D_e}\frac{C_e}{(C_{sat} - C_b)}$$

2. Release from Rods

When rods are being considered, the differential equation expressing the release can be solved, but the results cannot be stated in an explicit analytical form as was the case with flat plates. The equation relating the depth of the dissolving front to the release period can be obtained by making the assumption that accumulation of dissolved chemical within the matrix is negligible and that D_e remains constant:

$$\frac{D_e\theta}{r_o^2}\frac{(C_{sat} - C_b)}{C_e} = \left(\frac{D_e}{kr_o}\right)\left(\frac{z}{r_o}\right)\left(1 - \frac{z}{r_o}\right) + \frac{(1 - z/r_o)^2}{2}\ln\left(1 - \frac{z}{r_o}\right) - \frac{(1 - z/r_o)^2}{4} + \frac{1}{4}$$

The fraction of chemical released (f) is related to Z as:

$$f = \frac{\pi r_o^2 - \pi(r_o - z)^2}{\pi r_o^2} = 1 - (1 - z/r_o)^2$$

In well-stirred solutions, the first term on the right-hand side of the equation relating Z and θ may be ignored, and the fraction of chemical dissolved can be plotted against the term $(D_e\theta/r_0^2)$ $(C_{sat} - C_b/C_1)$. The calculations indicate that the chemical is fully released when:

$$\frac{D_e\theta}{r_o^2}\frac{(C_{sat} - C_b)}{C_e} = 0.25$$

or

$$\theta_{final} = \frac{r_o^2}{4D_e}\frac{C_e}{(C_{sat} - C_b)}$$

3. Release from Spheres

The release from spheres can be estimated in a manner similar to that used for cylinders. The distance of the dissolving front from the surface of the heads is related to the release period by:

$$\frac{D_e\theta}{r_o^2}\frac{(C_{sat} - C_b)}{C_e} = \frac{1}{3}\left(\frac{D_e}{kr_o}\right)\left[1 - \left(1 - \frac{z}{r_o}\right)^3\right] + \left(\frac{z}{r_o}\right)^2\left[\frac{1}{2} - \frac{1}{3}\frac{z}{r_o}\right]$$

When the mixture is well stirred, the first term on the right-hand side of the above equation can be ignored and the relationship is simplified to:

$$\frac{D_e\theta}{r_o^2}\frac{(C_{sat} - C_b)}{C_e} = \left(\frac{z}{r_o}\right)^2\left[\frac{1}{2} - \frac{1}{3}\frac{z}{r_o}\right]$$

The material is fully depleted when Z = 0 and

$$\frac{D_e\theta}{r_o^2}\frac{(C_{sat} - C_b)}{C_e} = \frac{1}{6}$$

or

$$\theta_{final} = \frac{r_o^2}{6D_e}\frac{C_e}{(C_{sat} - C_b)}$$

The fraction of chemical released at any instant can be estimated from the relationship between Z and θ. Here, the fraction released, f, is given by:

$$f = 1 - (1 - z/r_o)^3$$

ACKNOWLEDGMENT

This work was carried out in the Chemical Engineering Department of Dynatech R/D Company, Cambridge, Mass.

Chapter 10

ALTERNATIVES TO CONTROLLING DRUG RELEASE

Donald L. Wise and David Bergbreiter

TABLE OF CONTENTS

I. ALTERNATIVE CATALYSTS FOR POLYMERIZATION

Polylactic or polyglycolic acid formation is catalyzed by a variety of catalysts, however, in materials whose ultimate use is as a drug implant, some concern must be given to the nature of the catalyst. Tetraphenyltin is an example of an effective catalyst whose toxicity could pose a problem. Therefore, some common basic catalysts have been considered. The mechanism of polymer formation under these conditions is shown in Structure 1. In this scheme, some catalyst (Nu^-) that has an unshared pair of electrons and possibly a negative charge attacks the lactide or glycolide in an initiation step. Possible catalysts or initiators are a number of common bases. Sodium methoxide ($CH_3O^-Na^+$), sodium phenoxide ($C_6H_5O^-Na^+$), and *n*-butyllithium (n-$C_4H_9^-Li^+$) are examples of three bases that function in the same manner.* The Lewis acidity of the metal ion could also play an important part in the efficiency of polymerization. A more acidic metal ion than lithium, sodium, or potassium would be magnesium, zinc, or aluminum. These more-acidic metals would coordinate better to the carbon-oxygen double bond in the lactide and polarize it so that it would be more susceptible toward attack by the growing polymer chain. Examples of possible catalysts using this idea are magnesium methoxide [$Mg(OCH_3)^2$], zinc acetate [$Zn(CH_3CO_2)_2$], and aluminum methoxide [$Al(OCH_3)_3$].**

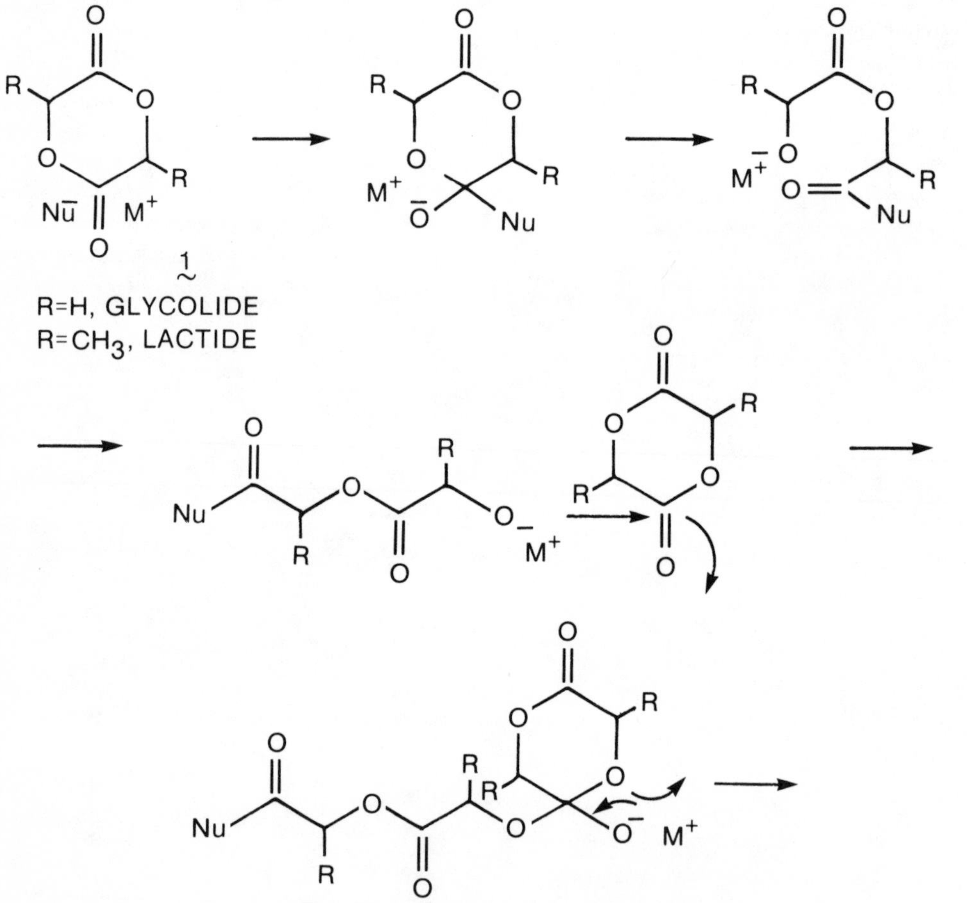

1

R=H, GLYCOLIDE
R=CH_3, LACTIDE

* These three bases are commercially available or could be prepared. Potassium alkoxides would also be suitable catalysts. Preparation of the alkoxides could be accomplished by addition of the corresponding alcohol to sodium or potassium hydride or to sodium or potassium amide. *n*-Butyllithium is sold by Alfa Inorganics.

** These three bases are commercially available from Research Organic/Inorganic Chemical Corp.

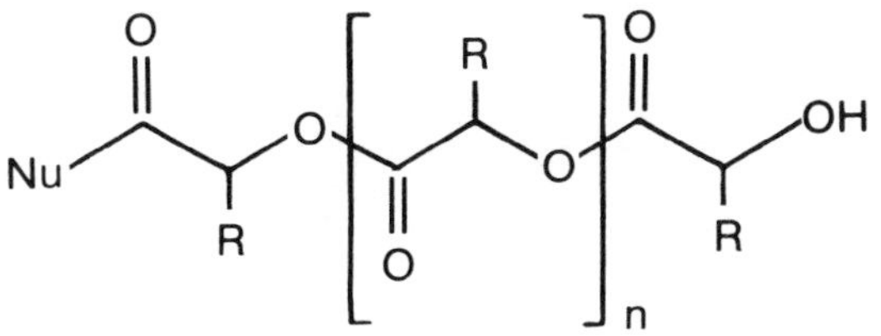

POLYMER

An important point with regard to all of these catalysts is that the polymerization will be sensitive to even small amounts of water. Presence of small amounts of water can reduce the molecular weight of the resultant polymer by protonation of the growing polymer chain. Shriver's book[1] (especially Chapters 7 and 8) is a standard reference for laboratory techniques for compounds or reactions that are air or water sensitive.

II. POLYMER CROSS-LINKING TO CONTROL DRUG RELEASE

Cross-linking of the polylactic/polyglycolic acid polymer is one means of controlling the release rate of a drug that is physically mixed with the polymer. Cross-linking should decrease the possibility that the drug could leach out of the polymer matrix. Cross-linking could also be an alternative to chemically binding the drug to the polymer. Any cross-linking agent will probably have some effect on the hydrolysis rate and on the physical properties of the polymer. However, the change in properties could be modulated by changing the amount of cross-linking agent and hence the amount of cross-linking. Biocompatibility of the resulting cross-linked polymer is essential as well. The possible cross-linking agents suggested are not listed as toxic in the *Merck Index*.

There are two possible approaches to cross-linking. The first approach and perhaps the easiest would be to do the cross-linking *in situ* (during the polymerization). To be effective as a cross-linking agent *in situ,* a chemical would have to have two functional groups, both of which could react with the growing polymer chain. Two possible cross-linking agents are shown below. 1,2,4,5-Benzenetetracarboxylic anhydride (Structure 2) has two anhydride groups and 1,2,7,8-diepoxyoctane (Structure 3) has two epoxy groups that can react with the growing polymer chain as in Structure 4.*

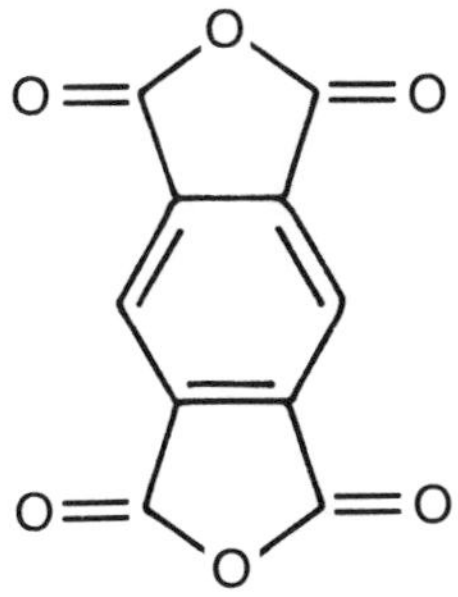

2

1,2,4,5 — BENZENETETRACARBOXYLIC ANHYDRIDE

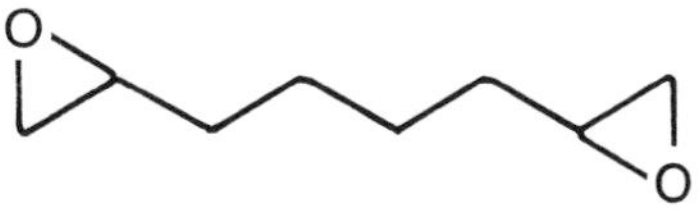

3

1,2,7,8 — DIEPOXYOCTANE

* Both chemicals are commercially available from the Aldrich Chemical Co.

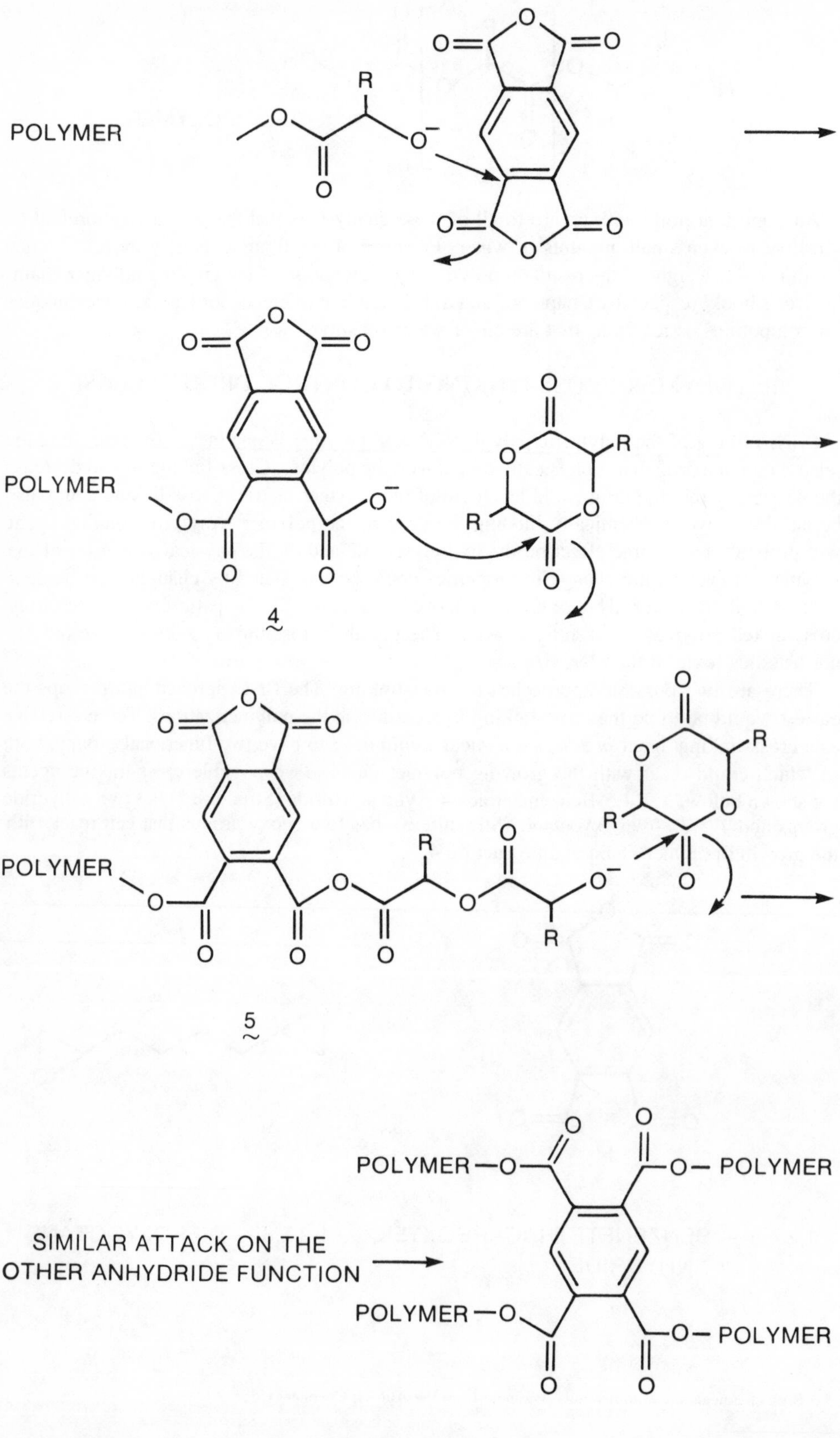

POLYMER

POLYMER

4

POLYMER

5

SIMILAR ATTACK ON THE OTHER ANHYDRIDE FUNCTION →

POLYMER—O … O—POLYMER

POLYMER—O … O—POLYMER

In Structure 4, the cross-linking agent is 1,2,4,5-benzenetetracarboxylic anhydride (pyromellitic anhydride). The cross-linking agent would be present during the polymerization to the extent of a few percent. One of the two anhydride groups would react with a growing polymer chain and incorporate itself into that chain. This process would liberate a free carboxylate anion (Structure 4) which could continue chain growth by reaction with another lactide (or glycolide) molecule. The resulting polymer (Structure 5) then has another anhydride group which could react with a different polymer chain to give cross-linking.

The second approach to cross-linking would be to incorporate as a copolymer some compound that has a reactive group that could serve as a cross-linking agent in a later step. Examples of two such compounds would be maleic anhydride and a 2-dodecen-1-ylsuccinic anhydride (Structure 6).*

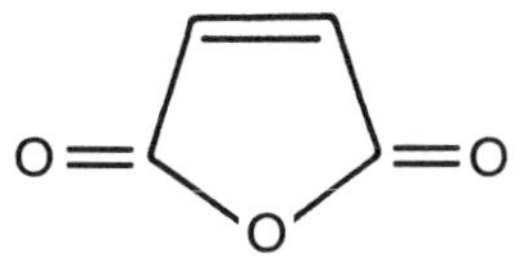

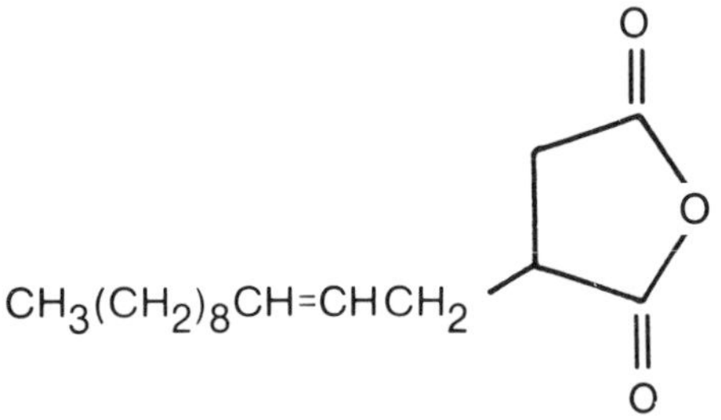

In this approach, the potential cross-linking agent would be copolymerized with the polylactic/polyglycolic acid to the extent of 1 or 2%. The resulting polymer would have an occasional carbon-carbon double bond in the polyester chain. Addition of a peroxide to the polymer and subsequent heating would produce free radicals which would add to these carbon-carbon double bonds. This would produce carbon radicals on one chain which could react with carbon-carbon double bonds on another chain to give cross-linked polymer. A very similar process is used to cross-link silicone rubber.[2,3]

III. CHEMICAL BINDING OF DRUGS TO POLYMER TO CONTROL RELEASE

Chemical binding of drugs to the polymer might result in better control of the drug release rate. In order to covalently bind some drug, the first consideration must be what functional groups are available on the drug as binding sites. In the case of the two morphine antagonists, Naloxone (Structure 7) and cyclazocine (Structure 8), the most reactive functional group is the phenolic hydroxyl (circled).

* Both of these chemicals are commercially available from the Aldrich Chemical Co.

• ACIDIC PROTONS

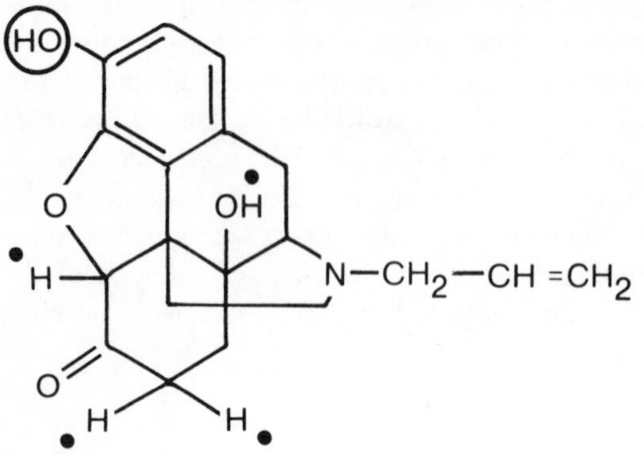

7 NALOXONE

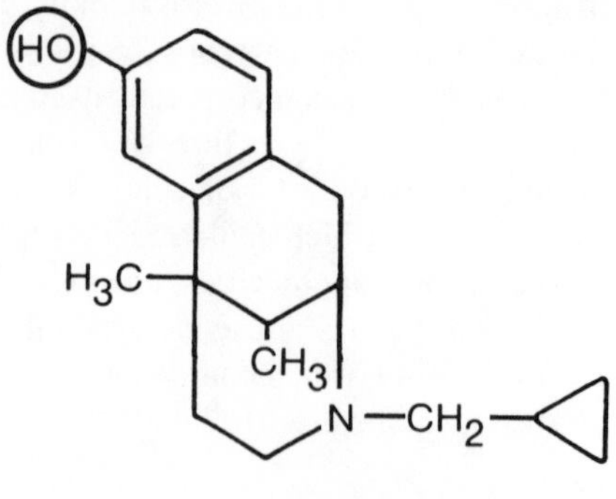

8 CYCLAZOCINE

The proton on this hydroxyl group is approximately a factor of 10^6 more acidic than any other proton in these two drugs. Therefore, addition of one equivalent of a base like ethoxide or methoxide will preferentially form the phenoxide. However, in Structure 7 there are four other protons that could be called acidic although they are much less acidic than the phenol. The problem here is that if they were pulled off they could produce a chemical change in the structure of the drug. For this reason, cyclazocine is the more suitable of the two drugs for chemical binding to the polymer. However, Structure 7 could still be tried. Chances of complications are just greater with it.

The two malaria-control chemicals, Structures 9 and 10, also differ in chemical complexity but not to the same extent as the morphine antagonists. In Structure 9 the functional group with the best potential for binding to the polymer is the carboxylic group (circled). The carboxylate anion from this group can be prepared with an alkoxide base or even a hydroxide base. It could also be esterified with an alcohol and an acid. The second malarial-control drug (Structure 10) has two acidic protons, but the hydroxyl proton H_A is about a factor of 10^{17} more acidic. Here the alkoxide could be prepared by reaction of Structure 10 with one equivalent of a strong base like sodium hydride or potassium hydride.

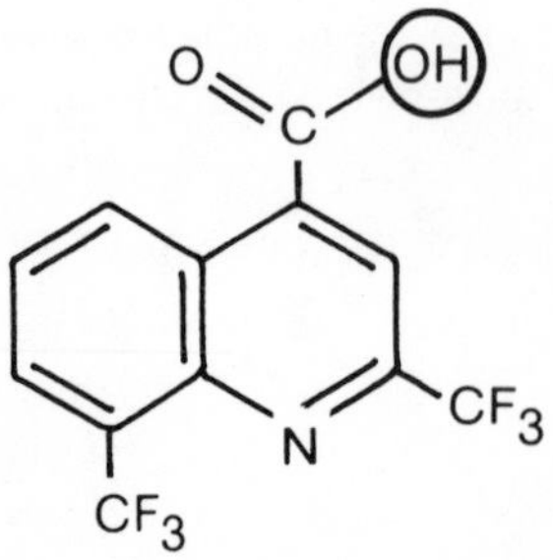

9

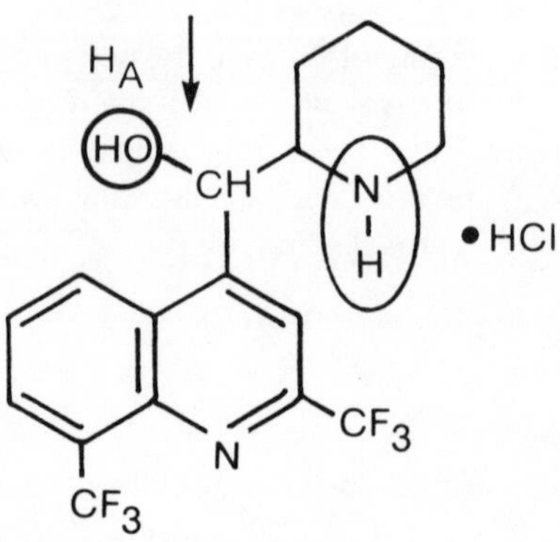

10

The steroid (Structure 11) is probably the most difficult of all four drugs with regards to chemical binding to a polymer. Here the best approach would probably be to try incorporating the drug physically in a cross-linked polymer rather than to try to covalently bind it. The best approach in this case would probably be to try and bind the drug by means of a readily hydrolyzable bond to the carbonyl group. A binding procedure using the acetate at C-17 might also be able to be developed.

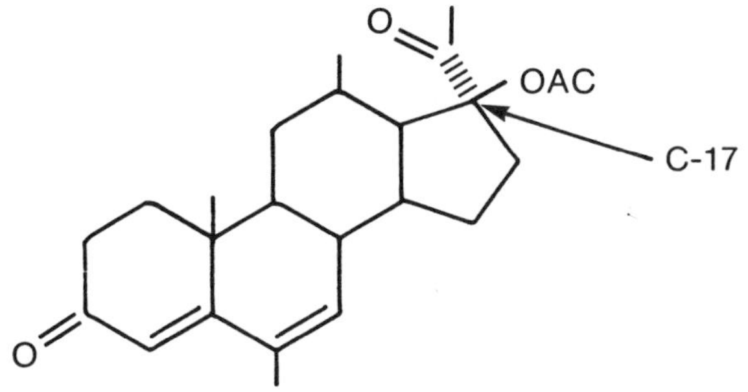

OAC

C-17

11

There are several possible procedures for chemical binding of these drugs. The drugs that can be made into alkoxide or carboxylate anions have the potential to be initiators in the polymerization of polylactic/polyglycolic acid. They could also be added to preformed polymer. In this case there would be some polymer degradation, but if the initial molecular weight was high it could work all right. Another possible procedure for Structure 9 would be to esterify the carboxylic acid and add it to the polymerization mixture. During the polymerization the growing polymer chain would attack this ester in a chain termination step to produce chemically bound drug and an alkoxide that would initiate further chain formation. Esterification of an acid is often conveniently accomplished by addition of alcohol and a catalytic amount of an acid such as p-toluenesulfonic acid to the acid to be esterified and then azeotroping away the water formed during the esterification. A similar idea to that proposed for Structure 9 would be to acetylate the alcohols in the other drugs and to add the acetates to the polymerization. As described above, the growing polymer chain could attack the acetate from the drug and free the drug as an alkoxide. The drug would then go on to initiate polymer formation. With this approach Structure 7 would be linked to two polymer chains (each hydroxyl) and Structure 10 might also be linked by both the nitrogen and the hydroxyl. A simple procedure for acetylation is that described by Fieser.[5]

In the case of the two morphine antagonists, a question has been raised about the way in which the drug would be hydrolyzed from the polymer. Because the bond between the drug and the polymer and the polymer ester bonds would hydrolyze at about the same rate, release of the drug could result. One way to get around this problem would be to bind the drug to the polymer with a bond that would hydrolyze much faster than the polymer. Examples of such linkages would be the groups shown below.

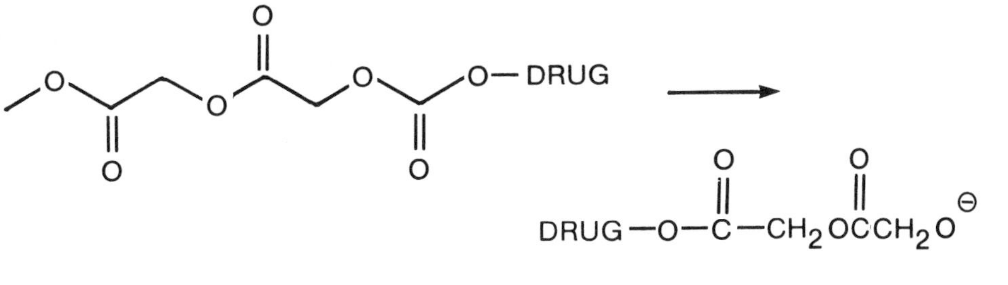

O—DRUG ⟶

$DRUG—O—\overset{O}{\overset{\|}{C}}—CH_2O\overset{O}{\overset{\|}{C}}CH_2O^{\ominus}$

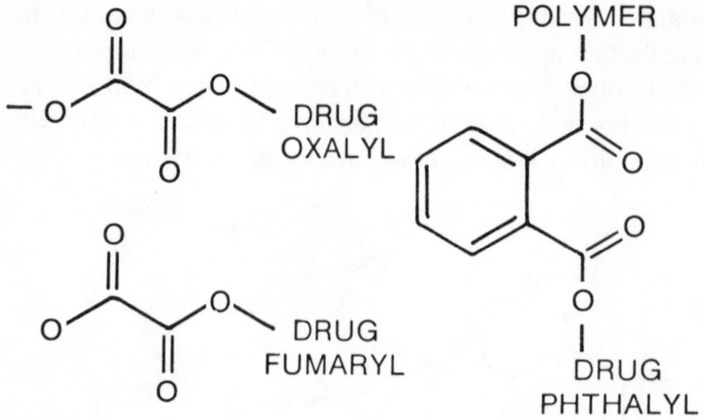

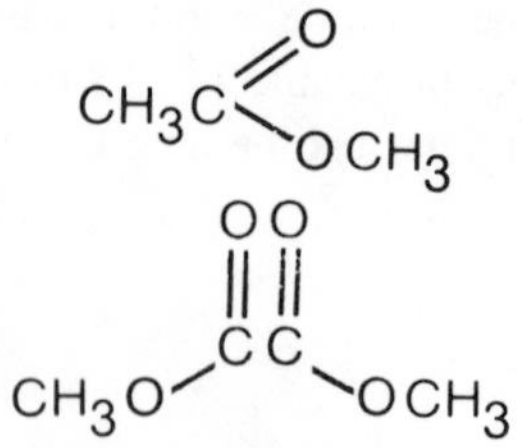

The alkaline hydrolysis rate — which shows the same effect of structure on rate as neutral hydrolysis — for Structure 12 vs. 13 is approximately 100,000 times faster for Structure 12.[17] The fumaryl and phthalyl groups should show similar effects, but the rate acceleration would probably not be nearly as much. The by-product of these linkages is biocompatible in the case of fumaryl. Oxalic acid and phthalic acid are both toxic in large amounts but should be biocompatible in this case because the amounts of oxalic and phthalic acid are small and are introduced over large periods of time. These types of linkages to the polymer would be prepared in the case of Structure 8 by adding the drug to an excess of the diacid chloride (e.g., oxalyl chloride). Evaporation under reduced pressure of the solution will remove the excess diacid chloride and give an aryl chloroglyoxalate (Structure 14) which, when added to a solution of the polymer, will react with the hydroxy end groups of the polymer to form a readily hydrolyzable bond.

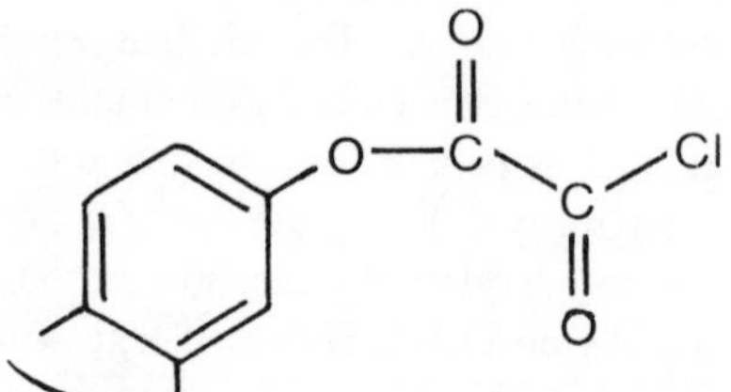

Incorporating drugs covalently in implants seems to be a very reasonable idea; initially it will be best to work with the most simple drugs. This way there will be less problem with changing the drug and evaluation of the technique may be easier.

IV. SUMMARY

A brief review was carried out on the potential for alternative factors influencing the sustained release of active agents from a polymeric matrix. Of importance for acceptance as an implant to humans, as well as on polymer molecular weight, a review of alternative catalysts was made. Further, the potential for cross-linking of the polymer to control release rate was explored. Also considered was the possibility of chemical binding of drugs to the polymer in order to further control drug release.

ACKNOWLEDGMENT

This work was sponsored by Dynatech R/D Company, Cambridge, Mass. when David Bergbreiter was a graduate student at the Massachusetts Institute of Technology, Cambridge.

REFERENCES

1. **Shriver, D. F.,** *The Manipulation of Air Sensitive Compounds,* McGraw-Hill, New York, 1969.
2. **Odian, G.,** *Principles of Polymerization,* McGraw-Hill, New York, 1970.
3. **Alliger, G. and Sjothun, I. J.,** *Vulcanization of Elastomers,* Reinhold, New York, 1964.
4. **Fieser, L. F.,** *Organic Experiments,* Raytheon Education Company, Lexington, Mass., 1968, 242.
5. **Hammett, L. P.,** *Physical Organic Chemistry,* McGraw-Hill, New York, 1940, 212.

Alternative Applications

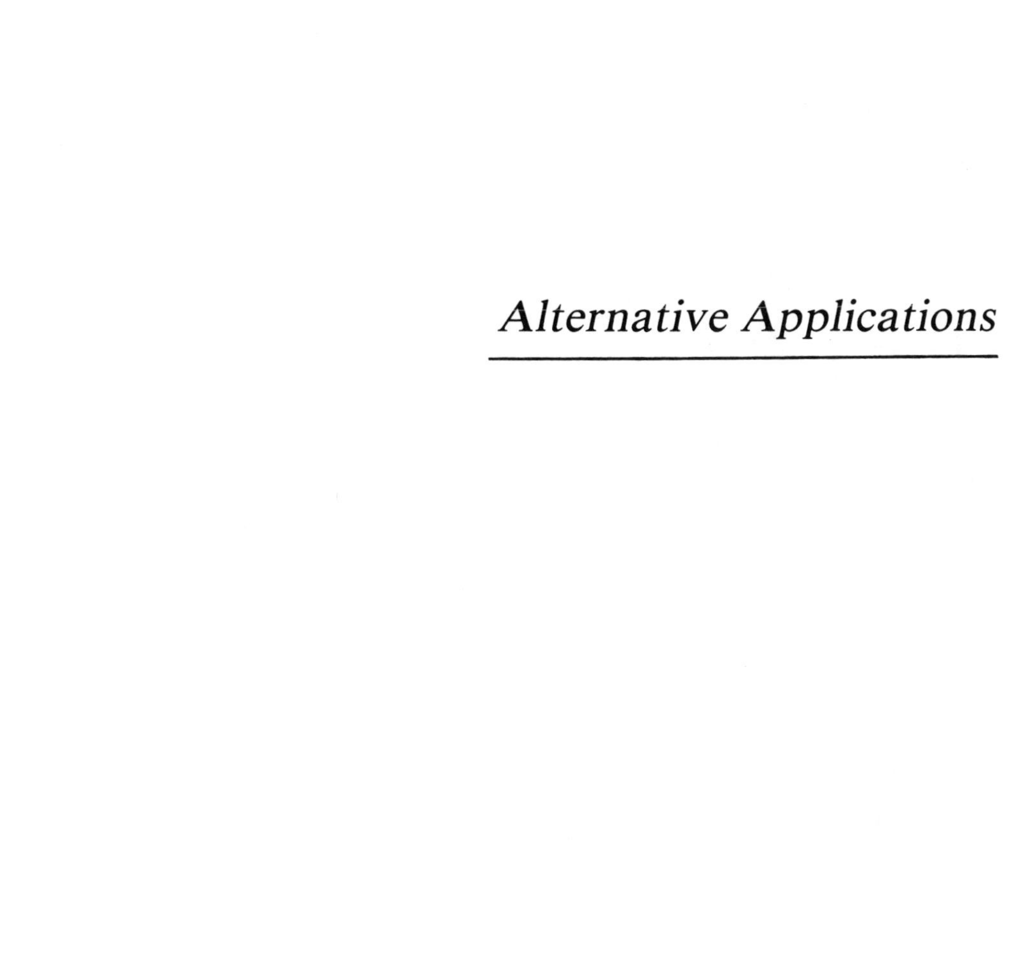

Chapter 11

EVALUATION OF REPAIR MATERIALS FOR AVULSIVE COMBAT-TYPE MAXILLOFACIAL INJURIES

Donald L. Wise, Ralph L. Wentworth, John E. Sanderson, and Stephen C. Crooker

TABLE OF CONTENTS

I. INTRODUCTION

The initial feasibility work to develop a repair material for avulsive combat-type maxillofacial injuries is described. A composition containing poly(propylene fumarate), an unsaturated cross-linkable polymer made from fumaric acid, one of the Krebs cycle acids, and propylene glycol, a commonly used diluent in parenteral drug formulations, along with benzoyl peroxide, vinyl pyrollidone, and an inert filler such as calcium sulfate (gypsum) has been shown to be easily workable by hand, to solidify in ~15 min at physiological temperatures, and to have physical properties suitable for the intended application. An additional component which may be required to provide adequate shelf life is a food grade antioxidant such as Tenox (TBHQ). Further, a medicament, growth factor, etc. may be incorporated into this formulation and be slowly released at a predesigned rate. The results obtained with this initial composition suggest that this material is ready for in vivo evaluation in a suitable animal model.

A. Present Status

Based on a feasibility program, a surgical repair material has been shown to be easily formulated, workable by hand to a "putty"-like consistency, to solidify in ~15 min at physiological temperatures, and to have physical properties suitable for the intended application of avulsive combat-type maxillofacial injuries. Incorporation of a sustained release medicament, growth factor, etc. into this "putty" is integral to the concept, but was not specifically evaluated at this time. The present feasible formulation — which demonstrates the concept but is not believed to be optional — is a composition containing: (1) poly(propylene fumarate), an unsaturated cross-linkable biodegradable polymer made from fumaric acid, one of the Krebs Cycle acids, and propylene glycol, a commonly used diluent in parenteral drug formulations, used in this case to form a polyester; (2) vinyl pyrollidone, a viscous liquid carrier, or solvent material having chemical unsaturation suitable for cross-linking; (3) an inert filler such as calcium sulfate (gypsum); and (4) benzoyl peroxide, a reagent capable of initiating cross-linking to the extent needed to convert the "putty" to a solid. An additional component which may be required to provide adequate shelf life is a food grade antioxidant such as Tenox (TBHQ). Further, as noted, medicaments for a number of purposes (bactericides, growth factors, etc.) may be incorporated into this formulation with the objective of being released in a predesigned manner. The results obtained with this composition to date suggest that this material is ready for in vivo evaluation in a suitable animal model. Clearly, continued research and development will be required but present results merit presentation.

B. Plans for Continued Work

Some of the work yet to be done is as follows. Foremost will be the practical evaluation of a range of filler loadings to achieve a suitable hand-workable putty that also has optional biodegradability and strength characteristics. Both inert inorganic salts and finely divided biodegradable polymers will be investigated. Further, the incorporation of a sustained release agent such as a growth factor will be investigated.

The use of copolymers of fumaric and succinic acids will be synthesized and evaluated. Here the objective will be to include succinic acid, having no cross-linking functionality, into the polymeric backbone along with the fumaric acid used presently which has cross-linking functionality on every mer unit. The result should be a tougher, more flexible, and less brittle polymer with lower inert filler loadings.

Several practical aspects of an optimal formulation will be investigated including shelf-life stability, sterility test, and formulation and packaging studies.

Of a more fundamental research nature, but with practical import, will be the careful determination of the heat of reaction of the surgical repair material. This information will be essential documentation to provide comparison of the present system with other surgical repair materials. Also of practical import will be the projection of scale-up methods.

C. Project Rationale

The potential of polymeric materials for surgical repair has been appreciated by surgeons, dentists, and medical researchers, and promising development has been reported. Some of the aims of work to date have been attainment of biodegradability, flexibility of formulation for tailoring at the surgical site, and achievement of ultimately acceptable esthetic results. The need for such materials is especially acute in the treatment of avulsive maxillofacial wounds in military situations. In these applications, there are encountered not only the exacting surgical demands of maxillofacial wound treatment, but the special logistical demands of military utilization. Thus the state of development of surgical repair materials to date, while promising, has not yet been brought to a satisfactory stage. Salient characteristics expected in the improved material include

1. Controlled biodegradability
2. Significant adherence to bone
3. A formable, moldable composition with acceptable working time
4. Development of adequate physical strength
5. Environmental stability
6. Incorporation of sustained release medicaments, growth factors, etc. into the repair material

The work described herein was based on the use of biocompatible, biodegradable polymers synthesized from substances occurring in the so-called Krebs cycle of metabolism. Chemical qualities of these polymers include the possibility of formulating them in a molecular weight range well-suited for preparing pastes or moldable putties. In addition, certain members of this class of polymers possess unsaturation, or potential for controlled cross-linking. Under proper control this cross-linking characteristic may be exploited to convert a formable mass to a rigid structure having good physical properties, but retaining the quality of biodegradability. Previous work to apply these materials to the sustained release of drugs has experimentally confirmed their biodegradability as well as revealing the preparative procedures required to provide the desired surgical repair materials. Separation of the desired fraction may be carried out by fractional precipitation. For example, a solution of polymer in methylene chloride blended with ethyl ether will yield a precipitate of high molecular weight polymer. The remaining low molecular weight material may also be recovered for use.

II. TECHNICAL DISCUSSION

The application of polymers and plastics to many areas of medicine and surgery has grown in several directions according to the primary technical needs to be met. Some needs emphasize permanence in the body environment. In other instances an impermanent quality is desired. Compatibility with tissues is a consideration in all cases, although total inertness is not vital in every instance. Additional properties of concern are physical strength or resilience and plasticity or formability. The permeability or diffusional transport characteristics of a material often are of primary concern. Such diverse needs can be met through application of materials chosen from the spectrum of polymer technology.

In the question of degradability, there exists at one extreme a demand for permanence, e.g., for uses in prosthesis such as heart valves or pacemakers. In instances such as fabricating a tissue-reinforcing network, a relatively undegradable material such as Mylar polyester may be chosen. At the other extreme, fairly prompt degradation may be desired. Degradable sutures are a prime example, and polyglycolic acid has emerged as a material of choice for preparation of degradable sutures. The related material, polylactic acid, has been applied extensively to the formulation of implants for sustained delivery of drugs for periods as short as a few weeks.

It has been postulated that the success of polylactic acid as an implant material tolerated by the tissues so well is due to the fact that the breakdown product of its hydrolysis, lactic acid, is a material naturally occurring in the body. The fact that no foreign substance or disruptive chemical is produced may be of primary importance in rendering polylactic acid innocuous when implanted in the tissues. This reasoning led to the search for other families of polymers possessing this trait, i.e., dissolution in the tissues to produce material normally present in the body. Success was met in this search when investigation was made of polymers prepared from the substances occurring in the so-called Krebs cycle of metabolism (otherwise termed the "citric acid cycle" or the "tricarboxylic acid cycle"). These polymers are polyesters prepared from such acids as citric, cis-aconitic, α-ketoglutaric, succinic, fumaric, malic, and oxaloacetic. These acids are reacted with physiologically tolerable polyol compounds, e.g., glycerol, glycerol esters, propylene glycol, mannitol, or sorbitol. Among these polymers are substances which have properties which fit them well for application as surgical repair materials. These properties are (1) susceptibility to preparation as a relatively low molecular weight viscous fluid suited for compounding as a paste, and (2) opportunity to formulate from monomers having vinyl unsaturation, permitting subsequent controlled cross-linking. These two qualities enable preparation of a moldable composition which can then be set to a firm form through the action of a cross-linking agent, as is the practice in preparing bone cements. These objectives are achievable in material having the quality of biodegradability.

A. Polymer Preparation

The specific polymer described herein was poly(propylene fumarate). The polymer is prepared through the reaction of propylene glycol and diethyl fumarate:

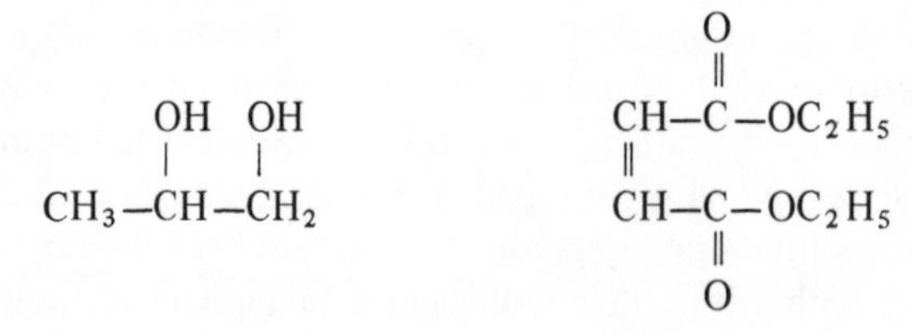

$$CH_3{-}\underset{|}{\overset{OH}{C}}H{-}\underset{}{\overset{OH}{\underset{|}{C}}}H_2 \qquad \begin{array}{l} \quad\ \ O \\ \quad\ \ \| \\ CH{-}C{-}OC_2H_5 \\ \| \\ CH{-}C{-}OC_2H_5 \\ \quad\ \ \| \\ \quad\ \ O \end{array}$$

Propylene glycol   Diethyl fumarate

Methods of preparation are suspension polymerization in silicone oil and bulk polymerization. In suspension polymerization, the polymer appears to form first in the oil phase, due to the solubility of diethyl fumarate in silicone oil. As the forming polyester reaches higher molecular weight, solubility in the glycol phase becomes favored and the site of polymer growth moves to the glycol. Polymerization is initiated at atmospheric pressure at a temperature of 180°C. An acid catalyst, e.g., p-toluene sulfuric acid, is used. Following about 90 hr under these initial conditions, the reactant mixture is exposed to vacuum at a pressure of 20 mmHg under reflux, and the polymerization is permitted to continue until the desired molecular weight is attained. Experience has shown that it is desirable to attain a temperature of 145°C while the polymerization mass is under reflux.

In the procedure of bulk polymerization, the reactants are heated at about 140°C. The distillate collected in this procedure is largely ethanol, but contains some diethyl fumarate. If a solid product is desired, heating is carried out to higher temperatures, up to 220°C with a distillation column attached. Final stripping is accomplished by application of vacuum.

In the procedures worked out for polymerization of propylene glycol and diethyl fumarate, a special concern has been avoidance of cross-linking of the fumarate position of the polymer. The procedures adopted avoid this, and regulation of molecular weight of the product is simply a matter of time held at elevated temperatures. When high molecular weight material is desired, the polymerization is permitted to proceed to a point where the product is a solid at room temperature, melting about 80°C. When a viscous fluid is required, polymer of this nature is produced through shorter treatment.

B. Principles of Formulation

The basis for the improved surgical repair material is fourfold:

1. A viscous liquid carrier material having chemical unsaturation susceptible to cross-linking
2. A filler material which will convert the liquid to a workable paste or putty suitable for emplacement by the surgeon
3. A reagent capable of initiating cross-linking to the extent needed to convert the putty to a solid
4. A medicament and/or growth factor for predesigned sustained release

These components must, of course, combine to produce a material having the biocompatibility and biodegradation qualities desired. It must adhere to bone and exhibit adequate physical strength.

The cross-linkable liquid medium is poly(propylene fumarate). Work has been done both with fluid, low molecular weight polymer, and with high molecular weight polymer dissolved in solvent. This liquid is converted to a paste or putty form through addition of a powdered filler material. It will be appreciated that if the liquid is blended with the powdered ingredients, a certain minimum proportion of liquid must be added to the powder before coherent mixture is obtained. If the proportion of fluid is then increased, the mass will take on plastic qualities, and it will exhibit a yield value, i.e., it will require some minimum force to deform it.

Still further addition of fluid will render the mixture more plastic and the yield value will decrease. A proportion of fluid finally will be reached at which the mass has no yield value. Such a mixture now may flow in the undisturbed state. The range of proportions of liquid and solid between establishment of coherence and loss of yield value is the plastic range of such mixtures. Within this range, useful workability will be found. However, within the plastic range there may exist compositions which will lose cohesion if deformed excessively or if deformed at an excessive distortion rate. Other compositions in the plastic range may possess little mechanical strength.

Another quality of such mixtures which will vary as the proportion of liquid is varied is the wetting of surfaces to which the mixtures are applied. Either the extent of wetting or the rate of wetting may change as the composition in the plastic range is changed. This property is of concern with respect to developing adhesion between bone and a surgical repair material.

In formulating to obtain a plasticity which will be totally satisfactory to surgeons using the proposed repair material, the principal variables of concern are the size, shape, and proportion of the particles of filler and cross-linking agent added to the liquid carrier material. Experience indicates that the finer the particle and the more asymmetric the particle shape, the more profound its influence on developing and changing plastic flow in mixtures with fluids. Thus, it may be necessary to have large proportions of large, spherical particles in order to obtain a plastic mixture. The effect on plasticity of changes in the proportions of such particles may be small. In contrast, low volumetric concentrations of fine, asymmetric particles may affect plasticity profoundly. Needle-shaped, platy particles, or agglomerations of spherical particles, e.g., are effective in developing plasticity of mixtures with fluids.

The chemical composition of the filler material is a further variable affecting performance. One approach considered in approaching the formulation was the use as filler of a powder, high molecular weight (i.e., solid) form of the poly(propylene fumarate). In this case the entire mass of the finished product may be composed of biodegradable polymer. A variation on this approach is the use of another biodegradable polymer as powdered filler. Polylactic acid was considered for this service.

An alternate choice in filler selection is used for a physiologically acceptable inorganic material. For some applications such inorganic filler could be a material not subject to dissolution. A fine silica is an example of such a material. In many instances, however, it will be desirable for an inorganic filler to disappear from the surgical site, just as the polymeric binding material is required to do. Candidate materials having this quality are calcium carbonate and calcium sulfate. A leachable filler material, whether organic or inorganic, provides another function to the repair composition. If the filler material is removed more rapidly than the polymeric matrix, there is created a porous structure into which tissue growth can proceed. Such ingrowth may be a useful contributor to therapy employing this repair material.

The final component of the mixture is an agent for converting the plastic material applied to the wound to a solid form. The conversion is carried out by initiating chemical cross-linking between the polyester molecules comprising the fluid component of the formulation. This cross-linking is possible due to the presence in these polyesters of vinyl unsaturation in the fumarate portion of the molecule. Addition to the mixture of a free radical generator, such as a peroxide, will lead to the desired cross-linking. Only a modest degree of cross-linking is desired, just sufficient to convert the mass from a plastic mass to a solid. The cross-linking must not be so extensive and thorough that the resulting solid becomes nonbiodegradable.

The action desired is very much like that obtained in the preparation and use of bone cements, e.g., those used to bond artificial hip joints to the femur. One such bone cement is prepared by mixing methyl methacrylate with benzoyl peroxide to form a reactive paste. Within a few minutes, the free radicals generated by the peroxide cause cross-linking of the unsaturated chemical bonds in the methyl methacrylate molecules and a solid mass results.

C. Filler Selection

Initial experiments to develop a filler for fluid poly(propylene fumarate) were made with polylactic acid. These experiments were unsuccessful, presumably because polylactic acid contains a hydrogen atom which may be readily extracted by free radicals generated by the cross-linking agent. This reaction consumes the cross-linking agent ineffectively.

High molecular weight (i.e., solid) poly(propylene fumarate) was investigated as a filler for the fluid, low molecular weight poly(propylene fumarate). At a loading of 30% by weight of solid powder, this composition provides a composition having suitable handling and molding properties. This composition is of further interest because a monolithic, unified, yet eventually degradable, structure may be created.

Further development was carried out with inorganic fillers having potential for degradation within the tissues. Fluid poly(propylene fumarate) loaded with up to 40% by weight of calcium carbonate has been cross-linked successfully to produce rigid materials. This appears to be the maximum level of $CaCO_3$ that can easily be worked by hand at room temperature. However, because of the density difference between calcium carbonate and PPF, the calcium carbonate represents less than 20% of the composition by volume. Higher filler loadings were obtained by warming the polymer to ~80°C before mixing in the filler. Sodium carbonate and sodium bicarbonate were investigated as fillers of potentially greater leaching rate. Warm blending followed by hand kneading was successful in increasing the loading level of these sodium carbonates to 70% by weight or slightly over 50% by volume. This material even after addition of a liquid initiator and accelerator had suitable handling properties. These fillers leached rapidly from the finished product; probably too rapidly for satisfactory functioning in vivo. The prospect remains to use a minor proportion of such fillers as a means for creating some degree of porosity early in the period following emplacement of the repair material. Filling of low molecular weight poly(propylene fumarate) with calcium sulfate at 40% by weight also gave a putty with suitable handling properties, and when cross-linked this formulation gave a material remarkably bone-like in appearance.

D. Cross-Linking Agents

In these studies, methyl methacrylate has been used as a control. Cross-linking studies are normally carried out in 16 × 150 mm test tubes in a 37°C bath. Under these conditions, methyl methacrylate containing 3.0% benzoyl peroxide and 0.5% *NN*-dimethyl aniline accelerator, polymerized in approximately 60 min. Poly(propylene fumarate), when the benzoyl peroxide is predissolved in a small amount of a *mutual* solvent, methylene chloride or acetone, cross-links somewhat faster than the methyl methacrylate under the same conditions. Unfortunately, filled samples of poly(propylene fumarate) prepared in this way produce only a rubbery material.

The effectiveness of a number of peroxide cross-linking initiators was investigated. The materials given trials were t-butyl hydroperoxide, t-butyl perbenzoate, and methyl ethyl ketone peroxide. None of these initiators alone produced cross-linking of fluid poly(propylene fumarate) sufficiently rapidly at 37°C. Addition to the formulations of initiators or promoters, such as *NN*-dimethyl aniline, *NN*-dimethyl-p-toluidine, or cobalt naphthenate enabled cross-linking to be achieved within 12 to 24 hr, but this is clearly unacceptable performance.

Since some of the initiator compositions used — particularly those based on methyl ethyl ketone peroxide — should have given almost explosive cross-linking rates, it became apparent that initiation was not the rate-limiting step. It appeared likely that free radical propagation was rate limiting. In order to test this hypothesis new formulations were prepared based on the use of high molecular weight poly(propylene fumarate) in conjunction with an unsaturated monomer acting as solvent. The principle is that reactive monomer can diffuse between the dissolved polymer chains to effect cross-linking in conjunction with initiator. At physiological temperatures in previous formulations employing low molecular weight polymer diffusion of radicals to sites of unsaturation is postulated to have been too slow to be useful.

Experiments to test this approach to putty formulation from high molecular weight poly(propylene fumarate) were carried out with the reactive monomers styrene, diethyl fumarate, and *N*-vinyl-2-pyrrolidone. Benzoyl peroxide is soluble in these substances. Compositions containing styrene and vinyl pyrrolidone were found to cross-link rapidly at physiological temperatures with benzoyl peroxide, the vinyl pyrrolidone without the use of an accelerator. The use of low molecular weight poly (propylene fumarate) in similar formulations also gave rapidly cross-linking formulations, but suffered from a lack of physical strength. Note that in the lattermost formulation fluid, low molecular weight poly(propylene fumarate) acted as solvent for initiator, but the solid high molecular poly(propylene fumarate) did not dissolve in the low molecular weight material.

E. Selected Composition and Properties

The investigations described have permitted selection of a composition suitable for surgical repair, specifically for maxillofacial injuries. The following composition will cross-link to a rigid mass in 15 min at 37°C and in approximately 30 min at room temperature. In 1 hr the surfaces exposed to air lose all traces of tackiness. Samples after 16 hr at 37°C are sufficiently hard that a saw is required to cut them.

The two parts of the composition are designated "putty" and "initiator". These two parts are intended to be blended by a surgeon at the time of use. On the basis of 100 parts by weight of each constituent, the formulation is as follows:

Constituent	Parts by weight
Putty composition	
Calcium sulfate dihydrate	68.2
High molecular weight poly(propylene fumarate)	22.6
Vinyl pyrrollidone	5.7
Initiator formulation	
Benzoyl peroxide	0.7
Vinyl pyrrollidone	2.8

The cured material has a hardness of about 84 Shore D (equivalent to 98 Rockwell C). This value is representative of other rigid polymers such as acrylic resins. Measurements of compressive strength were made on an Instron tester at a head speed of 0.1 in./min. These measurements ranged from 6435 to 7082 lb/in.^{2}. At a head speed of 1 in./min, the compression strength was measured to be 7950 lb/in.^{2}

The dissolution rate by hydrolysis of poly(propylene fumarate) has been measured in vitro through exposure of samples to pH 7 buffer solution at 37°C. In an experiment which may be cited as an example, 1/16-in. diameter spheres of poly(propylene fumarate) of molecular weight 34,000 required exposure in vitro for 180 days to reach complete dissolution. Analysis of the data obtained in these experiments indicated that the hydrolysis proceeded at the surface of the particles rather than within the particles. Other dissolution tests, performed with particles of different dimensions, confirmed this picture of the mode of the hydrolysis.

III. MATERIALS AND METHODS

A. Materials

Reagents used in the synthesis of poly(propylene fumarate) were readily obtained from commercial laboratory suppliers. Diethyl fumarate (Kodak® 1430), propylene glycol (Fisher P-354) and p-toluenesulfonic acid (Fisher A-320) were all successfully used as delivered without further purification. Initiators used in cross-linking studies — solid benzoyl peroxide (Alfa® 13633) and liquids such as t-butyl hydroperoxide, methyl ethyl ketone peroxide, di-t-butyl peroxide, and t-butyl perbenzoate (all from Lucidol®) were available for immediate use. Accelerators, also referred to as promoters, for the cross-linking initiators such as *N,N*-dimethyl aniline (Fisher A-746), *NN*-dimethyl-p-toluidine (Eastman® 646), and cobalt naphthenate (Pfaltz and Bauer C23710) were employed to help speed the cross-linking reaction. Polylactic acid and high molecular weight poly(propylene fumarate) were synthesized at Dynatech R/D Company, Cambridge, Mass. to be used as organic fillers. Inorganic fillers such as calcium carbonate (Fisher C-62), sodium bicarbonate (Fisher S-233), and calcium sulfate (Mallinckrodt® 4300) were employed to be easily leached from the cross-linked mixtures. Acetone and methylene chloride used as solvents for PPF, and anhydrous ether used for precipitation of high molecular weight-PPF, were likewise readily available from laboratory suppliers. *N*-Vinyl-2-pyrrolidinone was obtained from Aldrich Chemical and was normally used without purification. Tertiary butyl hydroquinone (Tenox TBHQ) used as an antioxidant was obtained from Eastman Chemicals.

B. Methods

Low molecular weight poly(propylene fumarate) was synthesized in a 1-ℓ flask fitted with a reflux condenser and a Barret Trap. As the ethanol is distilled and removed, it was collected from the receiver of the Barret Trap as a means of measuring completion of the reaction.

The apparatus used for synthesis of high molecular weight poly(propylene fumarate) was similar with the exception that instead of a Barret Trap and reflux condenser, the flask is fitted with a 25-cm Vigreaux distillation column and standard distilling head fitted with a drip tip collection adapter. The reaction is allowed to proceed until no more distillate is collected at the reaction temperature of 250°C. At this point, approximately 175 mℓ of distillate will have been removed from a 2-mol reaction (i.e., 344 g diethyl fumarate; 152g propylene glycol; 1g p-toluenesulfonic acid). The reaction mixture is then cooled to <100°C, the Vigreaux column is removed, and vacuum pump is attached to the system. The reaction mixture is then reheated to 220°C under full vacuum (~1 mm Hg) over a period of about 4 hr. At this time an additional 75 mℓ of distillate will have been collected. The reaction mixture is then cooled, dissolved in methylene chloride, and fractionally precipitated with ether in a separating funnel. The lower layer is washed with additional ether and dried under vacuum at room temperature to give a white to yellow powder melting at 80°C.

Cross-linking studies on unfilled PPF using liquid initiators are performed by weighing the desired amount of LMW-PPF, after warming in a water bath, into either nickel or stainless-steel 50-mℓ crucibles. The crucibles are placed on a hot plate and the PPF gently warmed until easily stirred. At this point the appropriate amount of promoter is added to the PPF and thoroughly mixed. The initiator is then added while the mixture is still warm and also thoroughly mixed. This warm mixture is then put into a small test tube for use in 37°C oil shaker bath or in an aluminum-foil weighing dish before placing the sample in a laboratory oven for elevated temperature studies.

Cross-linking studies are made in much the same manner for filled PPF samples. The PPF is added to the crucible, warmed and mixed with the promoter. Then the filler is gradually added and mixed thoroughly. When no more filler can be added because the mixture was too "stiff" to stir, the material is removed from crucible to a petri dish containing the remainder of the filler. The material is then kneaded by hand like bread dough to mix the remaining filler. The resulting ball of material is then weighed into portions needed for cross-linking studies. The appropriate amount of liquid initiator is added to the surface of the portion being cross-linked. The material is then worked by hand to mix the initiator with the sample thoroughly. The sample is then put into a test tube or an aluminum-foil weighing dish prior to being cross-linked.

Formulas containing only solid poly(propylene fumarate) may be mixed either of two ways. First, the PPF can be dissolved in the monomer component to form a plastic mass which is then filled by the kneading technique described earlier. Alternatively, the monomer component may be adsorbed on the filler prior to blending with the PPF. This method gives a dry powder precursor which does not form a plastic mass until the initiator monomer solution is added.

Cross-linking studies on these materials were carried out by packing the material in a large polyethylene pipet tip, usually with the assistance of vacuum. The pipet tip is then put into a test tube which is suspended in an oil bath at 37°C. Once cross-linked the pipet tip is split and the rigid sample is removed. The resulting cylinder is cut into discs with a hacksaw and then polished with emery cloth to remove sawmarks and to facilitate examination for uniformity.

Once synthesized, the poly(propylene fumarate) is characterized in several ways. Infrared spectra are obtained by running the liquid polymer on NaCl cells. Once the PPF is cross-linked, spectra are taken to compare relative intensity of the peak at ~1600 cm^{-1} (due to fumarate double bond) to that of the relative intensity of the same peak for the noncross-linked material. In most cases, the peak of cross-linked material is not significantly less intense than that of noncross-linked PPF. This indicates that the degree of cross-linking is low and probably not sufficient to destroy the inherent biodegradability of the polymer.

Another method of characterization that was performed is viscometry. These measurements are made at 24°C using a Brookfield LVF viscometer equipped with a #4 spindle at 0.3

rpm. Viscosity of lower molecular weight PPF is an important parameter to monitor because of the importance of the handling properties of the final composition.

Several attempts have been made to determine the number average molecular weight, Mn, for PPF by end group titration. Samples were dissolved in excess 1.0 *N* NaOH overnight and then back titrated with 1.0 *N* HCl solution to determine the apparent equivalent weight. None of these attempts gave satisfactory results. A more reliable determination of molecular weight was obtained by gel permeation chromatography using Waters® Styrogel® columns.

Another method to determine whether a cross-linked sample is sufficiently cross-linked to prevent biodegradation is to place a sample in a 1-ℓ flask with 250 mℓ of 1 *N* NaOH solution. The flask is fitted with a reflux condenser and heating mantle. Dissolution, as soon as heating is begun, suggests that the sample will be ultimately biodegradable at neutral pH and body temperatures.

In vitro leaching tests are made to determine biodegradability and rate of leaching of filler. Weighed samples are placed in stoppered 250 mℓ Erlenmeyer® flasks along with 200 mℓ of leaching solution, i.e., pH = 7 buffer, or pH = 1 buffer or in some cases distilled water. Recently 1.5-mm beads have been molded in a transfer mold and cross-linked at 37°C. Five of these beads are then placed in a 10 × 50 mm Whatman® cellulose extraction thimble and suspended in 50 mℓ of distilled water in test tubes. The test tubes are then placed in a 37°C shaker bath. The distilled water is checked regularly for pH and is changed when deviations from neutrality are observed or when a substantial precipitate is found with barium chloride.

IV. RESULTS AND DISCUSSION

A. Polymer Synthesis

Poly(propylene fumarate) is synthesized from diethyl fumarate and propylene glycol by transesterification using p-toluenesulfonic acid as a catalyst. Several runs have been made to produce a low molecular weight polymer for use as the fluid component of the composition. These materials were prepared initially by suspension polymerization in silicone oil, but better results have been obtained by bulk polymerization. Suitable material is produced for this application by removing 105 mℓ of distillate from a 1-mol reaction (172 g diethyl fumarate; 76 g propylene glycol; 0.5 g PTSA). This product has a viscosity of $\sim 1 \times 10^6$ cps when measured at 24°C using a Brockfield LV #4 spindle at 0.3 rpm.

The distillate is not all ethanol when collected in this manner. Infrared analysis indicates that the distillate, which comes over at 140°C, contains approximately 10% diethyl fumarate. This analysis is consistent with an estimate of the composition based on the vapor pressures of ethanol and diethyl fumarate at 140°C. Properties of several batches of low molecular weight PPF are shown in Table 1.

Loss of diethyl fumarate in the synthesis of low molecular weight poly(propylene fumarate) is not a serious problem, but it is where high molecular weight polymer is the goal. In order to synthesize solid, high molecular weight PPF for use as a filler in the composition, a distillation column is employed. When this is done, the distillate comes over at 78°C, indicating that it is nearly pure ethanol. Distillation is continued in this manner until the pot temperature reaches 250°C, about 5 hr. Then the column is removed and the remaining volatile components of the reaction mixture are stripped off under vacuum. After cooling, the resultant solid mixture is dissolved in methylene chloride and precipitated in diethyl ether. The precipitate is then dried under vacuum at room temperature for 48 hr, giving a yellow, free flowing powder which melted at about 75°C. The yield of final product is about 35%. The low molecular weight material remaining in solution may be isolated by evaporation and revacuum distilled to produce additional high molecular weight product.

Table 1
SUMMARY OF REACTION CONDITIONS AND PRODUCTS FOR LMW-POLY(PROPYLENE FUMARATE)

Run no.	Type	Reaction time (hr)	Maximum temperature (%)	Diethyl fumarate	Propylene glycol	Remarks
07778-1	SOS[a]	53	170—180	0.8	0.8	Opaque orange-yellow containing both viscous liquid and gel
011366	SOS	61	180	0.8	0.8	Orange-yellow, viscous tacky liquid; Mn $\cong$ 550 by end group titration
012407-1	SOS	80	170	0.8	0.8	Orange-yellow opaque liquid
012432-1	Neat	39	245	0.8	0.8	A red, clear liquid, extremely tacky and very viscous
012437-1	Neat	8.5	210	0.6	0.9	Light-yellow, clear liquid, least viscous of all runs
012709-1	Neat	19	239	0.76	0.76	Reddish-amber, clear liquid, not quite as viscous as run #012432-1.
013505-1	Neat	14	245	1.0	1.0	Reddish-amber, clear liquid

[a] Silicone oil suspension.

B. Filler Selection

Initial cross-linking studies on filled samples of PPF were run using polylactic acid as a filler. These experiments were unsuccessful, presumably because polylactic acid contains a hydrogen atom which should be readily extractable by a free radical.

Subsequently, as a result of the need for rapidly developing porosity in the material to facilitate intrusion of new tissue, inorganic fillers were investigated. PPF loaded with up to 40% by weight of calcium carbonate has been cross-linked successfully to produce rigid materials. This appears to be the maximum level of $CaCO_3$ that can easily be worked by hand at room temperature. However, because of the density difference between calcium carbonate and PPF, the calcium carbonate represents less than 2% of the composition by volume. In a final formulation, the filler should represent a higher volume percent of the composition to give the handling properties required for this application. Higher filler loadings were obtained by warming the polymer to ~80°C before mixing in the filler. At the same time, sodium carbonate and sodium bicarbonate were used to increase the leaching rate of the inorganic filler. Warm blending followed by hand kneading was successful in increasing the loading level to 70% by weight or slightly over 50% by volume. This material even after a liquid initiator and accelerator were blended in had suitable handling properties for maxillofacial reconstruction.

As the leaching results to be presented later will indicate, these fillers were leached too rapidly. The next inorganic filler to be tried was calcium sulfate. Filling of low molecular weight PPF with calcium sulfate at the same weight percentage as before also gave a putty with handling properties suitable for maxillofacial reconstruction and when cross-linked gave a material remarkably bone-like in appearance.

High molecular weight PPF has been investigated as a filler for low molecular weight PPF. Remarkably, this material gives a composition with suitable handling properties at a loading of about 30% This composition has other interesting properties, to be discussed later, which suggested that the ultimate composition would contain high molecular weight PPF along with the more rapidly leached inorganic fillers.

C. Cross-Linking Studies

In these studies, methyl methacrylate has been used as a control. Cross-linking studies are normally carried out in 16 × 150 mm test tubes in a 37°C bath. Under these conditions methyl methacrylate containing 3.0% benzoyl peroxide and 0.5% *NN*-dimethyl aniline accelerator polymerized in approximately 60 min. Poly(propylene fumarate), when the benzoyl peroxide is predissolved in a small amount of a mutual solvent, methylene chloride or acetone, cross-links somewhat faster than the methyl methacrylate under these same conditions. Unfortunately, filled samples prepared in this way produce only a rubbery material, possibly as a result of plasticization by the solvent. Attempts to remove the solvent after mixing but before cross-linking gave no significant improvement.

In order to overcome the apparent difficulties associated with the need to predissolve benzoyl peroxide, other initiators, particularly liquid initiators, were being investigated. The first of these to be investigated was t-butyl hydroperoxide (Lucidol® HEPV251). Although t-butyl hydroperoxide is one of the more thermally stable peroxide initiators, its use obviated many of the difficulties observed with benzoyl peroxide. When cross-linked at 210°C for 1 hr, a material of sufficient strength and rigidity for use in this, application was obtained. Similar results were obtained at 150°C for 1 hr. This was the first cross-linked material produced in this program that approaches the physical requirements for maxillofacial reconstruction.

In order to combine the rapid polymerization properties of benzoyl peroxide with compatibility advantages of t-butyl hydroperoxide, the primary initiator candidate then became t-butyl perbenzoate (Lucidol®); t-butyl perbenzoate is a "hybrid" of the two previous initiators.

Initial attempts at cross-linking both filled and unfilled samples of PPF using t-butyl perbenzoate as an initiator and *NN*-dimethyl aniline or *NN*-dimethyl-p-toluidine as promoters were not particularly successful. However, when cobalt napthenate was used as the promoter, or, if you will, accelerator, results were markedly improved. At a promoter concentration of 1.0% by weight (of total PPF content) and t-butyl perbenzoate at 2% unfilled samples of PPF cross-linked into a hard, rubbery solid in 20 min at ~110°C and the same result occurred at 37°C in less than 22 hr. Using the same conditions as above, hard, brittle samples were obtained at 110°C when the PPF had been filled with inorganic fillers such as $NaHCO_3$ or $CaSO_4$. However, due to handling problems, it was impossible to run these filled samples at 37°C. Similarly, PPF filled with powdered high molecular weight PPF cross-linked into a hard sample, looking like peanut brittle when cross-linked at 110°C for 20 min. When the above reactions were tried at 75°C, the samples obtained were hard and brittle only after being in the oven overnight.

Subsequently an extensive study was performed to develop a formulation based on t-butyl perbenzoate that would cross-link rapidly at 37°C. The results of many of these experiments are shown in Table 2. Based on these experiments it was concluded that the cross-linking times were 0 to 1 hr at 110°C, 2 to 5 hr at 60°C, and 12 to 24 hr at 37°C, and that the cross-linking times were relatively independent of the actual initiator formulation used.

Since some of the initiator compositions used — particularly those based on methyl ethyl ketone peroxide (Lucidol® DDM-9) — should have given almost explosive cross-linking rates, it became apparent that initiation was not the rate-limiting step. It appeared likely that free radical propagation may be rate limiting. In order to test this hypothesis new formulations were prepared based on the use of high molecular weight poly(propylene fumarate) in conjunction with an unsaturated monomer acting as solvent. The principle is that monomer can diffuse between the polymer chains to effect cross-linking, whereas diffusion was restricted at physiological temperatures in previous formulations employing low molecular weight polymer.

Experiments to test this approach to putty formulation from high molecular weight poly(propylene fumarate) were carried out with the reactive monomers styrene, diethyl fumarate, and *N*-vinyl-2-pyrrolidone. Benzoyl peroxide is soluble in these substances. Compositions containing styrene and vinyl pyrrolidone were found to cross-link rapidly at physiological temperatures with benzoyl peroxide, the vinyl pyrrolidone without the use of an accelerator. The use of low molecular weight poly(propylene fumarate) in similar formulations also gave rapidly cross-linking formulations, but suffered from a lack of physical strength. Note that in the lattermost formulation fluid, low molecular weight poly(propylene fumarate) acted as solvent for initiator, but the solid high molecular poly(propylene fumarate) did not dissolve in the low molecular weight material.

Samples in the form of disks have been prepared by solidifying the composition in a polyethylene tube. Once hard, the tube is removed and the cylinder of polymer is cut into disks approximately $^1/_2$ in. in diameter and 1/8 in. thick with a hacksaw. The surfaces of the disks were then polished with emery cloth.

The formulation is as follows:

Putty composition

$CaSO_4 \cdot 2H_2O$	12 g
HMWPPF	4 g
Vinyl pyrcllidone	1 g

Initiator formulation

Benzoyl peroxide	0.12 g
Vinyl pyrollidone	0.5 g

Table 2
CROSS-LINKING OF POLY(PROPYLENE FUMARATE) WITH t-BUTYL PERBENZOATE

Sample no.	t-Butyl perbenzoate concentration (%)	Promoter concentration	Filler concentration	Temperature (°C)	Reaction time (hr)	Results
013510-3	3.5	0.5% dimethyl aniline	62% $NaHCO_3$	108	1	Soft at oven temperature; hard and brittle at room temperature
013512-3	3.0	1% DMA	None	107	$1^1/_2$	Soft at oven temperature; hard and brittle at room tempeature
013514-1	2	0.5% cobalt naphthenate	None	108	$1^1/_2$	Rubbery at oven temperature; hard and brittle at room temperature
013516-2	3.5	0.5% CoN	71% $NaHCO_3$	108	$^1/_4$	Soft at oven temperature
					1	Hard at oven temperature
013518	3.5	0.5-pc CoN	71% $NaHCO_3$	108	2	Hard at oven temperature
013522-1	1	1% CoN	None	37	6	Soft
					22	Hard
013522-2	1	1% CoN	None	114	2/3	Rubbery
013524-1	2	1% CoN	None	37	18	Hard
013524-2	2	1% CoN	None	37	6	Soft
					18	Rubbery
013526-1	2	1% CoN	None	37	18	Hard
013526-2	2	1% CoN	None	110	$^1/_3$	Rubbery
013528-1	2	1% CoN	70% $NaHCO_3$	110	2/3	Hard, not brittle
013530-1	2	1% CoN	70% $CaSO_4$ $2H_2O$	110	$^1/_2$	Hard and brittle
013533-1	2	1% CoN	70% $CaSO_4$ $2H_2O$	75	2	Soft
					52	Rock hard
013541-1	2	0.6% CoN	36% HMW PPF	22	24	No reaction
013541-2	2	0.6% CoN	36% HMW PPF	108	$^1/_3$	Hard and brittle
013549-1	2	3% CoN	28% $NaHCO_3$	58	2	Rubbery

Table 2 (continued)
CROSS-LINKING OF POLY(PROPYLENE FUMARATE) WITH t-BUTYL PERBENZOATE

Sample no.	t-Butyl perbenzoate concentration (%)	Promoter concentration	Filler concentration	Temperature (°C)	Reaction time (hr)	Results
013954-1	4	3% CoN	62% $CaSO_4$ $2H_2O$	60	5	Rubbery
013970-1	4 (old sample)	2% CoN	None	110	$^1/_2$	Hard and brittle
013970-2	4 (new sample)	2% CoN	None	110	$^1/_2$	Hard and brittle
013974-1	2	3% CoN	50% HMW PPF	108	$^1/_2$	Hard and brittle

Table 3
RESULTS OF HARDNESS TESTS FOR POLY(PROPYLENE FUMARATE)

Reading no.	Hardness
1	81
2	85
3	86
4	86
5	82

Note: Average = 84 ± 2.3 These results are in the range of acrylics and other rigid polymers.

To the best of our knowledge, all of these components are physiologically acceptable, and we believe that this formulation offers a basis upon which optimization studies may be based. It has been demonstrated that the organic portion of the composition is completely dissolved by warm 1.0 *N* NaOH.

D. Physical Properties

Lot number 015451-1 of formulated poly(propylene fumarate) was cross-linked at 37°C. The resulting rod was removed 16 hr later, from the pipet tip and cut into five ~$^1/_2$ in. segments using a hacksaw. The ends of each piece were squared on a lathe using a facing tool. Each segment was measured for hardness using a Shore D-2 hardness tester. The results are given in Table 3.

The same samples were used to determine the compression strength of the material. The samples were measured using a Vernier caliper and were tested using an Instron tester at a head speed of 0.1 in/min. The results of these determinations are given in Table 4. Although these results are somewhat less than would be observed for acrylic bone cements, which would run approximately 10,000 psi under the same conditions, they are probably adequate for a temporary application such as maxillofacial injury repair. The strength could probably be improved by increasing the molecular weight of the polymer or by increasing the ratio of polymer to filler.

E. Leaching Studies

Beads 1.5 mm in diameter of calcium sulfate-filled poly(propylene fumarate) similar to the composition described were transfer molded and cross-linked at 37°C. Five beads were weighed into each of three Whatman® extraction thimbles and were suspended in test tubes of distilled water (50 mℓ). The tubes were put in a shaker bath at 37°C. After 16 days, a weight loss of 50% was detected by drying and weighing one set of beads. This weight loss is presumed to be a result of leaching of the calcium sulfate filler from the beads. It is interesting to note that the beads maintained their structural integrity even in the light of a 50% weight loss. This result suggests that the polymeric fraction of the composition is in the form of the continuous matrix surrounding the particles of calcium sulfate.

ACKNOWLEDGMENT

This work was carried out at Dynatech R/D Company under U.S. Army Medical R & D Command, Contract No. DAMD 17-80-C-0186 for the U.S. Army Institute of Dental Research.

Table 4
MECHANICAL PROPERTIES DATA REDUCTION SHEET

Material: Cross-Linked PPF Lot No. 015454-1
Conditioning: Specimens <24 hr old Test Mode: Compression Load Cell Range: 0-X-2000 lb
Chart Speed: 1 in/min Crosshead Speed: 0.1 in/min

Sample no.	Length (in.)	Width (in.)	Thickness (in.)	Area (in.^{2})	Gage length (in.)	Load (lb)	Strength (lb/in.$^{-2}$)	Deformation (in.)	Elongation (%)	Modulus (lb/in^{-2})	Comments
−A	0.510	0.435 0.450		0.154							Result not obtained
−B	0.475	0.459 0.471		0.170		1350	7950				Head speed, 1 in./min
−C	0.525	0.400 0.412		0.129		860	6667				0.1 in/min
−D	0.510	0.376 0.390		0.115		740	6435				0.1 in/min
−E	0.499	0.419 0.429		0.141		1000	7082				0.1 in./min

REFERENCES

1. **Perry, R. H. and Chilton, C. H.,** *Chemical Engineering Handbook,* 5th ed., McGraw-Hill, New York, 1373, 3.

Chapter 12

POLYESTERS FROM KREBS CYCLE MONOMERS AS VEHICLES FOR SUSTAINED RELEASE

Donald L. Wise

TABLE OF CONTENTS

I. ABSTRACT

Biocompatible polymers have been synthesized from monomers of all the basic metabolic pathways. Most recently, polyesters have been synthesized from selected monomers of the Krebs cycle. When incorporated with hydrocortisone (as a model drug) these polymers have shown striking uniformity of release rate and, especially, maintenance of this release until much of the drug was released. These new polymers have a substantial technical basis as sustained release vehicles.

II. INTRODUCTION

A universal problem in the administration of drugs is the regulation of the dosage delivered. It may be desirable to deliver a drug periodically to the system or to maintain it at a constant level. Protection of the drug against deleterious effects at a particular location, followed by delivery at another location, may be necessary. Practical matters, such as the frequency of injection, or pill consumption, may make storage of a supply within the system desirable. Often a balance must be maintained between therapeutic and toxic drug effects through dosage regulation. Requirements of this kind have resulted in much technical activity to devise improved and different means for regulating drug delivery.

An important category of dosage forms is sustained release of drugs delivered parenterally. Most frequently the objective in arranging sustained release within the body is to keep a constant level of medicament present within the system or available to it. Accordingly, the incorporation of medicaments into controlled release, tissue-absorbable preparations has been actively studied for many years. Two fundamentally different methods have been used to prolong the delivery of a therapeutic agent to the body fluids. One of these relies on chemical alteration of the agent so that its absorption by the body is delayed. An example of a material which makes use of this technique is controlled release sulfonamide. In the second method, the active agent remains chemically unchanged, but its availability to the body is delayed by physical means. For example, the agent may be mechanically dispersed in a matrix of therapeutically inert auxiliary ingredients which act as a binder for the medicament and which are slightly soluble in body fluids. Suspension of penicillin in a mixture of oil and beeswax is an example. Absorption of a drug on starch particles to form a slowly absorbed solid made injectable by suspension in oil or saline solution is another example. In general, such adjuvants are relatively weak in power of regulation.

A more positive approach to regulation is to surround or encapsulate a drug with a release-regulating material. A practical method for accomplishing this is the encapsulation of a drug within a shell of silicone rubber. Such a composition may be implanted within the body, and this procedure has been used to deliver steroid to the tissues through the mechanism of diffusion of steroid through the silicone rubber shell. It has already been demonstrated clinically that the implantation of suitable steroids contained within silicone rubber is an effective method of controlling conception.[1] This technique, using silicone rubber, also has been investigated.[2] as a means of delivering other therapeutic agents via implantation. A drawback of this otherwise effective procedure is the fact that after exhaustion of the active agent the silicone remains behind, requiring surgical removal in addition to the initial surgical placement.

A. Polyester Systems Available

Work has led to the development of new implantable drug delivery systems based on polymers which are slow to release the therapeutic agent. Implantable delivery systems currently under investigation offer the promise of controlled and sustained release of drugs.

The implantable material consists of a tissue-compatible, hydrolyzable polymer matrix in which drug is dispersed. The polymers are polyesters prepared from select natural metabolites, i.e., polymers prepared from monomers originating from any of the several major metabolic pathways of the human metabolism. The delivery system consists of the active agent dispersed in matrix form in these select polyesters. In an aqueous environment the physically entrapped drugs are released by diffusion. At the end of a designated period of time the active agent is gone. With appropriate polymer synthesis, the polymer can be designed to hydrolyze at a slower rate into metabolizable fragments. It appears most practical to have a system which permits uniform delivery of the drug from the polymer followed by complete hydrolysis within an additional period, preferably within one additional time span of the designed active agent delivery time.

A significant advancement in treatment techniques is suggested by the use of the implantable controlled release concept. As new, more potent drugs — which are effective in smaller doses — are introduced, a given portion of drug can provide longer protection when incorporated into similar size implants. More than one drug can be incorporated into a single implant so that treatment for a given period of time, using one kind of drug, can be automatically followed by treatment by a second drug or combination of drugs.

B. Specific Polymers

The technical basis which makes possible the preparation of new synthetic polymer matrices capable of slowly releasing medicaments is found in recent work on synthetic absorbable sutures prepared from natural metabolites. Long-standing dissatisfaction with catgut and other similar type suture materials stimulated investigation of synthetic replacements, particularly synthetic materials which may be absorbed by the body without tissues reaction. Signal success in this search has been attained through utilization of polylactic, polyglycolic, copolymers of lactic and glycolic acids, and the poly-γ-alkyl-L-glutamatic acids for this purpose. Further work has resulted in the synthesis of selected polyesters from monomers of the Krebs cycle. The rationale for this approach, the synthesis, and results using these new polymers as sustained release vehicles are presented.

The qualities which recommend these polymers, prepared from natural metabolites, for sutures and surgical repair materials, namely absorbability and innocuousness, recommend them and, potentially, other materials prepared from natural metabolites as implantable vehicles for drugs to be released within the body. In this system a suitable physiologically active substance is blended into a polymer matrix in such a way that the active substance is freed to the tissues within which a piece of such material has been implanted. Here, ready at hand then, is a basis for polymers which will lend themselves to additive incorporation and which will dissipate acceptably in body fluids.

III. TECHNICAL BASIS FOR POLYMERS FROM SELECTED NATURAL METABOLITES

Materials selected for use in vivo must be nonimmunogenic, nonthrombogenic, nonallergenic, and noncarcinogenic. One rational approach to the selection of substances having these qualities is to examine those compounds which are normally found in biosystems. If such compounds may be polymerized, especially into a polyester, the resulting polymer may then qualify for use as a matrix in sustained release drug delivery technology. The polymer itself must have several qualities:

1. The polymer must be innocuous to the tissues.
2. The polymer must be compatible with drugs to be incorporated within it.
3. The polymer must degrade through the action of substance present in the tissues at such a rate that satisfactory drug release occurs and the matrix ultimately disappears. If the polymer is a polyester, the product of such dissolution will be a compound normally present in the tissues, as noted above.

In a search for compounds to be considered as polymer candidates a systematic examination of the metabolic pathways may be expected to furnish a list of chemical entities normally encountered in the tissues. Such metabolic pathways include processes referred to by biochemists as (1) glycolysis, (2) amino acid metabolism, and (3) Krebs cycle (or the citric acid cycle, or tricarboxylic acid, or TCA-cycle). In each case relatively large molecules of a given class are converted in successive steps involving one or more electronic transitions at a time to simpler substances. Energy is extracted in the course of these transitions and the final products are suited for excretion. The interest is in identifying substances in this chain which are susceptible to polymerization and later dissolution to the original substance. In this way the biological system confronted with the degradation products of a matrix materials has accessible a disposal mechanism for dealing with the residue. Under these circumstances the impact on the system is minimal. A discussion of polymers prepared from these three major metabolic pathways is given in the following.

A. Polyesters from Monomers of Glycolysis

Most of the intermediates in glycolysis are phosphorylated compounds and as such these intermediates are not likely materials for polymerization. One of the end products of glycolysis, however, has already been demonstrated to be a satisfactory substance for incorporation within the body, namely, lactic acid. Another metabolite of this chemical classification, glycolic acid, has similar utility. Lactic acid, an α-hydroxycarboxylic acid, is produced during anaerobic or fermentative metabolism of glucose and as such is a normal product of muscle metabolism. (Physical exertion leads to fermentative metabolism in muscle.) For this reason its release by slow hydrolysis of polylactic acid is physiologically acceptable.

Since lactic acid is optically active[3] it is possible to prepare polylactic acid from both the dl-, D(−), and L(+) forms. Kulkarni and co-workers[4,5] prepared both forms of polylactic acid for evaluation as surgical repair materials. Poly(dl-lactic acid) melts at 60°C and is amorphous. The (L+) polymer, on the other hand, is crystalline and melts at 170°C. In keeping with these qualities the L(+) polymer was observed to be dissolved more slowly by tissue fluids than the dl-polymer. Both lactic acid polymers were found to be free of tissue reaction upon implantation. In use as pins for fracture repair, poly(dl-lactic acid) functioned satisfactorily and had virtually disappeared from the fracture site after 8 months.[5] The D(−) monomer is relatively costly and has received little attention for polymer synthesis.

Polyglycolic acid has found high favor as a suture material. From the manufacturers' standpoint the material is easy to form as filaments, and surgeons have been enthusiastic about both its functional characteristics and the lack of interaction with tissues.[6-9] The polyglycolic acid is a crystalline polymer melting at about 225°C. In early animal studies, using isotopically labeled polyglycolic acid, it was shown that the material is completely absorbed within 9 months following implantation. Upon further development it was found[9] that satisfactory sutures can be prepared from polyglycolic acid which is absorbed by animal tissues within 2 to 3 months.

The most probable mode of absorption of these polymers by tissue fluids is hydrolysis to the monomer acid, although it has been suggested[7] that esterase enzymes play a role. As indicated above, since both lactic and glycolic acids are naturally present in the tissues, mechanisms for their disposition are at hand, a factor which undoubtedly accounts in large degree for the lack of tissue reactivity. Indeed, the studies of polyglycolic acid sutures showed that the ultimate products of metabolism were excreted principally in the urine and as expired carbon dioxide, virtually none remaining in the tissues.

B. Polymers from Monomers of Amino Acid Metabolism

The next general class of metabolic intermediates is the amino acids. Amino acids are direct analogs of α-hydroxycarboxylic acids (such as lactic and glycolic acids). There are approximately 20 common amino acids which are found in proteins. Many of these have already been synthesized into synthetic protein-like polymers,[10-12] and one polyalkylamino acid, poly-γ-methyl-L-glutamate, is prepared and sold commercially (Ajicoat® sold by Ajinomoto Company, Tokyo). Its uses include synthetic leather and fabrics and surgical sutures. The use of polyamino acids as polymers for the controlled release of biologically active compounds appears promising for several reasons. The polymer and its hydrolysis products are biocompatible. The choice of amino acids, each with a unique functional moiety, allows the design of a wide variety of matrices for holding the compound to be released. Copolymers are readily synthesized such that the properties of two or more amino acids may be combined.

Glutamic acid is one of the least expensive amino acids available ($0.47/lb) as monosodium glutamate and is produced in the largest quantity (7,150,000 ton/year). Furthermore, polymers of glutamic acid and copolymers of glutamic acid and lysine are nonimmunogenic.[13] For these reasons its potential for use as a polymer for controlled release of physiologically active compounds is encouraging. Degradation products of the polymer are likewise physiologically acceptable.

Other polyamino acids with similar credits as poly glutamate are l-lysine and d,l-methionine. These also have unique side chains which would alter the character of the polymer from that observed for polyglutamate. Lysine has a net positive charge at physiological pH. Alanine and glycine are the amino acid analogs of the α-hydroxycarboxylic acids; lactic acid and glycolic acid on this basis show promise for use as implantable polymers.

The chemistry of polyamino acid synthesis is well established in the early chemical literature[14-16] and the patent literature.[17,18] The volume by Stahmann[12] is one of the most comprehensive collections of papers on polyamino acids.

Polyamino acids and particularly poly-l-glutamic acid is of interest for application as an implantable drug delivery system because it has been used for surgical sutures.[19,20] Small amounts of polyamino acids are commercially available from a number of biochemical supply houses. A patent[21] indicates that a large-scale, 50-kg synthesis is feasible. Polyamino acids have been extensively investigated as protein analogs and there is an extensive amount of literature about them. In the course of many of these investigations a considerable amount of information about the antigenic properties of polyamino acids has been obtained. Information[22] indicated that no homopolymer of an aliphatic amino acid has been prepared that is antigenic. However, the aromatic polyamino acids have an especially high degree of antigenicity associated with them. Perhaps the best evidence for the biocompatibility of poly-l-glutamic acid would be the fact that it has been used as a surgical suture.

An important aspect of polyamino acids that may have a bearing on their biocompatibility is their optical purity. In animal and plant proteins only L-amino acids occur. The effect of D-amino acids on the body is not clear. Fortunately, the polymerization procedure proceeds without racemization.

Hydrolysis rates of polyamino acids are slower than those of polyesters like polylactic or polyglycolic acid. Much of the data in the literature concerns itself with hydrolysis of polyamino acids by digestive enzymes. It was reported, however, that surgical sutures made from poly-L-glutamic acid hydrolyzed in 6 weeks, but these sutures were in the intestines of dogs where digestive enzymes could act on them. [20]

Perhaps the most accepted preparation of poly-L-glutamic acid is to proceed through the γ-alkyl-*N*-carboxyanhydride. This anhydride is prepared from the corresponding γ-alkyl-L-glutamic acid by addition of phosgene.* The syntheses of γ-methyl- or γ-ethyl-L-glutamic acid have been described.[23,24] Blount and Karlson[25] also described the preparation of γ-benzyl-L-glutamic acid.[26] Pravda's[23] synthesis of γ-ethyl-L-glutamic acid seems to be the most straightforward.

* γ-Benzyl-, γ-ethyl-, and γ-methyl-L-glutamic acids are commercially available from Sigma Chemical Co., St. Louis.

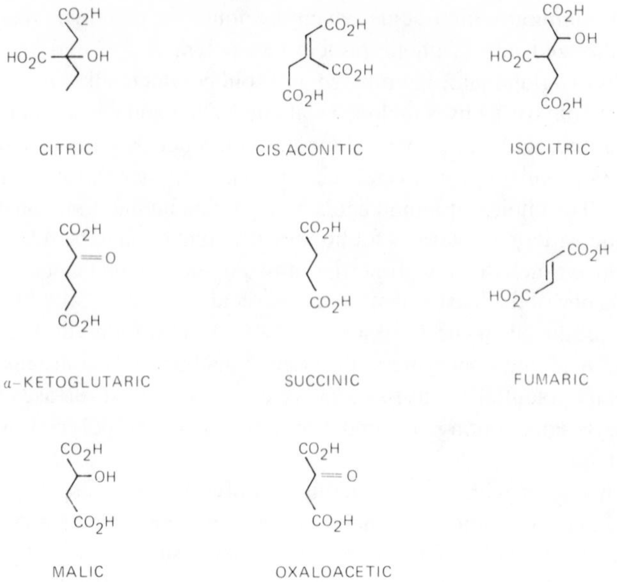

FIGURE 1. Acids in the Krebs cycle.

C. Polyesters from Monomers of the Krebs Cycle

For consideration to prepare polymers for use as implant material, there are several intermediates in the Krebs cycle or TCA cycle which have interesting properties. These are citric, isocitric, fumaric, and malic acids. All of these are di- or tricarboxylic acids, each with different degrees of functionality. Oxalacetate and α-ketoglutarate are keto analogs of amino acids and as such may be quite useful in the synthesis of amino acid-like polymers. It is not known whether homopolymers may be formed from these materials although the simple dicarboxylic acid, maleic acid (not known as originating as product of human metabolism, however), can be homopolymerized.[26] Since background literature is available on the preparation of synthetic polymers from monomers of this major metabolic pathway, an investigation was made to consider the potential for preparation of polymers from the Krebs cycle acids.

IV. POLYESTERS FROM MONOMERS OF THE KREBS CYCLE

It has been found that the hydrolysis of biocompatible polymers such as polyamino acids or polyalkylamino acids[27] and polylactic, polyglycolic copolymers of glycolic and lactic acid[28] containing physically entrapped or chemically bound drug molecules shows promise as a means of sustained release of these drugs. As described earlier these polymers are from two of the three major metabolic pathways. It should be possible to construct other such polymers from monomers of the third major metabolic pathway which can be broken down in the body by hydrolysis to give biochemically innocuous sideproducts. This third group, the di- and triacids of the Krebs cycle as listed in Figure 1, should be especially useful in this regard, since it offers a large variety of reactive functionalities as well as a range of physical properties.

Since all the compounds in the Krebs cycle contain at least two carboxylate groups, condensation polymerization of these acids with diols or diamines to yield polyesters of polyamides ought to be a feasible procedure (Figure 2). Unfortunately, the diols and diamines commonly used in industrial processes (such as ethylene glycol or p-phenylene diamine) are not found in the body; however, the industrial preparation of alkyd resins, commonly used in paints and enamels, involves the reaction of a diacid (phthalic acid) with a biologically

$$HO_2C\sim\sim\sim\sim\sim + HO\!-\!\!-\!OH \longrightarrow H_2O\ +$$

$$HO_2C\sim\sim\sim\sim\sim\overset{O}{\overset{\|}{C}}O\!\left[\!-O\overset{O}{\overset{\|}{C}}\sim\sim\sim\sim\sim\overset{O}{\overset{\|}{C}}O\!-\right]_n\!O\overset{O}{\overset{\|}{C}}\sim\sim\sim\sim\sim\overset{O}{\overset{\|}{C}}O\!-\!OH$$

$$HO_2C\sim\sim\sim\sim\sim CO_2H + H_2N\!-\!\!-\!NH_2 \longrightarrow H_2O\ +$$

$$HO_2C\sim\sim\sim\sim\sim\overset{O}{\overset{\|}{C}}N\left[-N\overset{O}{\overset{\|}{C}}\sim\sim\sim\sim\sim\overset{O}{\overset{\|}{C}}N-\right]N\overset{O}{\overset{\|}{C}}\sim\sim\sim\sim\sim\overset{O}{\overset{\|}{C}}N\!-\!\!-\!NH_2$$

FIGURE 2. Generalized polyester and polyamide formation.

common triol, glycerol, usually in the presence of a long-chain fatty acid. It is the feasibility of analogous reactions, involving the Krebs-cycle acids rather than phthalic acid, which will be explored in the following sections. Specific experiments conducted will then be discussed.

A. Background for Polymerization

The first alkyd-type polymers were prepared by Van Bemmelen,[29] who in 1856 heated together mixtures of succinic acid and glycerol as well as citric acid and glycerol, to form the insoluble materials succinin and citrin. Under most conditions of temperature and starting-material ratio, the polymers produced were jelly-like materials, These polymers, although easy to prepare, are probably gels such as those described by Kienle,[30-32] and thus would not be very useful. Kienle repeated the preparation of succinin and found that when the reaction was approximately 80% complete, the growing polymer chains suddenly congealed to an open, gelled state; this phenomenon was attributed to the high degree of branching in the growing polymer chains, made possible by the third hydroxyl functionality in glycerol (Figure 3). The prevention of gel formation is thus necessary for the preparation of satisfactory polymers.

Kienle et al.[31] found that heating these gels in a sealed tube at 150°C overnight resulted in "degelling"; although the physical properties of this "degelled" material are not described, it may well be a more-ordered material produced by ester-interchange reactions. Similarly, Arsem[34] has described a mixed polymer of succinic and phthalic acid with glycerol which is a nonfusible jelly that becomes plastic upon heating. Although phthalic acid would probably not be a feasible monomer for a biocompatible polymer, Arsem maintains that this procedure is applicable to a wide variety of diacids, including malic acid and succinic acid.

According to Sokolov,[34] the secondary hydroxyl group on glycerol reacts with phthalic anhydride only above 180°C; thus it ought to be possible to react succinic anhydride with equimolar quantities of glycerol below 180°C to form an essentially linear polymer by reaction predominantly at the primary hydroxyls. The secondary hydroxyl groups remaining could then be reacted at higher temperature with biocompatible monocarboxylic acids such as acetic, stearic, or oleic acid. Alternatively, a controlled degree of cross-linking could be achieved by reacting these secondary hydroxyls with a mixture of di- and monoacids; the greater the percentage of diacid in this mixture, the greater would be the extent of cross-linking in the finished material (Figure 4). Procedures somewhat similar to that described above (but usually utilizing temperatures above 180°C) are specified in a variety of patents;[35] although most of these reactions involve phthalic anhydride and various natural oils such as castor oil, similar reactions involving succinic anhydride and the monoacids mentioned above should be feasible. Other similar processes have been described for the formation of alkyd polymers with succinic acid.[36]

A third possible procedure involves the reaction of a diacid with a triester of glycerol (Figure 5). This procedure is called acidolysis; typical examples have been described by

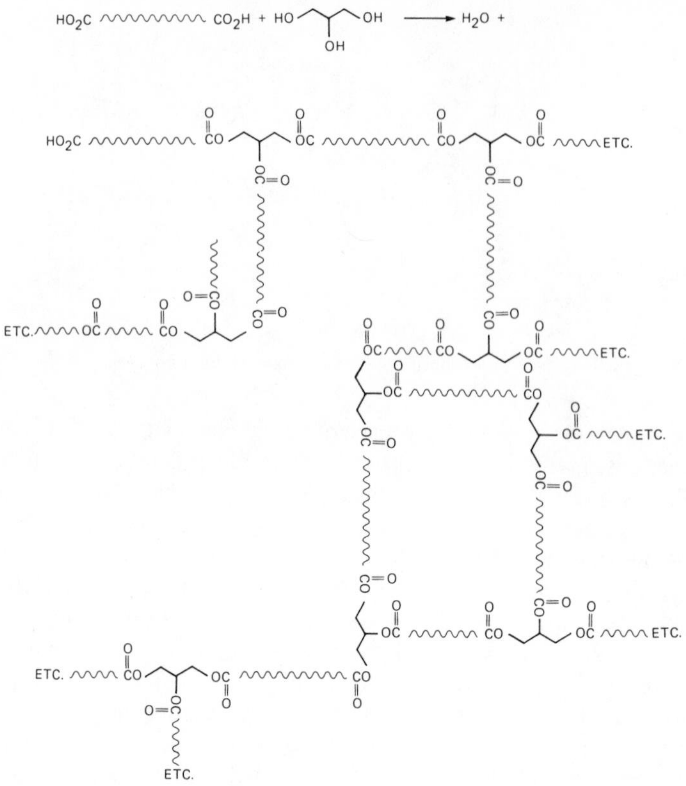

FIGURE 3. Gel formation with glycerol polyesters.

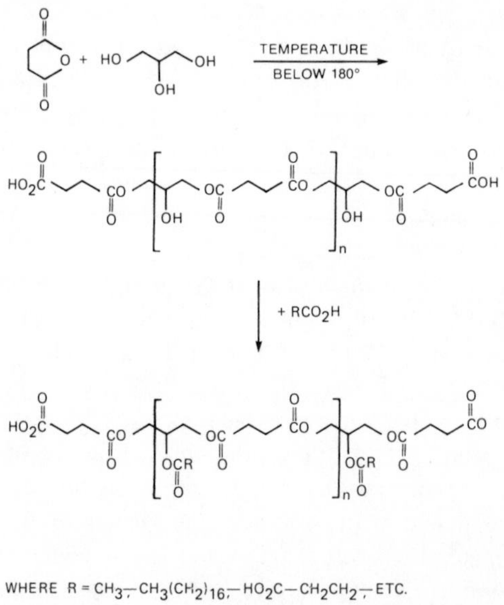

WHERE R = CH_3–, $CH_3(CH_2)_{16}$–, $HO_2C{-}CH_2CH_2$–, ETC.

FIGURE 4. Controlled glycerol polyesterification.

Carlston.[37] Commercially available (Fisher Chemicals) esters of glycerol such as triacetin, tristearin, or triolein could be used instead of the crude oils described in this article, and the Krebs cycle acids would of course be substituted for the phthalic acid isomers used by

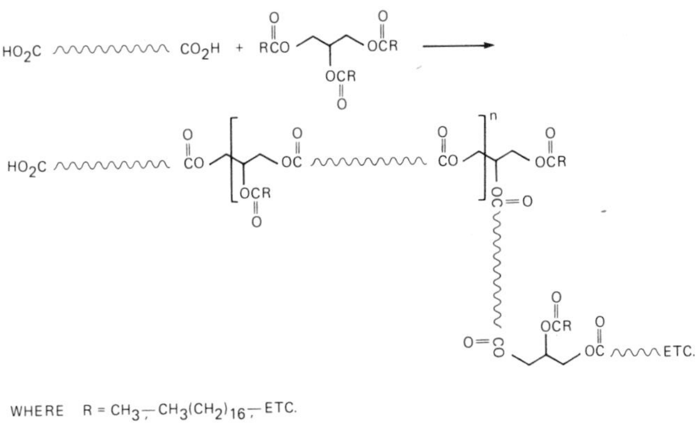

WHERE $R = CH_3-, CH_3(CH_2)_{16}-$, ETC.

FIGURE 5. Acidolysis.

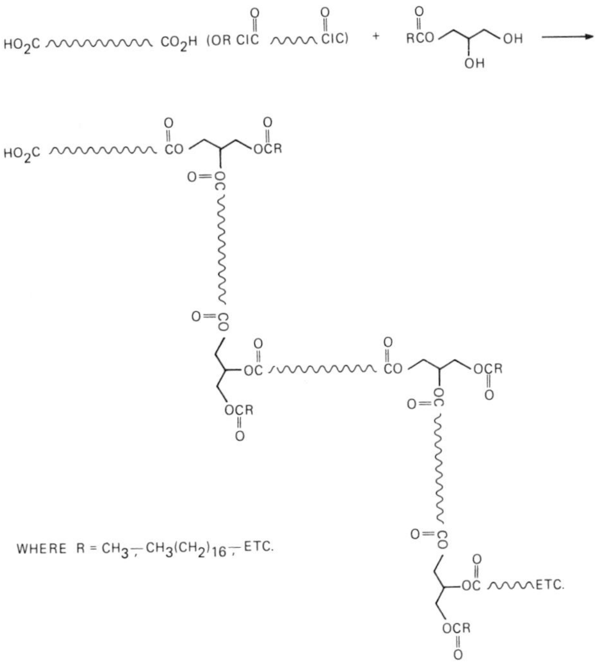

WHERE $R = CH_3-, CH_3(CH_2)_{16}-$, ETC.

FIGURE 6. Polyesterification of an α-monoglyceride.

Carlston. Since this procedure does not require the use of an acid anhydride, it should be applicable to a wider variety of the acids in the Krebs cycle.

A fourth procedure for the formation of alkyd polymers — alcoholysis — is most commonly used in the coatings industry. In the industrial process, a mixture of two thirds glycerol and one third oil (glycerol triester) is heated in the presence of a catalyst, equilibrating the mixture and forming predominantly glycerol a number of hours until polymerization is complete. More detailed experimental procedures are available,[38,39] but these industrial methods are far from optimal. First of all, the reaction of the triester with glycerol yields only about 44% monoester (instead of 100%)[40] use of commercially available (Fisher) monoacetin, monostearin, or monoolein in the reaction with the diacid should give a less-branched, more-linear polymer (Figure 6). However, these commercially available glycerides are generally esterified at an α-position, leaving one unreacted α-position as well as one

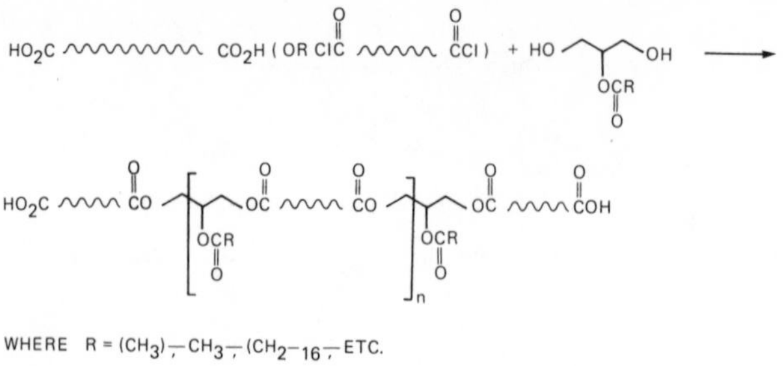

WHERE R = (CH_3)–, CH_3–, $(CH_2$–$)_{16}$–, ETC.

FIGURE 7. Polyesterification of a β-monoglyceride.

unreacted β-position available for polymerization. Because these two positions differ in reactivity toward esterification, growth of the alkyd polymer during polymerization may not be optimal. Reaction of a diacid with a β-monoglyceride (Figure 7) ought to yield a linear polymer with a longer chain length, since it involves reaction with two identical glycerol α-hydroxyl groups. Here again, a controlled degree of cross-linking could be obtained by adding a certain percentage of triacid or free glycerol. Fortunately, β-monoacetin, a monoacetate ester of glycerol, can be prepared in good yield.[41]

This preparation should also be applicable to the synthesis of β-monostearin and β-monoolein, the corresponding monoesters of glycerol and stearic acid and glycerol with oleic acid. These polymers could be prepared by bulk polymerization of equimolar quantities of glycerol monoester and succinic anhydride under conditions similar to those of the second step of alcoholysis[38,39] — heating with agitation from 130 to 230°C for 8 to 10 hr. Removal of water is necessary if a diacid is used rather than an anhydride; use of catalysts would also be important. Since esterification is acid catalyzed, a wide variety of catalytic agents are available for use. Sulfuric acid is commonly used as a polyesterification catalyst. A variety of metal-salts have been used as alcoholysis catalysts and it has been proposed that their catalytic activity carries over into the polyesterification process; their relative catalytic effectiveness has been determined.[42] p-Toluenesulfonic acid is probably the most effective catalyst for polyesterification; a variety of other aryl-sulfonic acids have also been used.[43]

Since polycondensation of Krebs diacids with β-monoglycerides is probably the most potentially useful route to the controlled polymerization of high molecular weight polyesters, it is worthwhile to explore briefly the possible variations on the procedure described above — the catalyzed bulk polymerization. Solution polymerization of these materials is also possible. The effect of temperature, catalysis, solvent choice, etc. in solution polyesterification reactions has been discussed.[44] In general, for the condensation of a Krebs cycle diacid such as succinic acid with a diol such as α- or β-monoacetin, the highest molecular weight polymers would be obtained with a water-immiscible solvent such as toluene or xylene, in the presence of a catalyst such as p-toluene sulfuric acid (approximately 1.5% by weight) at a temperature high enough to remove the water formed as side-product (since water will form an azeotropic mixture with these sorts of solvents, use of a Dean-Stark trap would probably be necessary to prevent excessive loss of solvent). Use of the more reactive succinyl chloride (Fisher) would allow the use of lower reaction temperatures and a wider variety of solvents (including those which are water miscible, since no water is liberated in this reaction). Hydrogen chloride would, however, be formed as a by-product, and would have to be removed by a suitable base — a tertiary amine such as triethyl amine. No catalyst is necessary for the acid chloride polymerization (Figure 8).

The condensation of diacid chlorides (such as succinyl chloride) with diols (such as α- or β-monoacetin) can also be effected by interfacial polymerization, in which an aqueous solution of diol reacts with an organic solution of diacid chloride at the interface between

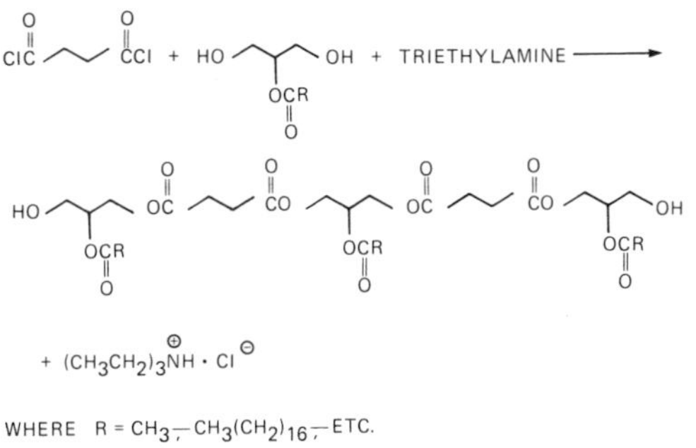

+ TRIETHYLAMINE →

+ $(CH_3CH_2)_3\overset{\oplus}{N}H \cdot Cl^{\ominus}$

WHERE R = CH_3—, $CH_3(CH_2)_{16}$—, ETC.

FIGURE 8. Polyesterification with a diacid chloride.

the immiscible layers; the film formed at the interface is continuously removed.[45,46] In a similar context, a threefold increase in the molecular weight of the polymer of phosgene and a diol was observed when the reaction was run in a two-phase system (organic solvent and aqueous sodium hydroxide) in the presence of a quaternary amine halide as compared to a homogeneous solvent system.[47] A similar effect could be expected for the reaction of succinyl or fumaryl chloride with α- or β-acetin.

If in fact these procedures do prove amenable to the preparation of suitable biocompatible polymers, a large number of possible modifications of the polymer structure should be feasible. Simple variation of the diacid monomers available from the Krebs cycle would of course change the physical properties of the polymer, as well as affect its biocompatibility and hydrolysis rates. Use of a small percentage of diacid instead of monoacid to block the "surplus" hydroxyl group in glycerol, as mentioned previously, allows control of the degree of cross-linking without inducing gelation. Variation of the monoacid at this "surplus" hydroxyl site allows some variety in the physical properties of the polymer; acetate ester polymers might be expected to be tighter and more compact, whereas stearate or oleate polyglycerides ought to be looser in structure but more hydrophobic, a factor which could significantly decrease hydrolysis rates. Furthermore, the use of an unsaturated diacid (fumaric acid or fumaryl chloride) and/or monoacid (oleic acid) provides a means of effecting cross-linking at carbon-carbon double bonds after polymerization is complete.

The inclusion of other biocompatible materials allows further variation of the polymer properties available. Polymerization of phthalic anhydride and glycerol in the presence of cellulose and cellulose derivatives yields a homogeneous material;[48,50] analogous products should result with succinic anhydride, and probably with succinic acid or other diacids as well. Also, glyceryl dilactate has been polymerized with a variety of diacids;[51] this procedure might also be applicable to many of the Krebs cycle diacids.

Finally, since many drugs have reactive hydroxyl, amino, or acid groups, it is possible that these could be chemically bound to the polymer matrix during polymerization, provided the reaction conditions were not too strenuous. The milder reaction conditions of the solution polymerizations would be best suited for this sort of reaction. Overall polymers from monomers of the Krebs cycle appear to merit development.

V. SPECIFIC EXPERIMENTS PREPARING POLYMERS FROM MONOMERS OF THE KREBS CYCLE

From the discussion in Section IV of the potential for synthesis of biocompatible polymers from monomers of the Krebs cycle, four experimental approaches for polymer synthesis were carried out. The following describes the approaches taken, the experimental work performance, and the results obtained. Suggestions for further work are included.

The first approach taken for polymer synthesis was that of acidolysis (see Figure 5 for proposed reaction mechanism). Several Krebs cycle acids were reacted with a triester. This consisted of the reaction of a diacid with a triester of glycerol. The Krebs cycle acids used were succinic, fumaric, and citric. Triacetin, a commercially obtainable triester of glycerol, was the triester used. These reactions were conducted through solution polymerization employing various reaction conditions.

Citric acid was found to be somewhat promising for formation of polyesters of suitable molecular weight for use as surgical implants. On the other hand, it is noted that succinic and fumaric acids do not show clear evidence of producing higher molecular weight polymers. Using fumaric acid did result in two promising materials. These polymers may be the result of the higher reaction temperature. However, the fact that the product was not rigid suggests that the polymers are of low molecular weight and thus following the present reaction procedure are unacceptable for implants. However, none of the results carried out to date using triacetin shows a polymer of sufficient molecular weight for immediate application as an implant material. This may, in part, be due to the relative unreactive state of triacetin.

The second approach to polymer synthesis with Krebs cycle acids involves the use of a monoester of glycerol instead of the triester. (See Figure 6 for proposed reaction mechanisms.) Succinic, fumaric, citric, and L-malic acids were reacted, using both solution and pearl polymerization, with monoacetin the commercial monoester of glycerol. The results are much more favorable than those using triacetin. Polymers were formed using both fumaric and citric acids. Several of the polymers formed from citric acid were combined with a drug and the release rate of drug evaluated, as will be described later.

These favorable results, noted for citric acid, were obtained by using α-monoacetin which has two hydroxyl groups of different reactivity which does not allow for optimal growth of the polymer. By using the β-form of monoacetin (presently not available commercially) longer linear chains of the polymer should be possible. The encouraging results obtained with the α-monoacetin suggest experimentation with the β-monoacetin.

The third approach (see Figure 4 for the proposed reaction mechanism) utilizes the anhydride of a Krebs cycle acid and glycerol. According to Sokolov[34] the second aryl hydroxyl group on the glycerol does not react at temperatures below 180°C. Thus, essentially linear polymers will be formed if the temperature is kept lower than 180°C since the reaction will be only with the primary hydroxyl groups. Succinic anhydride, reacted with glycerol by both solution polymerization and pearl polymerization, has been prepared. The hard yellow pearls obtained were combined with a drug, molded into a test form, and evaluated for its release rates as will be described.

Although experiments were not carried out, the succinic anhydride might be reacted with the β-monoacetin in order to assure a linear polymer. Concentrated sulfuric acid may be considered as a catalyst.

The fourth method involves the reaction of a diacid chloride with a diol such as α- or β-monoacetin (see Figure 8 for reaction mechanism). This approach has some advantages over the others presented. Specifically, water is not formed as a by-product of the reaction so that a water-miscible solvent may be used for the solution polymerization. Lower temperatures can be used because of the reactivity of the diacid chloride. Indeed, a catalyst may not be necessary. Further, the reaction time may be shorter. Succinyl chloride and α-monoacetin have been reacted in both solution and pearl polymerizations. Triethylamine has been added to neutralize the hydrogen chloride formed. The conditions used for reaction appear to have been too severe since the polymer formed was unsuitable. Even when the reaction was in an ice bath, the reaction was so rapid that the resulting polymer was unsuitable.

A number of possibilities exist to improve formation of polymer by this approach. Using β-monoacetin may result in a higher molecular weight polymer, although the application here does not appear to be so significant as with approach two or three discussed earlier.

The use of interfacial polymerization may increase the molecular weights substantially with approach four above. A small-scale interfacial polymerization was carried out using succinyl chloride and α-monoacetin; white brittle solid was formed at the interface. This technique of polymerization warrants much further study and development with this reaction system. It is also suggested that fumaryl chloride be used which may make tougher polymer than succinyl chloride since the double bond in a fumaryl chloride molecule restricts rotation.

In summary four experimental approaches to making polymers from Krebs cycle acids have been carried out and all look very promising for further work.

VI. DESIGN OF THE SUSTAINED RELEASE DELIVERY SYSTEM

The delivery system proposed consists of a tissue-compatible polymer matrix in which an active agent is dispersed. At the end of a designated period of time the active agent is gone. With appropriate polymer synthesis, the polymer can be designed to hydrolyze at a slower rate into metabolizable fragments. It appears most practical to have a system which permits uniform delivery of the drug from the polymer, followed by complete hydrolysis of the polymer within an additional period, preferably within one additional time span of the designed drug delivery time.

Several approaches to implant geometry, e.g., discs having specific concavities, have been suggested for achieving sustained release.[52] Using any one of the several techniques, the release rate of a drug by the polymer matrix can be adjusted so that it is relatively constant throughout the life of the sustained release device. The quantity of drug released per unit time can also be controlled. The more obvious methods of doing this are to vary the length of the cylinder implanted or increase the dosage per unit volume of the polymer matrix.

The amount of effective drug released by the implant is a function of the nature of the polymer, the weight fraction of drug in the polymer matrix, and the solubility and diffusivity of the drug in the fluids surrounding the implant. Drug loadings as high as 50% by volume in the polymer matrix are possible; however, at the 50% level, the drug may disrupt the polymer chains so that the polymer cannot crystallize. In this case, the resulting amorphous polymer will hydrolyze at a faster rate so that a lower drug weight fraction may be necessary to achieve the desired drug release rates.

Another method of dosage regulation is to change the hydrolysis characteristics of the base polymer. With a constant drug content, increasing polymer hydrolysis rate by lowering molecular weight will provide a higher dose rate. On the other hand, by partially cross-linking the polymer or by molecular chain extension, the rate of hydrolysis of the polymer can be decreased with a correspondingly lower dosage rate. Bonding of the chemical to functional side chains on the polymer is also a possibility for controlling drug delivery.

Time of treatment is obviously a function of size of the implanted cartridge, tailored to dosage rates as described above. At the end of a selected period, the cartridge has been totally absorbed by the body. As the end of the release period is approached, the dosage rate will drop rapidly. At this time, renewal of the implant may be indicated.

An alternative to a cartridge-type implant is an implant placed by injecting particles suspended in a suitable fluid carrier. In the fine particle/fluid system the polymer/drug material is prepared in the form of finely divided particles of the polymer/drug matrix, e.g., by spray drying a solution of the preparation. These fine particles may then be suspended in a fluid medium and injected into the patient. With a system of the fine particles of this kind, it is possible to obtain a higher dosage delivery rate than with the same polymer employed as a cartridge-type implant. This is due to the higher surface area per unit weight achieved with fine particles. Following are sample engineering calculations for a typical particle/fluid medium delivery system.

A. Engineering Calculations of the Release Rate

For calculation purposes it will be assumed for the polymer/drug matrix that (1) the particles of polymer/drug are perfect spheres, (2) the particles are all of uniform size and (3) the particles are 15 μm, i.e., uniform spheres of 15 μm in diameter. On this basis it may be calculated what particular release rate is required in order to design the specific polymer. The rate of polymer/drug release per unit surface area may be defined as (1/A) (dN/dt). Here A is the exposed surface area of a particle, N is the mass of the particle, and t is the time. For a spherical particle the mass may be related to the volume, V, and density, ρ as follows:

$$(1/A)\ (dN/dt) = (\rho/A)\ (dV/dt)$$

Since the area of a sphere of diameter, D, is πD^2, and the volume is $(\pi/6)D^3$, then

$$(1/A)\ (dN/dt) = (\rho/\pi D^2)\ d\ (\pi D^3/6)/dt$$

and

$$(1/A)\ (dN/dt) = (\rho/2)\ (dD/dt)$$

Over a specific release period, if linear dissolution is assumed, then the release rate per unit surface area may be expressed incrementally as follows:

$$(1/A)\ (dN/dt) = (\rho/2)\ (\Delta D/\Delta t)$$

For the design conditions of a 15-μm diameter particle and an estimated 1000-day-sustained release period the term $\Delta D/\Delta t = 1.5 \times 10^{-6}$ cm/day. The density term, ρ, using a typical polymer specific gravity, is 1.4 gm/cm^3. Thus the term (1/A) and (dN/dt) = 0.001 mg/day/cm^2 surface area; this is the sustained rate from the exposed surface area on which to base polymer design.

A mathematical description of the behavior of the proposed delivery system is of interest. If the model involving superficial dissolution postulated is valid then the mass of a polymer pellet can be shown to decrease linearly with time. On the other hand, if water penetration into the polymer is rapid, the chemical degradation of the polymer might be expected to occur throughout its cross-section. This degradation may or may not be catalyzed by the degradation products and a simple model is postulated which indicates the behavior under either case.

B. Specific Features of Proposed System

The matrix utilized in these compositions dissolves at a regulated rate when implanted, leaving no residue when metabolized. The matrix thus serves to contain and withhold the active substance before and during use. The active substance is physically integrated into the polymer/active substance, yet the combination does not constitute a new chemical entity. The matrix is harmlessly dissipated at the end of use. In other systems the additives simply act as carriers, or if the active substance is contained, the matrix persists in the body after treatment, frequently without having furnished all the active ingredients, and ultimately must be surgically removed.

C. Practical Techniques for Preparing Drug/Polymer Matrix

Techniques for blending an active substance into the polymer vary. For example, supercooled solutions of polymer/drug have been prepared by a hot melt vacuum blending technique followed by a quick quench at −40°F. For this system the drug is considered to be molecularly dispersed in the polymer. Another technique for incorporating the drug into the polymer is by selection of a compatible solvent system. If a solvent for both chemical and polymer is found, then upon removal of the solvent a well-integrated drug/polymer matrix results. If the drug is not soluble in the polymer/solvent system, then care must be taken to achieve reduced particle size of the drug. Ball milling for 3 days has been required to achieve micron-sized particles of drug integrated into the polymer. Direct high temperature/high pressure molding of powdered polymer and powdered active substance has been carried out.

Once the blended polymer/drug system has been prepared, techniques can be employed to form molded plates or cartridges for testing. The importance of careful molding techniques is to be stressed. For example, trace amounts of residual solvent may alter the overall hydrolysis characteristics of the polymer, perhaps by modifying the permeabilities of the polymer. For this reason, care should be taken to vacuum mold (to 0.1 Torr) all sample plates.

Once the blending of the polymer and active substance has been carried out, there are available high speed production processes which lend themselves to the production of variable concentration gradient and constant area drug delivery systems discussed above.

A cylindrical implant can be produced using techniques similar to those used in the wire coating industry. A fine thread of pure polymer can be passed through successively more dilute dispersions of drug in a solution of the polymer. After drawing the coated thread through dies to control the thickness of each coating, the coated thread can be dried in towers as it passes continuously from dispersion until a ''wire'' of the desired size is produced. The wire can then be cut into segments of the required size to provide the needed dose rate.

The cylindrical structure can be extruded using conventional plastics technology. In this process, a mixture of powdered drug and polymer is fed to the screw of an extruder. As it passes down the screw, the powdered drug is intimately mixed with the polymer which becomes molten. At the end of the screw, the compound is forced through a die to form the desired shape.

Flat films or discs of the polymer-active substance mixtures can be solvent cast or made by other standard plastic film production techniques. Conventional spray drying equipment can be used with success to obtain fine particles of polymer active substance material. Overall, there appear to be practical techniques for preparing any polymer/active substance delivery system on a large scale.

VII. SPECIFIC IN VITRO RESULTS

Following are examples of specific experiments carried out to demonstrate the sustained delivery of active substances for polymers synthesized from nomomers of the Krebs cycle. The active substance selected for all these experiments was hydrocortisone (11β, 17α, 21-trihydroxy-4-pregnene-3, 20-dione). The medical application for hydrocortisone in humans is in adrenocortical hormone therapy. A veterinary application is for ketosis in cows. However, the selection of hydrocortisone was made only to furnish a model active substance having application to demonstrate this treatment technique in humans and animals.

In Table 1 are summarized the release rates of this active agent (hydrocortisone) from the select polymer matrices. The active agent was ^{14}C labeled and release rates were evaluated by radioactive scintillation analysis of solution in which the polymer/active substance is placed. The preparation and testing procedures are as follows.

The hydrocortisone was dissolved in a solvent (ethyl alcohol) and a small amount of ^{14}C-labeled hydrocortisone added; the solvent was removed under vacuum leaving a material of uniform radioactivity. The radioactivity was determined by combustion analysis. The hydrocortisone content of the test samples was determined by adding a measured amount of labeled hydrocortisone to the polymer (nonradioactive). The finely divided hydrocortisone

Table 1
RELEASE RATES OF A REPRESENTATIVE ACTIVE AGENT (HYDROCORTISONE) FROM POLYMERS PREPARED FROM KREBS CYCLE MONOMERS

Identification no.	12971-1	12971-2	12972-1	12972-2
Hydrocortisone content (% by weight)	16.7	33.3	20.0	33.3
Sample size (GM)	0.2610	0.2590	0.6283	0.2702
Solution volume, mℓ (solution was pH 7 buffer @ 37° in an agitated bath)	50	50	50	50
Days from placement in test solution				
4	31.0	18.4	16.6	22.8
8	42	21.7	18.8	25.6
9	70.9	28.7	27.4	39.1
11	72.1	32.8	30.0	41.6
15	75.4	38.2	33.2	45.7
17	80.9	43.5	35.3	47.8
19	90.5	53.3	43.3	56.7
24	94.3	57.4	47.4	61.2
26	96.1	59.3	49.5	61.0
29	94.2	61.7	51.1	65.4
32	95.7	66.7	56.0	70.2
36	95.3	70.7	65.0	74.8
40	95.5	75.8	70.7	80.8

and the polymer were mixed by rolling a jar containing them for several hours so that they became uniformly blended. Some of this mixture was cintered and some was mulled to form test samples. When the polymer was quite hard the cintering procedure was used; when the polymer was soft and rubber-like, mulling was used to blend the polymer and drug.

Cintering is a fusing of drug and polymer through heat and pressure. It uses a specially designed stainless-steel mold with two brass dies. The polymer and drug at either 20 PHR (16.7% by weight active agent) or 50 PHR (33.3% by weight active agent) were placed between the brass dies. This assembly was heated to 150 to 200°C and pressure applied. A small thick disc resulted. Mulling is a procedure for blending together two materials by rubbing — in this case the hydrocortisone was mulled by hand into the selected polymers resulting in a uniform, soft matrix of polymer/hydrocortisone. The resulting samples, either cintered or mulled, were weighed and placed in 50 mℓ of pH 7 buffer (phosphate) in an agitated constant temperature bath at 37°C. Periodically (daily) samples were taken from the buffer solution (solution changed weekly). Samples were evaluated by radioactive scintillation analysis to determine the amount of hydrocortisone released.

The results of this testing are given in Table 1. It is to be noted that sustained release of a representative active agent (hydrocortisone) was achieved over the test period. Figures 9 and 10 are plots of the data of Table 1.

ACKNOWLEDGMENT

This work was carried out at Dynatech R/D Company, Cambridge, Mass.

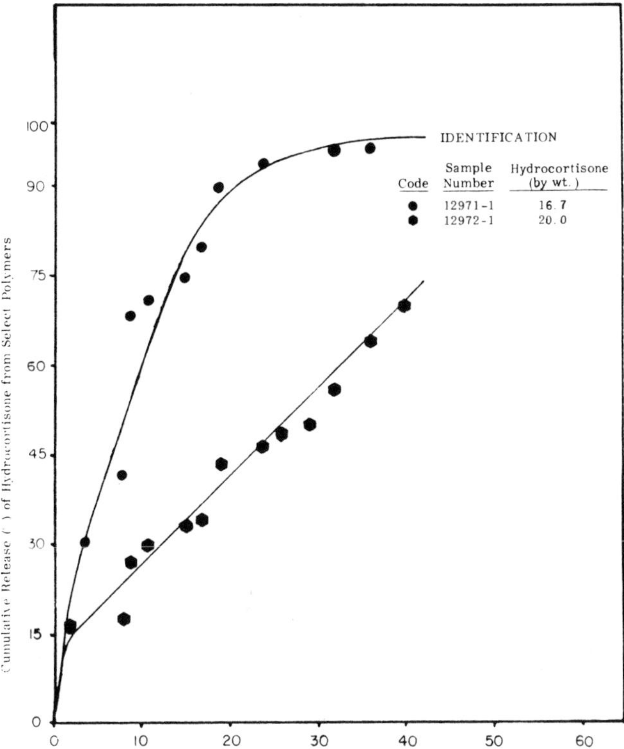

FIGURE 9. Days from insertion in test solution.

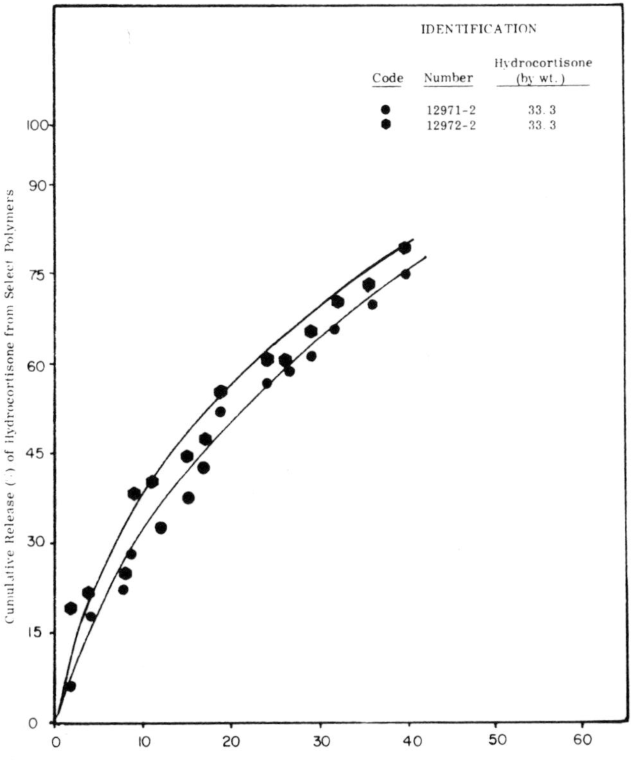

FIGURE 10. Days from insertion in test solution.

REFERENCES

1. **Croxatto, H., Diaz, S., Vera, R., Etchart, M., and Atria, P.,** *Am. J. Obstet. Gynecol.*, 105, 1135, 1969.
2. **Folkman, J. and Long, D. M.,** *J. Surg. Res.*, 4, 139, 1964.
3. **Lockwood, L. B., Yoder, D. E., and Zienty, M.,** *Ann. N.Y. Acad. Sci.*, 119(3), 854, 1965.
4. **Kulkarni, R. K., Pani, K. C., Neuman, C., and Leonard, F.,** *Arch. Surg.*, 93, 838, 1966.
5. **Kulkarni, R. K., Moore, E. G., Hegyeli, A. F., and Leonard, F.,** *J. Biomed. Mater. Res.*, 5, 169, 1971.
6. **Morgan, M. N.,** *Br. Med. J.*, 2, 308, 1969.
7. **Kelly, R. J.,** *Rev. Surg.*, March-April, 142, 1970.
8. **Herrmann, J. B., Kelly, R. J., and Higgins, G. A.,** *Arch. Surg.*, 100, 468, 1970.
9. **Frazza, E. J. and Schmitt, E. E.,** *J. Biomed. Mater. Res. Symp.*, 1, 43, 1971.
10. **Astbury, F. R. S., Dalgliseh, C. E., Darmon, S. E., and Sutherland, G. B. B. M.,** *Nature (London)*, 162, 596, 1948.
11. **Hill, R.,** *Fabrics from Synthetic Polymers*, Elsevier, New York, 1953.
12. **Stahmann, M. A.,** *Poly-Amino Acids, Polypeptides, and Proteins*, University of Wisconsin Press, Madison, Wisconsin, 1962.
13. **Katz, D. H., Davie, J. M., Paul, W. E., and Benacerraf,** *J. Exp. Med.*, 134, 201, 1971.
14. **Hanby, W. E., Waley, S. G., and Watson, J.,** *Nature (London)*, 161, 132, 1948.
15. **Farthing, A. C.,** *J. Chem. Soc.*, 3213, 1950.
16. **Woodward, R. B. and Schramm, C. H.,** *J. Am. Chem. Soc.*, 69, 1551, 1947.
17. **Woodward, R. B.,** U.S. Patent 2,657,972, 1953.
18. **Kaczalski, E.,** U.S. Patent 2,578,428, 1951.
19. **Miyamae, T., Mori, S., and Takeda, Y.,** U.S. Patent 3,371,069, 1968; *Chem. Abstr.*, 68, P89882p, 1968.
20. Courtaulds Ltd., Belg, 636,530 (1963); *Chem. Abstr.*, 62, 4184b, 1965.
21. Ashai Chemical Industry Co., Br. 1,252,869 1971; *Chem. Abstr.*, 76, 73022n, 1972.
22. **Fasman, G. D., Ed.,** *Poly-Amino Acids*, Marcel Dekker, New York, 1967, 621.
23. **Pravda, Z.,** *Collect. Czech. Chem. Commun.*, 24, 2083, 1959.
24. *Nipon Nogei Kagaku Kaishi*, 34, 782, 1960; *Chem. Abstr.*, 59, 6509a, 1963.
25. **Blount, E. R. and Karlson, R. H.,** *J. Am. Chem. Soc.*, 78, 941, 1956.
26. U.S. Patent 3,557,065.
27. U.S. Patent Application, Dynatech R/D Co., January 1973.
28. U.S. Patent Application, Dynatech R/D Co., January 1974.
29. **Van Bemmelen, J.,** *J. Prakt. Chem.*, 69, 84, 1856; See also Translations of sections on glycerine and some glycerine derivatives, *Beilstein's Handbook*, 4th ed., Glycerine Research Council, New York.
30. **Kienle, R. M. and Hovey, A. G.,** *J. Am. Chem. Soc.*, 51, 509, 1929.
31. **Kienle, R. M., van der Menlen, P. A., and Petke, F. E.,** *J. Am. Chem. Soc.*, 61, 2258, 1939.
32. **Kienle, R. M. and Petke, F. E.,** *J. Am. Chem. Soc.*, 62, 1053, 1940.
33. U.S. Patent 1,098,776.
34. **Sokolov, L. B.,** *Synthesis of Polymers by Polycondensation*, Israel Program for Scientific Translations, Jerusalem, 1968.
35. U.S. Patents 1,098,728; 1,098,777; 1,119,592; 1,141,944.
36. British Patent 336,645 (*Chem. Abstr.*, 25, 2013); U.S. Patent 2,218,553 (*Chem. Abstr.*, 35, 1145).
37. **Carlston, E. F.,** *J. Am. Oil Chem. Soc.*, 37, 366, 1960.
38. **Martens, C. R.,** *Alkyd Resins*, Reinhold, New York, 1961, chap. 8.
39. **Chen, L. W. and Kumanotani, J.,** *J. Appl. Polymer Sci.*, 9, 3649, 1965.
40. **Seavall, A. J.,** *J. Oil Col. Chem. Assoc.*, 42, 319, 1959.
41. **Bergman, M. and Carter, N. M.,** *Z. Physiol. Chem.*, 191, 211, 1930.
42. **Astbury, F. R. S., Dalgliseh, C. E., Darmon, S. E., and Sutherland, G. B. B. M.,** *Nature (London)*, p. 68, 1948.
43. French Patent 698,795 (*Chem. Abstr.*, 25, 3503).
44. **Morgan, M. N.,** *Br. Med. J.*, 1969.
45. **Morgan, M. N.,** *Br. Med. J.*,1969.
46. **Gould, R. F., Ed.,** *Advances in Chemistry*, American Chemical Society, Washington, D. C., 1962, chap. 14.
47. **Morgan, M. N.,** *Br. Med. J.*, p. 96, 1969.
48. British Patent 376,332 (*Chem. Abstr.*, 27, 4110).
49. U.S. Patent 2,022,011 (*Chem. Abstr.*, 30, 538).
50. Canadian Patent 365,559 (*Chem. Abstr.*, 31, 4418).

51. **Stearn, J. T., Makower, B., and Groggins, P. M.,** *Ind. Eng. Chem.*, 32, 1335, 1940.
52. **Cooney, D. O.,** *AICHE, J.*, 18, 446, 1972.

Chapter 13

INITIAL STUDIES ON SUSTAINED RELEASE OF A (MODEL) BACTERICIDE FROM A BURN-WOUND COVERING

Joseph D. Gresser

TABLE OF CONTENTS

I. ABSTRACT

The objective of the work described is to cover — immediately postburn — the burn-wound area with a slightly viscous fluid; within approximately 30 sec after application this fluid is formed into a nonsticky plastic film that adheres to the burn-wound area. This conformable and adhering plastic covering is to have the pervaporation rate of human skin. A polymeric material with the pervaporation rate (water transport) of human skin is desirable in order that (1) fluid exudate does not build up under this covering and (2) extensive water loss does not occur. Simply keeping the burn wound clean is another objective of the proposed covering. Further, sustained release of a bactericide (examples include sulfadiazine and penicillin) from the covering into the burn wound is also integral to this immediate postburn covering.

II. INTRODUCTION

The area of burn-wound covering has received significant medical and scientific attention. For standard civilian and conventional military situations involving a severely burned patient, the current procedure is to immediately — usually within 24 hr and certainly never greater than 48 hr — bring the severely burn-wounded patient to a burn/trauma center. Here the third degree burn wound is excised and a covering is applied. Much research and development has been devoted to these postexcision burn-wound coverings. These coverings are well-developed, although challenging research problems still exist. For *immediate* emergency treatment of the civilian or military burn wound, however, essentially no satisfactory medical procedure exists.

One of the reasons there is no standard and accepted covering material for immediate postburn treatment is that the severely burned patient is airlifted or transported to a burn trauma center so rapidly. However, there may be situations where this modern, efficient treatment system may not be able to function. In this case, the only choice available today is keep the patient quiet and wrapped in a blanket — often with fatal results. Clearly this cannot be tolerated by a modern military force.

An immediate postburn treatment can be useful in two situations. In the first, it would be a temporary covering to prevent infection, water loss, and penetration when the patient cannot be immediately evacuated, and has to wait for up to 24 to 48 hr for hospital treatment. In the second, it would also serve as a protective covering, but for a protracted time. In these cases, the incorporation of a sustained release bactericide into the covering will be most desirable.

III. OVERVIEW OF BURN-WOUND COVERINGS

It has long been recognized that burn wounds cause severe systemic and local disturbances of tissue metabolism and morphology. Thus, there have been many efforts to make artificial skins and to help nature do her work a little faster or better. These effects have focused mostly on postexcision coverings and treatment, although there has been a small amount of work on immediate postburn coverings. This situation has arisen because the burn victim is so easily removed to a trauma center where standard treatment can begin immediately.

After the burn patient is brought in, the eschar must be surgically (or otherwise) removed and the wound closed by some sort of postexcision covering. The optimal material is an autograft, but its applicability is limited because of trauma and lack of enough healthy donor-site skin in severe burn patients. Thus, a number of postexcision coverings, both temporary and absorbable, have been developed. The ideal covering regulates the environment of the wound site to permit, or even accelerate, eventual formation of normally structured skin.

The properties necessary in such a covering are listed below, in approximate order of importance:

- Sine-qua-nons
  - Adherence
  - Barrier to bacteria (total) and water (partial)
- Extremely important
  - Nonantigenic, nonallergenic
  - Elastic and flexible, but strong enough to be secured as necessary
  - Available
- Rather important
  - Sterilizable
  - Capable of indicating infection beneath
  - Not easily bacterially degradable
  - Minimizing of scar formation
- Useful
  - Incorporable by the body, at a controllable rate
  - Accelerative of wound closure
  - Allowing control of infection without removal; implies permeability to antibacterials
  - Restorative or normal skin function
  - Inexpensive

In addition, general systemic benefits enjoyed by the patient over less ideal coverings might include reduction of the usual heat losses due to water evaporation at an open burn site; possible reduction of metabolism to more nearly normal levels; and earlier resumption of mobility. Even though significant advances have been made recently, the state of the art is still far from such a single covering, or method of treatment.

It is to be noted that the burn wound is in an unstable condition for up to several days postburn, and immediate protection of the site to prevent dehydration and bacterial contamination may be of considerable clinical value, both to the burn site locally and systemically by lessening fluid losses. Although there have been some attempts made at an immediate postburn covering, none has been satisfactory. Possibilities examined up to the present have included dry and wet films and foams of various materials, applied as wipe-ons, spray-ons, and slap-ons.

A topical literature study focused on coverings firm and adherent enough to be used without additional dressings, and included dry (nongel type) films, biological gels (gelatin and gelatin/pectin materials), synthetic hydrogels, odd materials such as complex ionic gels, and adhesives. This distinct lack of any satisfactory immediate postburn covering has led to the development of the immediate postburn wipe-on type coverings concept, described as follows.

A. Preparation of Gelatin Films

Early experiments indicated that gelatin could be used to advantage as a wipe-on covering in first-aid treatment of burns. Gelatin solutions were shown to be capable of cross-linking by addition of formaldehyde, and to form flexible, water-resistant barriers. The rate of cross-linking was sufficiently slow that after addition of the cross-linking agent, the still-liquid mixture could easily be wiped or brushed onto a surface. These experiments also showed that glycerol, when added to the gelatin solution prior to the addition of the formaldehyde, served as a plasticizer for the insolublized film. Films incorporating glycerol remained supple and flexible for many days, while those without glycerol became brittle within 24 hr. Work has expanded on these observations with these results:

1. Measured water vapor transmission through glycerol plasticized films
2. Demonstrated sustained release of phenolphthalein from these films
3. Tested adherence of two wipe-on formulations on burned rats

B. Equilibrium Properties of Cross-Linked Gelatin Films

The purpose of these experiments was twofold: first, to measure the quantity of water loss from the insolubilized films immediately after formulation, and second, to measure the rate of water vapor transmission through these films after they have reached an equilibrium moisture content.

One formulation, plasticized with glycerol, was tested. Samples were made by incorporating formaldehyde and glycerol into aliquot portions of a stock solution. This stock solution (014958-1) was made by dissolving 20.0 g of Hormel® GP-4 gelatin in 50.0 mℓ of distilled water. Five films were cast in petri dishes from this stock. Three petri dishes had diameters of 8.9 cm each, two of 9.7 cm each. The film formulation was as follows:

Stock solution 014958-1	10.0 mℓ
Formaldehyde, 37% aq.	1.0 mℓ
Glycerol	1.0 mℓ

A record was kept of weight loss until equilibrium was reached. This is reported in Table 1. At equilibrium, films had lost 62.6 ± 1.1% of their initial weight.

Film thicknesses were also measured at equilibrium. The mean film thickness of the 8.9-cm diameter films was 0.52 ± 0.08 (S.D.) mm. The mean film thickness of the 9.7-cm diameter films was 0.33 ± 0.07 (S.D.) mm. Dimensional data for each film are also recorded in Table 1.

The equilibrium water content may be estimated reasonably well. The total volume of gelatin solutions is additive: in work reported below a volume of 170 mℓ was recorded for a solution of 48 g of GP-4 gelatin in 120 mℓ of water. Thus, the solids content of 10 mℓ of Stock 014958-1 will be (2/7)10 = 2.86 g. The glycerol content (1.0 mℓ) is therefore 1.26 g. The total nonvolatile weight, excluding cross-linking moieties from the formaldehyde is therefore 2.86 ± 1.26 = 4.12 g. The observed mean weight of these films at equilibrium was 3.97 ± 0.15 g. Therefore, we conclude that the equilibrium water content of these films is negligible.

C. Water Vapor Transmission through Equilibrated Cross-Linked Gelatin Films

After films 014958-1A through -1E had equilibrated in air, the rate of water vapor transmission through these was measured. The apparatus employed was the Payne Permeability Cup, with 3.5 cm diameter. These cups are equipped with a flange extending around the cup rim and a washer with internal and external diameters matching the cup rim diameter and the flange diameter. Each cup was filled with 10.0 mℓ of distilled water. Films were sealed to the flange and washer with high vacuum silicone grease to insure no air or moisture leaked past the films. Measurements of weight were taken periodically. Between weighings, cups were stored at 35°C. The weights of water lost through these films are shown in Table 2.

From data reported in Table 2 it is possible to calculate the rate of water vapor transmission through each film. The calculation is made by use of the following formula:

$$R = \frac{w\ell}{tA}$$

where R = rate of water vapor transmission ($g/hr^{-1}/cm^{-1}$); w = water loss (g) in time, t; t = time (hr); A = film area (cm^2); and ℓ = film thickness (cm). Rates, calculated for each increment of time for each film, are reported in Table 3. The mean value for all films and all increments is $(6.981 \pm 1.945)\ 10^{-4}$ $g/hr^{-1}/cm^{-1}$. The rate reported for human skin is 14.58×10^{-4} $g/hr^{-1}/cm^{-2}$.[1] Thus, a thickness of gelatin, equivalent in the rate of moisture transmission, would be 4.7 mm.

Table 1
WEIGHT LOSS AND DIMENSIONS OF CROSS-LINKED GELATIN FILMS

	Weight loss in grams of films				
Time (hr)	**014958-1A**	**014958-1B**	**014958-1C**	**014958-1D**	**014958-1E**
1.5	1.57	1.44	1.44	1.58	1.54
65.5	7.11	7.36	6.77	6.10	6.29
71.5	7.05	7.33	6.75	6.07	6.26
Final film weight	4.05	4.20	3.86	3.87	3.88
Weight loss (%)	63.5	63.6	63.0	61.1	61.7
Film thickness (mm)	0.52 ± 0.05	0.60 ± 0.03	0.45 ± 0.07	0.40 ± 0.01	0.27 ± 0.01
Film diameter (cm)	8.9	8.9	8.9	9.7	9.7

Note: Mean film weight = 3.97 ± 0.15 (S.D.) g; mean percent weight loss = 62.6 ± 1.1 (S.D.) %; mean film thickness (8.9 cm diameter) = 0.52 ± 0.08 (S.D.) mm; mean film thickness (9.7 cm diameter) = 0.33 ± 0.08 (S.D.) mm.

Table 2
WATER VAPOR TRANSMISSION THROUGH CROSS-LINKED GELATIN FILMS AT 35°C (FILM AREA = 9.621 cm^2)

	Weight loss in grams through films				
Time (hr)	**014958-1A**	**014958-1B**	**014958-1C**	**014958-1D**	**014958-1E**
17.5[a]	2.1070	1.7186	2.6511	—	—
18.8	—	—	—	2.709	2.157
25.0	3.1947	2.5959	3.6529	—	—
41.0[b]	4.8955	4.3652	5.7890	—	—
43.5	—	—	—	5.420	4.168
47.8[c]	5.5135	5.2472	6.7460	—	—
Mean thickness (mm)[d]	0.574 ± 0.039	0.762 ± 0.031	0.508 ± 0.051	0.442 ± 0.034	0.335 ± 0.070

[a] All films are buckled inward. Films -1A and -1B are more uneven than -1C, which is more smoothly concave inward.
[b] All films are smoothly concave inward.
[c] Film -1A is almost flat. Films-1B and IC are concave inward.
[d] Film thickness after measurements. Note that these values differ from equilibrium values.

Table 3
RATE OF WATER VAPOR TRANSMISSION (g/hr^{-1}/cm^{-1})

Time	**014958-1A**	**014958-1B**	**014958-1C**	**014958-1D**	**014958-1E**
17.5[a]	7.183×10^{-4}	7.778×10^{-4}	7.999×10^{-4}	—	—
18.8	—	—	—	6.620×10^{-4}	3.995×10^{-4}
25.0	8.652	9.264	7.053	—	—
41.0	6.342	8.758	7.049	—	—
43.5	—	—	—	5.042	2.835
47.8	5.422	10.273	7.431	—	—

Note: These values are calculated for each increment of weight loss and time. Ex.: the rate of water vapor transmission reported for film -1A at 41.0 hr was calculated as follows:

$$R = \frac{w\ell}{\tau a} = \frac{(4.8955 - 3.1947)(0.0574)}{(41.0 - 25.9)(9.621)} 6.342 \times 10^{-4}$$

[a] Using film thickness after measurements.

D. Sustained Release of Phenolphthalein — a Soluble Model Compound — from Cross-Linked Gelatin Films

Protective barriers over burned skin should minimize water loss, but not prevent it entirely. Results reported herein suggest that cross-linked gelatin may be a simple and effective means of approximating the normal rate of water loss through skin.

A second function, however, is suggested by the susceptibility of wounds, including burns, to sepsis. Microorganisms trapped between the burned surface and the barrier can proliferate in such an environment. It is therefore desirable to incorporate into the wound covering an antibiotic, using the term in its most general sense.

We tested the feasibility of the concept by including in the formulation phenolphthalein, a soluble and easily identifiable indicator of molecular weight 318.33. A film was prepared

Table 4
SUSTAINED RELEASE OF PHENOLPHTHALEIN

Time (hr)	Absorbance at 546 mm	Released (mg)	Released (%)
2.75	0.049	0.27	8.1
21.25	0.096	0.52	15.6
46.75	0.092	0.50	15.0

Note: Initial film thickness = 0.43 ± 0.07 mm; final film thickness = 0.78 ± 0.20 mm.

and allowed to equilibrate as previously described. It was then immersed in distilled water and held in a shaker bath at 37°C. Aliquot samples of the water were removed periodically and the phenolphthalein contents analyzed spectrophotometrically as a function of time.

The film (Film 014959) was cast in a 9.7-cm diameter petri dish. The recipe for that film was as follows:

Stock solution 014958-1	8.0 mℓ
Glycerol	1.0 mℓ
Phenolphthalein solution	1.0 mℓ
37% Aqueous formaldehyde	1.0 mℓ

To make the phenolphthalein solution 0.10 g of the indicator was dissolved in 10.0 mℓ of ethanol and then diluted to 30 mℓ with distilled water. Thus, the indicator concentration was 3.33 g/ℓ. A spectrum was taken of the phenolphthalein between 450 and 580 nm. To do this the phenolphthalein solution was diluted with 0.1 *N* NaOH in two steps to a final concentration of 3.41×10^{-2} g/ℓ (0.5 to 3.05 mℓ and 0.2 mℓ of this to 3.2 mℓ). The spectrum revealed a single maximum at 546 mm with a specific absorbance of 3.66×10^4 mℓ/g^{-1}/cm^{-1}.

After casting, the film was allowed to come to constant weight prior to taking any further measurements. The weight record was as follows:

Time (hr)	0	88.3	94.3	~142
Weight (g)	7.65	3.58	3.61	2.44
% Loss of weight at ~142 hr (%)	68.1			

The film was immersed in 200 mℓ of distilled water and the flask was placed in a gently agitated shaker batch at 37°C. Periodically 0.5-mℓ aliquot samples were withdrawn and diluted with 4.0 mℓ of 0.1 *N* NaOH. The absorbance, A, at the wavelength maximum was measured and the quantity of phenolphthalein in solution calculated from the following equation.

$$w = AV/\epsilon d$$

where w = weight of phenolphthalein (mg); A = absorbance; V = volume of solution (200 mℓ); ϵ = specific absorbance (3.68×10^4 mℓ/g^{-1}/cm^{-1}); and d = path length = 1.0 cm. These data are presented in Table 4.

Although recovery of phenolphthalein is only about 15% in two days with half of that released within the first 3 hr, this experiment clearly demonstrates that sustained release from gelatin is possible. The remaining phenolphthalein is retained. Quite possibly, some of it has been covalently attached to the cross-linked polymer. It should be stressed, however,

Table 5
EXPERIMENTAL DESIGN[a] AND INDIVIDUAL RESULTS (LB/IN. × 10[3]) FOR IN VIVO EVALUATION OF GELATIN-BASED BURN COVERING

	Control				Experimental			
Formulation	**014969-1**		**014969-2**		**014969-1**		**014969-2**	
Covering removed after 2 hr	C-1	1.30**	C-4	4.08	E-1	20.88	E-4	12.08
	C-2	5.94	C-5	10.11	E-2	11.79	E-5	6.97
	C-3	7.55	C-6	3.54	E-3	16.69	E-6	17.53
Covering removed after 24 hr	C-7	20.20	C-10	28.08	E-7	12.79	E-10	9.33
	C-8	14.79	C-11	19.65	E-8	20.74	E-11	24.84
	C-9	—	C-12	83.58	E-9	34.58	E-12	14.45

[a] Numbers following rat identification (the C- or E-designations) are V results calculated for each rat in lb/in. adherence.
[b] All results are to be multiplied by 10^{-3} to obtain adherence in lb/in.

that this experiment was conducted with a dry film; in actual use, the water content of the film will initially be much higher. This will probably facilitate drug release in the absence of chemical alteration of the drug.

E. In Vivo Evaluation of the Gelatin-Based Wipe-On Burn Covering

Two formulations were evaluated on burned rats using unburned rats as controls. Wistar (CD-1) rats of either sex weighing between 150 and 200 g were obtained from Charles River Breeding Laboratories, Cambridge, Mass.

Stock solutions of each formulation were made up according to the following recipes.

Stock solution no.	**014969-1**	**014969-2**
Hormel® GP-4 gelatin (g)	48.0	48.0
Distilled water (mℓ)	120.0	120.0
Gycerol (mℓ)	17.0	34.0

The volume of gelatin solution before addition of glycerol was in each case ~170 mℓ, allowing an estimate of the gelatin content of films to be made.

In this experiment, 24 rats were used. 12 were reserved for controls and 12 were burned. The latter are termed the experimentals. Six controls received formulation 014969-1 and six received formulation 014969-2. A similar division was made of the experimentals. In order to observe difference in ease of removing the burn coverings, six controls and six experimentals were stripped of their coverings on the same day of application about 2 hr later. Coverings were removed from the remaining animals about 24 hr after application. The experimental matrix described above is summarized in Table 5. In this table are also included adherence results for individual animals.

Animals were prepared for the experiment as follows. All were anesthetized with 50 mg/kg of Nembutal®. Their backs were shaved and then depilated with Nair®. Burns were administered by pipeting 1.5 mℓ of ethanol into an ellipical dam (major axes: 3 × 7 cm) held against the rat's back. The alcohol was ignited and allowed to burn until none remained. This technique achieves a reasonably uniform second- to third-degree burn. After burning, 10.0 mℓ of the stock solution was rapidly mixed with 1.0 mℓ of 37% aqueous formaldehyde.

The still-liquid mixture was brushed evenly over the burned area and a strip of gauze lightly pressed into it. To insure that the gauze was thoroughly imbedded in the gelatin, some of the gelatin solution was brushed over the gauze. The gauze was Hospital Brand®, 44 × 36 mesh USP Type 1. Control rats were covered in an identical manner.

Coverings were removed from 12 animals after 2 hr. These 12 included 6 controls, 3 of which had received Formulation 014969-1 and 3 of which, Formulation 014969-2. Of the remaining 6 experimentals, 3 had received Formulation 014969-1 and 3 Formulation 014969-2.

After 24 hr the remaining 12 animals were stripped of their coverings. Treatment regimes were as above. Prior to cover removal, animals were housed in individual cages and allowed food and water *ad libitum*. Overnight, only one animal, C-9, had pulled its cover off and was lost to the experiment.

Coverings were removed as follows. Anesthetized animals were held on a specially constructed board mounted in an Instron Tensile Tester. Table 6 presents the mean adherences of the coverings on the test animals.

The maximum observed mean adherence was 0.0271 lb/in. for the 24 hr control with Formulation 014969-2. However, differences between the 24 hr controls and experimentals do not appear to be significant. At 2 hr, however, the experimentals of both formulations showed greater adherence than did the controls of either formulation.

Although controls at 24 hr of either formulation adhere more strongly than did the controls at 2 hr, this difference was much less pronounced with the experimentals.

Gelatin films adhered well to the contours of the animals' backs, and were removable with no injury to either the burned or unburned tissue. Mean values are given in Table 7, although it should be stressed that the reported materials were placed in full excision wounds, not burned skin.

ACKNOWLEDGMENT

This work was carried out at Dynatech R/D Company, Cambridge, Mass. under Office of Naval Research Contract No. N00014-81-C-0468; this contract followed earlier work, under ONR Contract No. 00014-73-C-02010.

Table 6
MEAN ADHERENCE OF GELATIN FILMS (LB/IN)

	Control		Experimental	
Formulation	**014969-1**	**014969-2**	**014969-1**	**014969-2**
2 hr	$(4.93 \pm 3.25)10^{-3}$	$(5.91 \pm 3.65)10^{-3}$	$(16.45 \pm 4.55)10^{-3}$	$(12.19 \pm 5.28)10^{-3}$
24 hr	$(17.50 \pm 3.83)10^{-3}$	$(27.10 \pm 7.02)10^{-3}$	$(24.02 \pm 10.91)10^{-3}$	$(16.21 \pm 7.90)10^{-3}$

Note: In all cases, 3 rats were used in each determination, except for the 24-hr pull of control Formulation 014969-1, for which 2 animals were used.

Table 7
GELATIN FILM ADHERENCE

Material	Time (hr)	Condition	Adherence[a]
014969-1	2	Control	4.93
014969-1	24	Control	17.50
014969-1	2	Burned	16.5
014969-1	24	Burned	24.0
014969-2	2	Control	5.91
014969-2	24	Control	27.10
014969-2	2	Burned	12.2
014969-2	24	Burned	16.2

[a] All results are to be multipled by 10^{-3} to obtain adherence in lb/in.

REFERENCE

1. **Tregear, R. T.,** *Physical Functions of Skin*, Academic Press, New York, 1966; Rollhauser, H., *Jahrbuch*, 90, 249, 1950.

Chapter 14

POLYALKYLAMINO ACIDS AS SUSTAINED RELEASE VEHICLES

Donald L. Wise and Oliver Midler

TABLE OF CONTENTS

I. INTRODUCTION

A general class of metabolic intermediates is the amino acids. Amino acids are direct analogs of α-hydroxycarboxylic acids (such as lactic and glycolic acids). There are approximately 20 common amino acids which are found in proteins. Many of these have already been synthesized into synthetic protein-like polymers.[1-3] The use of polyamino acids as polymers for the controlled release of biologically active compounds appears promising for several reasons. The polymer and its hydrolysis products are biocompatible. The choice of amino acids, each with a unique functional moiety, allows the design of a wide variety of matrices for holding the compound to be released. Copolymers are readily synthesized such that the properties of two or more amino acids may be combined.

Glutamic acid is one of the least expensive amino acids available and is produced in the largest quantity. Furthermore, polymers of glutamic acid and copolymers of glutamic acid and lysine are nonimmunogenic.[4] For these reasons its potential for use as a polymer for controlled release of physiologically active compounds is encouraging. Degradation products of the polymer are likewise physiologically acceptable.

Other polyamino acids with similar credits as polyglutamate are l-lysine and d,l-methionine. These also have unique side chains which would alter the character of the polymer from that observed for polyglutamate. Lysine has a net positive charge at physiological pH. Alanine and glycine are the amino acid analogs of the α-hydroxycarboxylic acids, lactic and glycolic acid, and on this basis show promise for use as implantable polymers.

The chemistry of polyamino acid synthesis is well established in the early chemical literature[5-2] and the patent literature.[8,9] The volume by Stahmann[3] is one of the most comprehensive collections of papers on polyamino acids.

Polyamino acids and particularly poly-L-glutamic acid is of interest for application as an implantable drug delivery system because it has been used for surgical sutures.[10,11] Small amounts of polyamino acids are commercially available from a number of biochemical supply houses. A recent patent[12] indicates that a large-scale, 50-kg synthesis is feasible. Polyamino acids have been extensively investigated as protein analogs and there is an extensive amount of literature about them. In the course of many of these investigations a considerable amount of information about the antigenic properties of polyamino acids has been obtained. Earlier information[13] indicated that no homopolymer of an aliphatic amino acid had been prepared that was antigenic. However, the aromatic polyamino acids have an especially high degree of antigenicity associated with them. Perhaps the best evidence for the biocompatibility of poly-L-glutamic acid would be the fact that it has been used as a surgical suture.

An important aspect of polyamino acids that may have a bearing on their biocompatibility is their optical purity. In animal and plant proteins only L-amino acids occur. The effect of D-amino acids on the body is not clear. Fortunately, the polymerization procedure proceeds without racemization.

Hydrolysis rates of polyamino acids are slower than those of polyesters like polylactic or polyglycolic acid. Much of the data in the literature concerns itself with hydrolysis of polyamino acids by digestive enzymes. It was reported, however, that surgical sutures made from poly-L-glutamic acid hydrolyzed in 6 weeks, but these sutures were in the intestines of dogs where digestive enzymes could act on them.[11]

Perhaps the most accepted preparation of poly-L-glutamic acid is to proceed through the γ-alkyl-*N*-carboxyanhydride. This anhydride is prepared from the corresponding γ-alkyl-L-glutamic acid by addition of phosgene. The syntheses of γ-methyl- or γ-ethyl-L-glutamic acid have been described.[14,15] Blount and Karlson also described the preparation of γ-benzyl-L-glutamic acid.[16] Pravda's synthesis[14] of γ-ethyl-L-glutamic acid seems to be the most straightforward.

A. γ-Alkyl L-Glutamate (NCA) Synthesis and Polymerization

The synthesis of γ-methyl-L-glutamate *N*-carboxyanhydride from L-glutamic acid was carried out. The γ-methyl-L-glutamate NCA was polymerized using the method described in the following.

Synthesis of the γ-ethyl-L-glutamate (NCA) was also carried out using the γ-methyl L-glutamate procedure and substituting ethanol for methanol.

B. Mechanism of the Synthesis of γ-Methyl L-Glutamate (NCA) from L-Glutamic Acid

The γ-methyl L-glutamate *N*-carboxyanhydride (4-substituted oxazolidine 2-5 dione) was first prepared by Leuchs in 1906. A summary of syntheses is presented in *Synthesis and Chemical Properties of Poly-α-Amino Acids* by Katchalski and Sela, Weizmann Institute of Science, Rohovot, Israel. Early syntheses used phosgene gas as a reactant. In order to avoid using the hazardous gas, a synthesis method proposed by Hanloy et al.[17] was used. The method required many refinements before good yields and high quality product were obtained. The procedure is presented later and a discussion of the mechanism follows.

The synthesis is a three-step process: (1) making the γ-methyl ester of L-glutamic acid, (2) making γ-methyl *N*-carbobenzyloxy L-glutamate from the γ-methyl ester, and (3) converting the *N*-carbobenzyloxy to the *N*-carboxyanhydride.

1. Step 1

The L-glutamic acid;

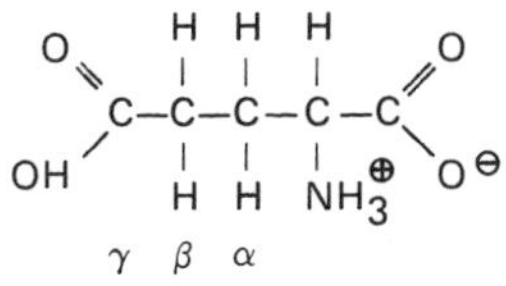

$$HO(O{=})C-CH_2-CH_2-CH(NH_3^{\oplus})-C({=}O)O^{\ominus}$$

γ β α

is converted to the γ-methyl ester:

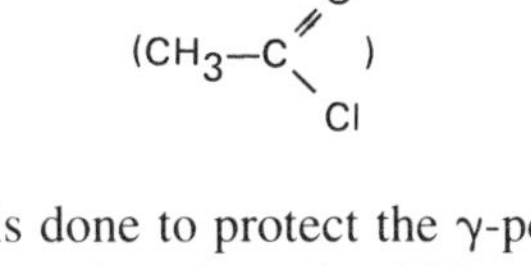

$$CH_3O(O{=})C-CH_2-CH_2-CH(NH_3^{+})-C({=}O)O^{\ominus}$$

by acetyl chloride

$$(CH_3-C({=}O)Cl)$$

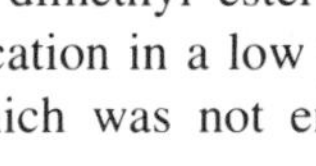

in an excess of methanol. This is done to protect the γ-position during subsequent steps. It was first thought that a short reaction time should be used to prevent formation of the dimethyl ester. However, a high percentage of starting material remained. Ultimately a 20-hr reaction period was found to yield high quality γ-methyl ester which required only one recrystallization. Large amounts of dimethyl ester did not form because the amino acid function is protected against esterification in a low pH system.

Another possible problem — which was not encountered — is the formation of the hydrochloride salt of the acid:

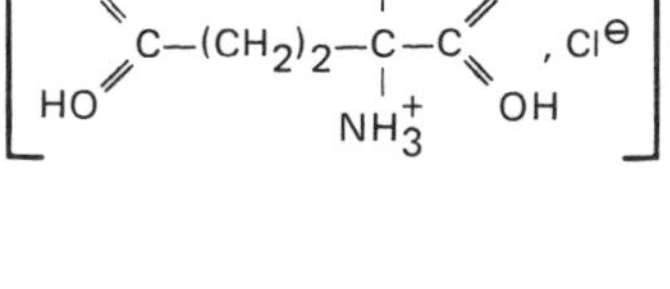

$$\left[HO(O{=})C-(CH_2)_2-CH(NH_3^{+})-C({=}O)OH\ ,\ Cl^{\ominus}\right]$$

It is believed this did not form because the mixture was not shaken once the reagents were added.

Once made, the γ-methyl ester is kept from precipitating out of the HC1 solution by formation of a hydrochloride salt soluble in methanol. Since the ester is sensitive to hydrolysis in the hot water-pyridine solution, care should be taken to perform the step promptly.

2. Step 2

The γ-methyl *N*-carbobenzyloxy L-glutamate is made in the second step. Initially a reaction was tried which led to an amide by action of an acid chloride on an amine (amine acylation):

$$R{-}C(=O)Cl + R{-}NH_2 \rightarrow \left[R{-}C(OH)(Cl){-}HNR^1 \right] \rightarrow R{-}C(=O){-}NH{-}R^1 + HCl$$

However, good yields were not obtained.

Good yields were obtained using benzyl chloroformate and taking advantage of the amine function on the glutamate. That mechanism will not work, however, if the glutamate is in the zwitterion form:

$$-C(H)(NH_3^{\oplus}){-}C(=O)O^{\ominus}$$

since the pair of electrons on the nitrogen are blocked. Thus Na HCO_3 is added to raise the pH in order to maintain the amine function:

$$\rightarrow -C(H)(\bar{N}H_2){-}C(=O)O^{\ominus} + H^{\oplus}$$

and permit attack on the carbon of the C = O with positive polarization:

$$C_6H_5{-}CH_2{-}O{-}\overset{+\delta}{C}(Cl)=\overset{-\delta}{O} + CH_3O{-}C(=O){-}(CH_2)_2{-}C(NH_2){-}C(=O)O^{\ominus} \longrightarrow CH_3O{-}C(=O){-}(CH_2)_2{-}C({-}C(=O)O^{\ominus}){-}N(H){-}C(=O){-}O{-}CH_2{-}C_6H_5$$

γ—METHYL N-CARBOBENZYLOXY L-GLUTAMATE

The product is an oil rather than crystals. The oily liquor is washed with ether and then acidified to release the γ-methyl *N*-carbobenzyloxy L-glutamate from the alkaline water where it was kept in solution under the ionized form:

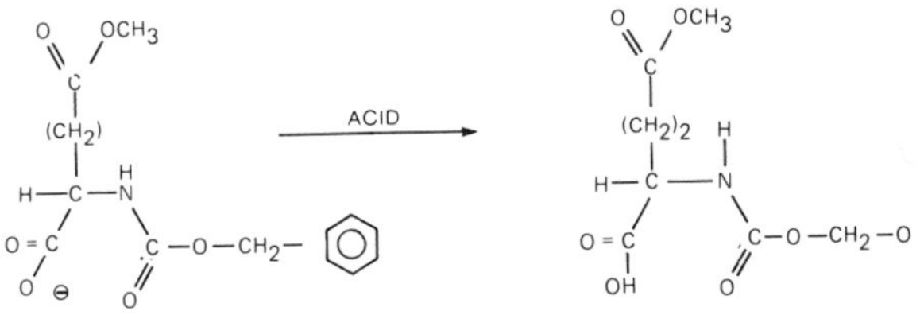

Unfortunately this product does not crystallize but turns into an oil which is extracted with methylene chloride. In order to purify the oily substance, it must be converted into its dicyclohexylamine salt:

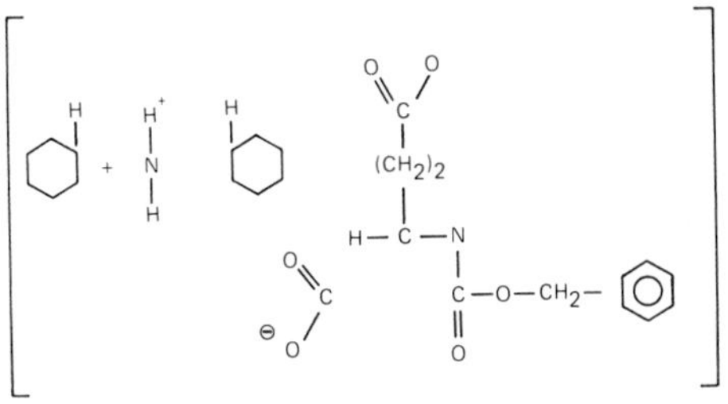

which crystallizes easily in ether. The salt is then recrystallized from boiling methanol by the addition of ether.

The purified salt is reconverted to the original product by addition of 0.5 *M* citric acid. The reaction is carried out in ether in which the salt is insoluble. The product is obtained as an oil which crystallizes easily. The crystals can be recrystallized from CCl_4.

3. Step 3

The starting material is the γ-methyl *N*-carbobenzyl L-glutamate. The reagent used is phosphorous pentachloride which first reacts on the acid function, as usual:

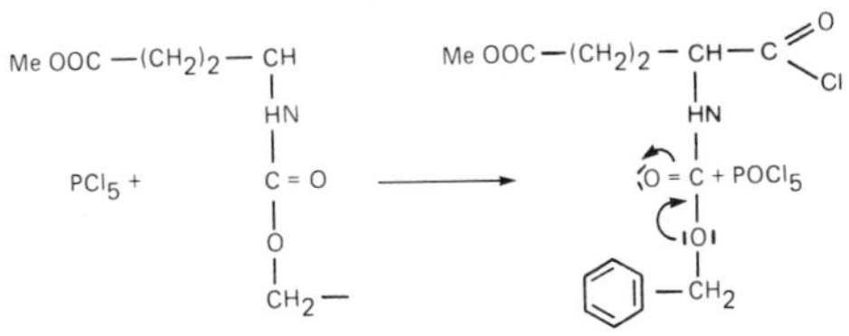

However, this last molecule has resonance form:

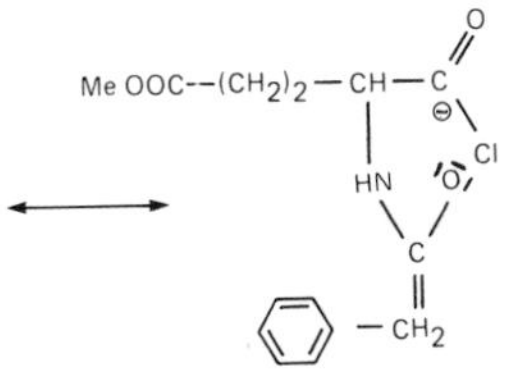

and the ⊖ charge is able to displace the C1 of the acid chloride:

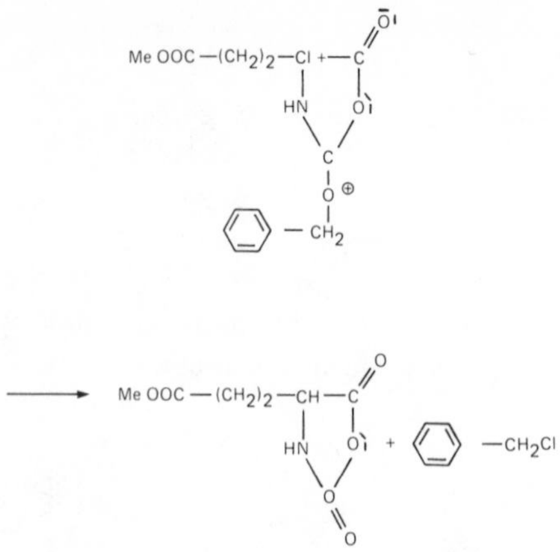

Me OOC —(CH$_2$)$_2$—Cl +—C(=O|)—O|; HN; C; O ⊕; ⬡ — CH$_2$

⟶ Me OOC —(CH$_2$)$_2$—CH—C(=O)—O| + ⬡ —CH$_2$Cl; HN; O; O

The final product is then recrystallized to a fine 99 to 100°C melting point. For successful polymerization all the phosphorous must be removed.

II. PROCEDURE FOR SYNTHESIZING γ-METHYL L-GLUTAMATE FROM L-GLUTAMIC ACID

A. Preparation of the γ-Methyl L-Glutamate

In a hood, distill acetyl chloride until 100 mℓ of pure (b.p. 51 to 52°C) liquid is obtained. Meanwhile, cool 1250 mℓ of dry methanol (methanol stored at least 2 days over molecular sieves) in a 2 ℓ Erlenmeyer® flask by keeping the bottom of the flask in a dry ice-acetone mixture. Slowly add the 100 mℓ of acetyl chloride to the methanol (this should be done in a hood). Stopper the flask and allow the mixture to warm to room temperature. The stopper should be kept on during the warming up, but removed from time to time to release the pressure caused by expanding gases.

When the solution has reached room temperature, add 184 g of L-glutamic acid to the flask with a powder funnel. Shake the flask vigorously for 1 to 2 min (further shaking increases the possibility of precipitation of the hydrochloride which could stop the esterification). Separate the liquid from any undissolved solids by filtration or decantation. Let the mother liquor sit for 20 hr at room temperature in a stoppered 2-ℓ Erlenmeyer® flask. Then add 75 mℓ of pyridine. Shake the flask and set aside for 48 hr at room temperature.

After 48 hr filter the crystals from the solution with a Buchner® funnel and a medium coarse filter paper (e.g., Whatman® #1). Save the mother liquor.

Dry the crystals on the filter paper at room temperature. Then scrape the crystals from the paper and dry them at room temperature in a dessicator under vacuum. Evaporate the two thirds of the solvent from the mother liquor with rotary evaporation. Collect the crystals by filtration.

B. Recrystallization of the γ-Methyl L-Glutamate

This is the delicate part of the procedure. The crystals can only be recrystallized from water. However, they are very sensitive to hydrolysis in the high pH environment caused by the pyridine. Also the presence of unreacted L-glutamic acid will cause complications.

The γ-methyl-L-glutamic powder must be completely dry. Let "m" be weight of the powder. In a 2-ℓ Erlenmeyer® flask, heat 1.5 × "m" mℓ of distilled water to 65 to 75°C with a hot plate equipped with a magnetic stirrer. On another hot plate (in a hood) bring to a boil 6 × "m" mℓ of methanol. Use boiling chips. Add the powder to the warm water stirring continuously with the magnetic stirrer. All of the powder should dissolve. If not, add more water until the total volume of water added is 2 × "m" mℓ. Any remaining undissolved solid is probably L-glutamic acid which must be removed. Filter the solution with a heated (70°C) Buchner® funnel using Whatman® #4 filter paper.

To the clear solution add 3 vol of boiling methanol for every volume of water. Crystallization should occur. Let the mixture cool to room temperature; then place in a 0°C refrigerator overnight. Filter the crystals from the mother liquor; dry them; and take a melting point (175 to 176°C required). If the crystals are not pure, repeat the crystallization procedure.

The purified product should be kept in the freezer at -20°C until needed.

III. PROCEDURE FOR SYNTHESIZING γ-METHYL *N*-CARBOBENZYLOXY L-GLUTAMATE FROM γ-METHYL L-GLUTAMATE

A. Preparation of γ-Methyl *N*-Carbobenzyloxy L-Glutamate

Dissolve 58.4 g of sodium bicarbonate in 360 mℓ of distilled water using a magnetic stirrer-equipped hot plate. Do not heat over 40°C.

Transfer the solution into a three-neck round bottom provided with a mechanical stirring system and a 250-cc addition funnel (pressure equalized if possible) and place in a ice water-NaCl bath. The stirrer is turned on and 53.4 g of pure γ-methyl L-glutamate is then added through the third neck with a powder funnel. Meanwhile the addition funnel has been filled with 60 cc of benzyl chloroformate (Aldrich Chemical Co., Boston). When all the glutamate is added and when the round bottom is cool, the benzyl chloroformate is added in 5 fractions — as equivalent as possible — every 3 min.

After 2 hr the ice-NaCl bath is removed and the reaction is allowed to continue for 2 more hours at room temperature (stirrer still on).

B. Extraction of the γ-Methyl *N*-Carbobenzyloxy L-Glutamate

The liquid from the above reaction is poured into a separatory funnel and washed twice with ether (1 vol ether: 4 vol reaction liquor). This removes organic by-products (e.g., excess benzyl chloroformate). Save the ether layers. Acidify the water layer with 1 *N* HC1 until the pH = 1. A whitish oil will form in the water. The oil is extracted from the emulsion by washing three times with methylene chloride (1 vol methylene chloride: 3 vol emulsion). Save the acid layer. Combine the methylene chloride solutions and dry by the addition of anhydrous magnesium sulfate. Filter the solution into a *tared* round bottom flask. Remove the methylene chloride with a rotary evaporator. A thick yellow oil is the desired product.

C. Purification of the γ-Methyl *N*-Carbobenzymloxy L-Glutamate

1. Formation of the Dicyclohexylamine Salt

In order to purify the oil, it is necessary to convert it to a salt; recrystallize the salt and then reconvert the salt back to the oil.

To do this dissolve the oil in anhydrous ether (5 cc of ether per gram of oil). Distill 1.1 mol of dicyclohexylamine (181 mol wt) for every mole of oil (295 mol wt). Dissolve the amine in a volume of anhydrous either equal to that used to dissolve the oil. Add the amine-ether solution to the oil-ether solution. Stir the solution at least 4 hr in the hood (overnight stirring is more desirable).

The crystals are collected by filtration using a Buchner® funnel and Whatman® #4 paper. Dry under vacuum at room temperature.

2. Recrystallization of the Salt

Let "m" equal the weight of the crystals. Bring to a boil 1.2 × "m" mℓ of methanol on a stirrer-provided hot plate. Slowly add the crystals to the methanol. Filter any undissolved solids from the solution using a heated (65°C) Buchner® funnel and Whatman® #4 paper. Allow the solution to cool to room temperature. In a hood, carefully add 4 vol of anhydrous

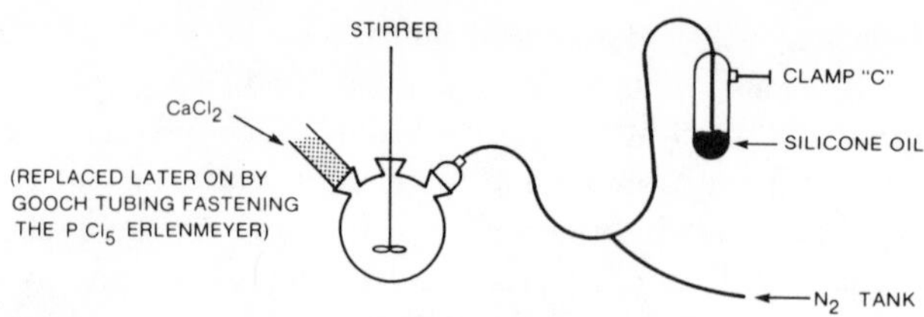

FIGURE 1. Reaction vessel.

ether for every volume of methanol. Let the solution cool to room temperature then put in the 0°C refrigerator. Seed crystal can be added to facilitate crystallization. Filter the crystals from the mother liquor. Evaporate the mother liquor with a rotary evacuator.

This might yield more crystals. Dry the crystals under vacuum at 45°C. Take the melting point; it should be 149 to 150°C. If not, perform the recrystallization again.

3. Reconversion of the Salt to the γ-Methyl N-Carbobenzyloxy L-Glutamate

Make a suspension of the salt with anhydrous ether (15 mℓ of ether per gram of salt). Add 0.5 *M* citric acid (192 mol wt) until there are 3 mol of citric acid per mole of salt. Stir at room temperature with a magnetic stirrer. When all the solids are dissolved, transfer the solution to a separatory funnel. (Clean separating funnel with chromic acid cleaning solution before using.)

The citric acid (lower layer) is collected and saved. The ether layer is washed twice with 0.5 *M* citric acid — about 1 *M* equivalent per washing. Combine the citric acid layers. Extract with ether using one fourth of the acid volume. Combine both ether layers.

Wash the ether layers twice with distilled water to remove all the citric acid. Dry the ether with anhydrous magnesium sulfate; filter with Whatman® #4 paper and collect in a tared flask. Remove the ether with the rotary evaporator. The pure oil will remain.

This oil is then crystallized using the following procedure. Cover the oil with about $^1/_2$ in. of hexane. Using a glass rod scratch the bottom of the flask below the hexane. The oil will agglomerate and form gummy chunks which will eventually crystallize. If this does not work add some seed crystals and resume triturating. Recrystallize with hot CCl_4.

IV. PROCEDURE FOR SYNTHESIZING γ-METHYL *N*-CARBOXYL L-GLUTAMATE ANHYDRIDE FROM γ-METHYL *N*-CARBOBENZYLOXY L-GLUTAMATE

In the hood, set up the apparatus as shown in Figure 1. When clamp C is closed the system is maintained at $^1/_4$-in. silicon oil pressure with the nitrogen purge. Once the nitrogen pressure is established, heat the glassware to drive out moisture. The nitrogen must remain during the cooling period to prevent condensation of moisture in the system.

When the system has cooled, quickly add 1050 mℓ of anhydrous ether (use a *new* container); then reestablish the nitrogen purge. Add 59.1 g of γ-methyl *N*-carbobenzyloxy L-glutamate. Start the stirrer. After the crystals dissolve, position an ice bath around the flask.

Weigh 45.4 g of phosphorous pentachloride into a *dry* Erlenmeyer®, flask as quickly as possible. Stopper the flask. Attach the flask to the three-neck flask in place of the $CaCl_2$ tube by means of gooch tubing. This enables one to add the phosphorous pentachloride without contacting outside moisture. Close clamp C. This will expand the gooch tubing and the pentachloride is added in 0.5-g portions. The addition should take about 30 min.

When the pentachloride addition is completed continue stirring the mixture and maintain the ice bath for 30 min; then remove the ice bath and allow the reaction mixture to warm

Table 1
POLY-γ-BENZYL-L-GLUTAMATE

Sample no.	12914-4	12912-2
Hydrocortisone (% by wt)	167.7	33.3
Designation of polymer synthesis	Poly-γ-benzyl-L-glutamate	Poly-γ-benzyl-L-glutamate
Form tested	Molded plates	Molded plates
Technique used	Molding	Molding
Sample size	Approximately 0.03 g	Approximately 0.03 g
Solution volume	50	50

Days from placement in bath	Cumulative release (%)	Days from placement in bath	Cumulative release (%)
11	14	1	3
39	18	15	14
55	21	25	15
70	23	35	17
80	26	37	18
90	27	50	20
		70	20
		90	22

for 30 min. Add a straight reflux condenser between the three-neck flask and the nitrogen stopcock. Purge the system with N_2 for 1 min. Replace the gooch tubing with a stopper. Set up a heating mantle. Reflux the system for 1 hr.

Stopper the two side necks of flask and remove most of the ether from the reaction system with a rotary evaporator. Crystals will appear. Add 3 to 5 mℓ of *dry* ethyl acetate and heat the flask with a heat gun to dissolve the crystals. (Do not boil.) Transfer to an Erlenmeyer® and add an equivalent volume of dry petroleum ether. Stopper the Erlenmeyer®. The product will crystallize in the −20°C freezer or, if not, in the dry ice box.

Recrystallize the crystals in the same way: dissolve in ethyl acetate, add an equal volume of petroleum ether, cool, and filter. Melting point is 99 to 100°C. The crystals should be used as quickly as possible. Store in the dry ice box.

V. PREPARATION AND TESTING OF POLYMER/DRUG MATRIX

Following are examples of specific experiments carried out to demonstrate the sustained delivery of active substances from polyamino acids and polyalkylamino acids. The active substances selected for all these experiments was hydrocortisone (11β, 17α, 21-trihydroxy-4-pregnene-3,20-dione). The medical application for hydrocortisone in humans is in adrenocortical hormone therapy. A veterinary application is for ketosis in cows. However, the selection of hydrocortisone was made only to furnish a model active substance having application to demonstrate this treatment technique in humans and animals.

In Table 1 and Figure 2 are summarized the release rates of this active agent (hydrocortisone) from the select polymer matrices. The active agent was ^{14}C labeled, and release rates were evaluated by radioactive scintillation analysis of solution in which the polymer/active substance is placed. The preparation and testing procedures are as follows.

The hydrocortisone was dissolved in a solvent (ethyl alcohol) and the ^{14}C-labeled hydrocortisone added; the solvent was removed under vacuum, leaving a material of uniform radioactivity. The hydrocortisone content of the final test samples was regulated by adding a portion of this blend to nonradioactive polymer by solvent blending or by mixing powders and then molding. For example, to solvent blend, the samples of poly-γ-benzyl-L-glutamate

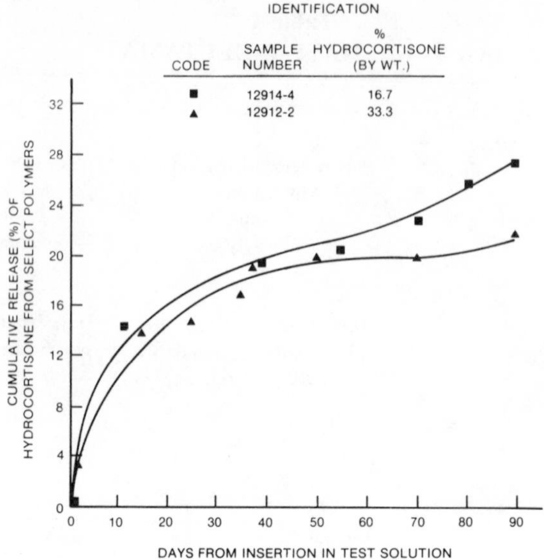

FIGURE 2. Release of hydrocortisone from a selected polyalkylamino acid.

and the hydrocortisone were dissolved in a common solvent (solvent = 50 mℓ methylene chloride, 10 mℓ acetone, 10 mℓ methanol, 5 mℓ water) yielding a clear solution. This solution was cast on a glass modeling plate and the solvent permitted to evaporate. The films were removed and evacuated under vacuum (0.1 Torr) overnight. The material was then vacuum molded at 95 to 105°C in a specially designed stainless-steel mold with a brass die designed to produce molded plates (1 cm × 4 cm × 1 mm). The molded plates of polymer/active substances at either 20 PHR (16.7% by weight active agent) or 50 PHR (33.3% by weight active agent) were quite flexible. These plates were placed in 50 mℓ of pH 7 buffer at 37°C. Aliquots (2 mℓ) were taken twice weekly and the solution was changed weekly. Radioactive scintillation was carried out on the samples of solution; the results are listed in Table 1 and Figure 2. After several weeks the molded plates appeared relatively intact, indicating the potential for reasonable longer-term service as a practical implantable delivery system.

For powder blending of the hydrocortisone/polymer (the polyamino acids in this case) the finely divided active hydrocortisone and the finely divided polymer were mixed by rolling a jar containing them for several hours so that they became uniformly blended. The mixture was then molded in a mold press at temperatures from 200 to 230°C. Testing procedure followed as described above.

For one polymer (poly-L-glutamic acid) the active agent and polymer were dissolved in the solvent system — 40 mℓ methylene chloride, 50 mℓ acetone, 10 mℓ water, and films cast. The films were clear and the system appeared to be a good film former. The films, when placed in pH 7 buffer at 37°C, were found to have completely fragmented within 24 hr. The solution was then evacuated under vacuum (0.1 Torr) at 70°C giving a similar film as initially cast. This film was again placed in pH 7 buffer at 37°C and it was observed to immediately fragment. Such a polymer/active agent system may have application as an enteric coating or an intravaginal coating or any application where very short-term release is desired.

With respect to the results of the sustained release tests it is seen that release of the active agent from the polymer/active agent matrix did occur over a period of time. In every respect, the results demonstrate the sustained release of active agents from polyamino acids and polyalkylamino acids.

An array of pure polyamino acids, copolymers of various polyamino acids, and polyalkylamino acids appear suitable for application as implantable systems for the sustained release of active substances. Cross-linking of the polymer to increase the content of the active substance and to further control the release may be carried out. Bonding of the active substances to the polymer may further enable more close regulation of the release or protection of the active substance.

ACKNOWLEDGMENT

This work was carried out at Dynatech R/D Company, Cambridge, Mass. on an independent research and development project as well as under the sponsorship of the National Institute on Drug Abuse (NIDA) Contract HSM-42-73-267 (HD).

REFERENCES

1. **Astbury, F. R. S., Dalgliesh, C. E., Darmon, S. E., and Sutherland, G. B. B. M.,** *Nature (London),* 162, 596, 1948.
2. **Hill, R.,** *Fabrics from Synthetic Polymers,* Elsevier, New York, 1953.
3. **Stahmann, M. A.,** *Poly-Amino Acids, Polypeptides, and Proteins,* University of Wisconsin, Press, Madison, 1962.
4. **Katz, D. H., Davie, J. M., Paul, W. E., and Benacerraf,** *J. Exp. Med.,* 134, 201, 1971.
5. **Hanby, W. E., Waley, S. G., and Watson, J.,** *Nature (London),* 161, 132, 1948.
6. **Farthing, A. C.,** *J. Chem. Soc.,* 3213, 1950.
7. **Woodward, R. B. and Schramm, C. H.,** *J. Am. Chem. Soc.,* 69, 1551, 1947.
8. **Woodward, R. B.,** U.S. Patent 2,657,972, 1953.
9. **Kaczalski, E.,** U.S. Patent 2,578,428, 1951.
10. **Miyamae, T., Mori, S., and Takeda, Y.,** U.S. Patent 3,371,069, 1968; *Chem. Abstr.,* 68, P89882p, 1968.
11. **Courtaulds Ltd.,** Belg. 636,530, 1963; *Chem. Abstr.,* 62, 4184b, 1965.
12. Ashai Chemical Industry Co., Brit. 1,252,869, 1971; *Chem. Abstr.,* 76, 73022n, 1972.
13. **Fasman, G. D., Ed.,** *Poly-Amino Acids,* Marcel Dekker, New York, 1967, 621.
14. **Pravda, Z.,** *Collect. Czech. Chem. Commun.,* 24, 2083, 1959.
15. *Nippon Nogei Kagaku Kaishi,* 34, 782, 1960; *Chem. Abstr.,* 59, 6509a, 1963.
16. **Blount, E. R. and Karlson, R. H.,** *J. Am. Chem. Soc.,* 78, 941, 1956.
17. **Hanloy, W. E., Waley, S. G., Watson, J.,** Synthetic polypeptides, *J. Chem. Soc.,* p. 3239, 1950.

Chapter 15

A NEW COMPOSITE MATERIAL FOR FIXATION OF ORTHOPEDIC SURGICAL IMPLANTS

Donald L. Wise and John B. Gregory

TABLE OF CONTENTS

I. INTRODUCTION

Terms used to describe nonmetallic materials which bond other materials (both metallic and nonmetallic) are an indication of their various compositions and functions. Overall, "glue" and "adhesive" describe nonmetallic materials in which attachment to a surface involves principally molecular attraction. On the other hand, "lutes" and "cements" act principally through mechanical interlocking and may function also as gap-filling agents. The technological use of such terms is often arbitrary since no practical surface is completely smooth and an element of mechanical interlocking is present in all adhesive joints. Both adhesion and mechanical interlocking are useful mechanisms of bonding under biological conditions.

The principal use of cements and adhesives in bone has been for the joining and fixation of fractures, the repair of defects, and the fixation of prostheses. The use of cements in this connection dates back to the 19th century when a bone glue composed of colophony, pumice, and plaster of paris was used to fix joint replacements made of ivory. Over the years moldable polymeric materials which may be shaped and placed *in situ* have been developed.

It is interesting to note that the first application for a new biocompatible material is usually in the dental area. For example, only fairly recently has polymethylmethacrylate bone cement been used extensively in orthopedic surgery, especially femoral endoprostheses. However, it has been the primary constituent of the majority of artificial dentures for approximately 40 years. The material has also been used by neurosurgeons to form replacements for skull defects (cranioplasty). Polymethylmethacrylate cement is conventionally prepared as a powder/liquid system. The powder is essentially polymethylmethacrylate in the form of a mixture of fine particles containing about 1% benzoyl peroxide. The liquid is methylmethacrylate monomer containing approximately 1% of dimethyl paratoluidine and less than 0.01% of polymerization inhibitor. The monomer (liquid) and polymer (powder) are usually mixed in proportions of 1:2 by weight. Concurrent dissolution of part of the polymer in the monomer and polymerization of the monomer through the peroxide amine system occur. The consistency of the mixture changes from a slurry to a moldable "dough" after a few minutes. Polymerization of the monomer occurs quite rapidly, involving a significant heat of reaction and a corresponding temperature rise of the material to 100°C or greater which also results in some loss of the methylmethacrylate monomer. Within about 6 to 10 min the polymerization is complete, resulting in a hard, rigid, white bone-like mass having a basic structure of the original polymer granules cemented together by newly formed polymer.

The outstanding mechanical strength parameters and physical characteristics of polymethylmethacrylate cement for application to orthopedic surgery have, to date, offset concern about the effects of the exothermic reaction of the *in situ* polymerization and the toxicity aspect represented by the evolution of the monomer. On the other hand, as new biocompatible materials begin to compete with respect to the mechanical and physical properties of polymethylmethacrylate, then the undesirable features of this material may provide a basis for recommending its discontinuation.

A potential candidate for replacement of polymethylmethacrylate bone cement is another powder/liquid material — polycarboxylate. As the early application of polymethylmethacrylate was in the dental area, so this new material, polycarboxylate, has been applied first to dental repair. This new material is known to set and no temperature rise is noted. On the other hand, only with special care can polymer molecular weights be obtained which result in high compression and tensile strengths. It was proposed to add to the powder chopped fibers or small spherical particles of a reinforcing material. This reinforcing material is also a relatively new biocompatible polymer — poly-ε-caprolactone. Cross-linking of the two polymers for added strength appears to be practical. Polycarboxylate cement, reinforced with a suitable form of poly-ε-caprolactone, may provide for unique overall superior characteristics as a bone cement. Further, in corporation of an antibiotic or growth factor into the bone cement for purposes of sustained release is integral to this system. In the following is discussed the technical background of these materials.

II. POLYCARBOXYLATE CEMENT

Polycarboxylate cements were developed by D.C. Smith, Professor of Dentistry, University of Toronto, for application to dental repair.[1] A British patent describing the preparation of polycarboxylate cements (zinc oxide/polyacrylic acid) was awarded to Prof. Smith in 1969 assigned to the National Research Development Corporation.[2] The development and properties of these cements have been discussed further by Smith.[3-5] An excellent review article by Smith[6] discusses early clinical results, especially those involving orthodontic appliances in which the stainless-steel orthodontic brackets were directly bonded to the teeth.[7-10] has described 5 years of experience in general practice when the polycarboxylate cements were used for cementation of gold inlays, full crowns, or metal-ceramic bridge work. Overall the work reported in the literature using polycarboxylate cements appears to be directly addressed to applications for dental repair, although Smith[6] cites possible application to repair of surgical defects.

The polycarboxylate cements are powder-liquid materials. The powder is a modified zinc oxide similar to that already used in other dental cements. The liquid is a solution of prepolymerized polyacrylic acid in water. Polyacrylic acid is a glass-clear solid prepared from acrylic acid (CH_2=CHCOOH) and having the repeating mer unit:

$$\left[\begin{array}{l} -CH_2-CH- \\ \qquad\quad | \\ \qquad\ COOH \end{array}\right]_{\eta}$$

When an approximately 40% solution of polyacrylic acid (of an appropriate molecular weight) in water is mixed with an appropriate amount of zinc oxide powder (containing less than 10% magnesium oxide), the resultant paste sets to a hard mass which may be made virtually insoluble in water. Setting, not a reaction involving heat evolution, is due to a chemical bonding in which zinc ions link adjacent polyacrylic acid molecules producing a large cross-linked structure. The acid groups in the long chain molecule also have the capacity to chelate to calcium and other metals of suitable chemical reactivity. Thus, if the freshly prepared paste-like cement is placed on a clean calcific or suitable metal surface, it will set through both cross-linking and through bonding to the underlying surface by chelation. These two bonding mechanisms are shown below:

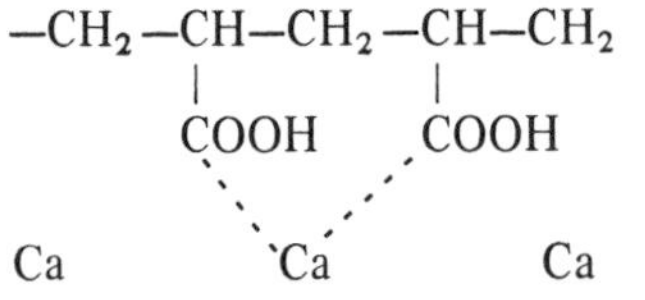

```
–CH2–CH–CH2–CH–CH2                 –CH–CH2–CH–
      |       |                     |       |
     COOH    COOH                  COOH    COOH
        `.  .'                         `Zn'
Ca       Ca        Ca              COOH    COOH
                                    |       |
                                   –CH–CH2–CH–CH2–

Chelation to surface                 Cross-linking
```

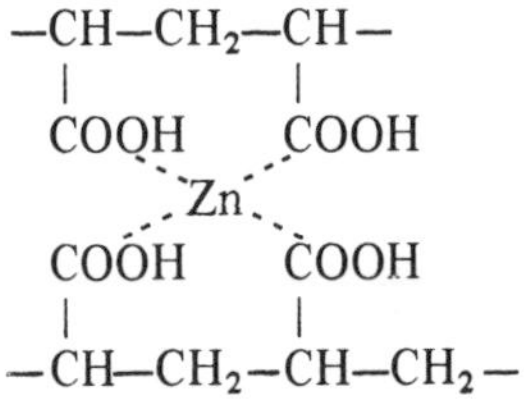

The potential to form these two types of bonds is considerable since each molecule has many functional carboxyl groups. The polyacrylic acid will also complex and bond with protein.[4]

It is of interest to note that the basic powder and liquid components may be varied to produce cements with physical properties and strength characteristics over a wide range.

For example, the reactivity of the zinc oxide powder can be adjusted to give a specific setting time. The molecular weight and the concentration of the polyacrylic acid may also be varied to provide for a selected viscosity and ultimate strengths. By control of these variables it has been possible to obtain dental cements ranging from fluid rapid-setting mixes, appropriate for root canal therapy, to viscous putty-like material suitable for periodontal packs.[4]

The polycarboxylate cements have been prepared with compressive strengths up to 20000 psi and tensile strengths of 2000 psi; further, these materials gain strength rapidly attaining 75% of the 24-hr value in 15 min and 90% within an hour.[4] Smith reports[4] that both tensile and compressive strength increase slightly on storage in water and cite that reports on weakening of the material in water by Mortiner and Tranter[13] were due to faulty preparation techniques. Clearly the possibility of water solubility and cement life is a concern but since development and testing of this material is so recent no long term, i.e., greater than 5 years, results are available. Incorporation of an antibiotic or growth factor is a further potential advantage.

III. POLY-ϵ-CAPROLACTONE REINFORCEMENT MATERIAL

The recent advent of sutures[14,15] and surgical materials[16,17] based on synthetic polymers, as well as the work on lutes, glues, cements, and adhesives discussed earlier, has resulted in a keen interest in other potential nontoxic synthetic polymers for application as implantable material. Investigations have also recently been initiated on the suitability of poly-ϵ-caprolactone[18] for applications as an implantable material. This material is not yet completely characterized for in vivo applications, but it has been shown to be virtually nonbiodegradable[19,20] and in vivo results at this present time which respect to strength and nontoxicity are outstanding.[21] In addition, it has recently been shown to have potential as a burn covering or wound dressing.[22]

Although poly-ϵ-caprolactone has only recently been demonstrated to be a satisfactory substance for incorporation within the body and for topical applications on exposed tissue, this linear polyester was synthesized by Carothers and Arvin[23] many years ago, and a patent was later awarded to Carothers for this synthesis[24] in 1937.

Poly-ϵ-caprolactone is characterized by the repeating unit:

$$(\mathrm{O{-}(CH_2)_5{-}\underset{\underset{\displaystyle O}{\|}}{C}{-}})$$

A low molecular weight polymer was described by Carothers et al.[25] but more recent studies have shown that high molecular weight polymers are readily prepared.[26] Catalysts used in the polymerization are well suited for applications where biocompatibility is important. For example, polymerization of ϵ-caprolactone catalyzed by both dibutylzinc and triisobutylaluminum has been carried out.[27] Calcium salts, also suitable as a catalyst for preparation of implant materials, have been investigated as catalysts.[28]

From the standpoint of careful evaluation of physical properties of poly-ϵ-caprolactone, a substantial background is available.[27,29,30] The polymerization reaction is also well characterized. The catalyst (initiator), catalyst concentration, and type of end group have been found to be extremely important with respect to the thermal and hydrolytic stability of poly-ϵ-caprolactone.[31]

Clearly, a very substantial technical background is available on the polymerization mechanisms and physical characterization of poly-ϵ-caprolactone and a very complete summary of this lactone is presented by Lundberg and Cox.[32]

Extensive animal studies on poly-ε-caprolactone have been carried out at the U.S. Army Medical Bioengineering Research and Development Laboratory, Ft. Detrick, Md.[18-21] The application of this polymer is as a surgical repair material. In one study[18] poly-ε-caprolactone was found to have essentially no change over long periods of time when implanted in rats.

The U.S. Army Medical Bioengineering Research and Development Laboratory continued with the in vivo testing of poly-ε-caprolactone, and results are encouraging. Research workers at Ft. Detrick indicated that poly-ε-caprolactone is stronger than either Dacron® or nylon and, further, it is more tissue compatible than nylon.[21]

IV. POLYMETHYLMETHACRYLATE CEMENT (MMA CEMENT)

At the present time, the most commonly used orthopedic implant cement or lute is a mixture of powdered methylmethacrylate or methylmethacrylate copolymer containing benzoyl peroxide with promoter and a liquid monomer consisting largely of methylmethacrylate. This cement when mixed initially forms a soft dough which is easily handled by the surgeon and when cured it has physical properties which are close to those required for an ideal bone cement. The major drawbacks to this combination are that the polymerization of the methylmethacrylate monomer is strongly oxothermic (a rise to 80°C is typical)[33] so that it is impossible to keep the temperatures in the bone cavity below those that will cause some bone tissue destruction. Also, the heat of reaction causes considerable loss of monomer to the surrounding tissues. As a result of the heat and absorbtion of monomer, a significant amount of bone adjacent to the cement is killed and must be absorbed and replaced by new bone before the implant fixation attains its maximum strength. Also the monomer in the blood stream can cause acute cardiovascular collapse.

To avoid the problems with MMA cement, it was proposed to study a novel composite formed by combining polycarboxylate cements developed by Prof. Smith, with fibers or pellets of a poly-ε-caprolactone polymer earlier, this polymer has a high degree of tissue compatibility[18-21] and should reinforce or strengthen the polycarboxylate cements.

V. EXPERIMENTAL

The procedures given in British Patent 1,139,430[2] for making powders of zinc oxide and solutions of polyacrylic acid produced material which seemed comparable in behavior to the powders and liquid in the commercial dental carboxylate cements. A polymer was synthesized of ε-caprolactone of sufficiently high molecular weight so that it could be spun into fibers which were easier to chop cleanly than fibers made from the poly-ε-caprolactone made commercially which had a lower molecular weight. Poly-ε-caprolactone beads were not made because little adhesion was found between the poly-ε-caprolactone fibers and the zinc carboxylate cement. Fibers would be expected, and were found, to strengthen the cement because of their ability to spread the load, however, little, if any, reinforcement might be expected from, beads.

The physical property data were of particular interest in indicating the good prospects for this new composite material for the fixation of surgical implants. A sample met the tentative specification for compressive strength and came close to meeting the requirement for diametral tensile strength. The modulus of elasticity in compression was considerably higher than that of MMA cements. A typical modulus value for MMA is 33,500 psi,[34] whereas a number of the samples tested had moduli of over 100,000. Thus, the new combination was better than MMA in this respect since the ideal bone cement should have a modulus between that of bone and metal, i.e., 2.2×10^6 to 2.8×10^6 psi.

The properties of the zinc oxide powder and solution of polyacrylic acid prepared were comparable to those of three commercial dental carboxylate cements tested. The major problem encountered with both the commercial cements and with the cements made from ingredients synthesized was the short pot life. In order to get them into the mold, the cements had to be mixed at 4°C. When kept at this temperature, they were easily worked, although they tended to stick to the tools. However, when one of the cements was gathered into a mass in order to place it into the mold either with a spatula or a syringe, it soon became slightly warm and then set up rapidly over a period of about 1 min. Since the gelled material does not stick to itself very well, it was difficult to mold specimens without flaws. The pot life of carboxylate cements was increased to three times that of the commercial cements, but in order to have a cement which could be handled at ambient temperatures, another tenfold increase in pot life was needed. If this were achieved, there should be no problem in meeting the physical property requirements of the proposed specification for bone cements. The physical properties of all the specimens would have been considerably better if the test specimens had been flaw free.

It should be noted that these cements did generate some heat when they set. However, the amount of heat generated was small in comparison to that generated by MMA cement. Typical peak temperature for MMA was 80°C,[33] whereas the peak temperature for a carboxylate cement was 44°C. This small amount of heat should not destroy the adjacent bone surface. Further, since there is no monomer present in the carboxylate cement, no tissue damage from that source will occur with carboxylate cements, whereas it is a serious problem with MMA cement.

An attempt was made to improve the properties of the mixture of zinc oxide powder and polyacrylic acid solution by using a powder liquid ratio of 2:1, but this decreased the pot life so much it was not possible to mold samples.

In order to lengthen the pot life, the zinc oxide was replaced both by magnesium oxide and by tricalcium phosphate. But when these modified powders were mixed with solution 23608, the combination had a shorter pot life than when all zinc oxide was used. The longest pot life achieved was using zinc oxide which was calcined at 1000°C for 24 hr including the 8 hr warm-up time. Longer zinc oxide calcining times and/or higher calcining temperatures should give a further increase in pot life. It appears that what is needed is a method for increasing the crystal size and decreasing the activity of the zinc oxide so the zinc ions are not released so rapidly. Zinc oxides of near-colloidal dimensions were used so a considerable increase in particle size was possible before having difficulty in achieving a homogeneous mixture with the polyacrylic acid.

The adhesion of the poly-ϵ-caprolactone fibers to the zinc carboxylate matrix is capable of improvement although probably not necessary to meet the strength requirements of the cement. The fibers can be treated with minute quantities of the various silane adhesion promoters of the type so successfully used in other fiber reinforced plastics, or the ϵ-caprolactone can be copolymerized with other monomers which will promote the adhesion by providing groups with which the polycarboxylate adhesive will react. Further, an available silane adhesion promoter such as 3-glycidoxypropyltrimethoxy silane may be used. If the fiber is treated with this material, the silane should react with the fiber providing glycidyl groups to react with the carboxy groups along the polyacrylic acid chain.

VI. CONCLUSIONS AND RECOMMENDATIONS

The combination of poly-ϵ-caprolactone fiber and zinc carboxylate cement has been shown to have the potential for meeting the physical property requirements of an orthopedic bone cement. It has the following advantages over the currently used MMA cement:

1. Much lower exotherm — low enough so bone destruction will be eliminated
2. Higher modules of elasticity

3. Absence of methyl methacrylate monomer and concomitant dangers of cardiovascular collapse during surgery, a constant threat with MMA cement
4. Incorporation of an antibiotic and/or growth factor for sustained release appears practical

Because of the potential of the combination for being a superior replacement for MMA cement and the number of potential means for improving the present inadequate pot life, further work is recommended. The chief emphasis should be the investigation of methods for increasing the pot life of the cement so that it will be practical for a surgeon to work with.

Incorporation of an antibiotic and/or growth factor should be carried out and the sustained release evaluated.

VII. SUMMARY

A composite material of polycarboxylate cement reinforced with a suitable form of poly-ϵ-caprolactone such as chopped fibers or small spheres was investigated for preparation and testing as a bone cement for fixation of orthopedic surgical implants such as femoral endoprostheses. Incorporation of an antibiotic or growth factor into this bone cement for sustained release is integral to the concept.

Polycarboxylate is a powder/liquid cement having a successful early record in dental application. It is formed when an aqueous solution of prepolymerized polyacrylic acid is mixed with zinc oxide which then sets through a mechanism of cross-linking and chelation to the surface. As a result, no temperature rise in the material nor evolution of any component is experienced. Poly-ϵ-caprolactone is a well-known polymer having especially outstanding strength characteristics and is shown to have excellent potential for biological applications.

All pertinent reference materials on these materials are presented and discussed. A limited but comprehensive preparation and testing program was conducted in order to appropriately evaluate this composite material.

ACKNOWLEDGMENT

This work was carried out at Dynatech R/D Company, Cambridge, Mass.

REFERENCES

1. **Smith, D. C.,** *Br. Dent. J.*, 125, 381, 1968.
2. British Patent 1,139,430.
3. **Smith, D. C.,** *Dent. Clin. North Am.*, 15, 3, 1971.
4. **Smith, D. C.,** *J. Can. Den. Assoc.*, 37, 22, 1971.
5. **Mizrahi, E. and Smith, D. C.,** *Br. Dent. J.*, 127, 410, 1969.
6. **Smith, D. C.,** *Biomed. Eng.*, 108, 1973.
7. **Mizrahi, E. and Smith, D. C.,** *Br. Dent. J.*, 130, 132, 1971.
8. **Mizrahi, E.,** *J. Den. Assoc. South Afr.*, 27, 279, 1972.
9. **Phillips, R. W., et al.,** *J. Am. Dent. Assoc.*, 81, 1353, 1970.
10. **Beagrie, G. S., et al.,** *Br. Dent. J.*, 132, 351, 1972.
11. **McLean, J. W.,** *Br. Dent. J.*, 132, 9, 1972.
12. **McLean, J. W.,** *J. Br. Endoscopy Soc.*, 20, 1971.
13. **Mortiner, K. V. and Tranter, T. C.,** *Br. Dent. J.*, 127, 365, 1969.
14. **Kulkarni, R. K., Pani, K. C., Neuman, C., and Leonard, F.,** *Arch. Surg.*, 93, 839, 1966.
15. **Hermann, J. B., Kelly, R. J., and Higgins,** *Arch. Surg.*, 100, 486, 1970.

16. **Kulkarni, R. K., Moore, E. G., Hegyeli, A. F., and Leonard, F.,** *J. Biomed. Mater. Res.*, 5, 169, 1971.
17. **Ruderman, R. J., Hegyeli, A. F., Hattler, B. G., and Leonard, F.,** *Trans. Am. Soc. Artif. Intern. Organs*, 18, 30, 1972.
18. **Ruderman, R. J., Bernstein, E., Kairinen, E., and Hegyeli, A. F.,** *J. Biomed. Mater. Res.*, 7, 215, 1973.
19. **Dillon, J. G.,** USAMBRL MR 24-71, MR 1, 3, 4, 6, 10, 1972.
20. **Brandes, G., et al.,** U.S. Army Medical Bioengineering Research and Development Laboratory, Ft. Detrick, Md., unpublished report.
21. **Wade, C. W. R.,** personal communication.
22. Development of a Synthetic Polymer Burn Covering, Contract #N00014-73-C-0201 with the Office of Naval Research, Dynatech R/D Co., Cambridge, Mass.
23. **Carothers, W. H. and Arvin, J. A.,** *J. Am. Chem. Soc.*, 51, 2560, 1929.
24. **Carothers, W. H.,** U.S. Patent 2,071,250, 1937.
25. **VanNatta, F. J., Hill, J. W., and Carothers, W. H.,** *J. Am. Chem. Soc.*, 56, 455, 1934.
26. **Cox, E. F. and Hostetler, F.,** U.S. Patent 3,021,310, 1962.
27. **Lundberg, R. D., Koleske, J. V., and Wischmann, K. B.,** *J. Pol. Sci.*, 7, 2915, 1969.
28. **Wilfong, R. E.,** *J. Pol. Sci.*, 54, 385, 1961.
29. **Koleske, J. V. and Lundberg, R. D.,** *J. Pol. Sci.*, 7, 795, 1969.
30. **Koleske, J. V. and Lundberg, R. D.,** *J. Pol. Sci.*, 7, 897, 1969.
31. **Brode, G. L. and Koleske, J. V.,** *J. Macromol. Sci. Chem.*, A6(6), 1109, 1972.
32. **Lundberg, R. D. and Cox, E. F.,** Lactones, in *Kinetics and Mechanism of Polymerization*, Vol. 2, Frisch, K. C. and Roger, S. L., Eds., Marcel Dekker, New York, 1969.
33. **Milne, I. S.,** *Anaesthesia*, 28, 538, 1973.
34. **Haas, S. S., et al.,** *J. Bone Jt. Surg.*, 57A, 3, 1975.

Index

INDEX

A

B

C

N

O

P

V

W

Z